SPEECH AND HEARING SCIENCE:
Selected Readings

Edited by
Norman J. Lass, Ph.D.
West Virginia University

MSS Information Corporation
655 Madison Avenue, New York, N.Y. 10021

This is a custom-made book of readings prepared for the courses taught by the editor, as well as for related courses and for college and university libraries. For information about our program, please write to:

MSS INFORMATION CORPORATION
655 Madison Avenue
New York, New York 10021

MSS wishes to express its appreciation to the authors of the articles in this collection for their cooperation in making their work available in this format.

Library of Congress Cataloging in Publication Data

Lass, Norman J   comp.
    Speech and hearing science: selected readings.

    1. Speech, Disorders of — Addresses, essays, lectures.
2. Hearing disorders — Addresses, essays, lectures.
3. Speech — Addresses, essays, lectures. 4. Hearing —
Addresses, essays, lectures. I. Title. [DNLM: 1. Hearing
— Collected works. 2. Speech — Collected works.
WV501 L346s 1974]
RC423.L35   612'.78'08   73-21984
ISBN 0-8422-5154-5
ISBN 0-8422-0377-X (pbk.)

CONTENTS

INTRODUCTION

The readings in this book are intended to expose the reader to a number of contemporary areas of investigation in the speech and hearing sciences. Whenever appropriate, a chronological ordering of the readings within each subtopic is employed in an attempt to provide a meaningful progression of ideas.

The readings in *TEMPORAL ASPECTS OF SPEECH* are concerned with the production and perception of speech rate. The relationship of diadochokinetic rate, speaking rate, and reading rate, as well as a comparison of temporal speech characteristics of picture-elicited and topic-elicited speech, are explored. Also included in this section are discussions of the following topics: the importance of pause time in perceptual judgments of speech rate; a comparison of the perceptual rate judgments of experienced and inexperienced listeners; the significance of the duration of the silent interval as a perceptual cue for speech pauses; the effect of morphological and syntactic boundaries on the temporal structure of spoken utterances; and the relationship between the production and perception of speech rate, as established by psychophysical procedures.

In the *TIME-COMPRESSED SPEECH* section, the readings deal with various methods for controlling the rate of recorded speech, with special emphasis on the *sampling technique*. A thorough review of the literature on time-compressed speech, as well as the importance of the variables of age and hearing status of the listener, and a comparison of listening rate preferences for oral reading and impromptu speaking tasks, are also discussed.

The phenomenon in which continued listening to recorded repetitions of a stimulus produces perceptual illusory changes in listeners is the subject of discussion in the *VERBAL TRANSFORMATION EFFECT* section. The readings in this section are concerned with the implications of this perceptual phenomenon toward a better understanding of the speech perception process and the auditory perceptual mechanisms responsible for this effect. Also discussed is the importance of the variables of meaningfulness and phonetic complexity of the auditory stimuli; the phonetic vs. non-phonetic training of the listeners; the consistency of reported verbal transformations; and the effectiveness of non-speech stimuli in eliciting this phenomenon.

7

The readings in *ORAL SENSATION AND PERCEPTION* provide the reader with an orientation to the *servosystem model* of speech production, and a discussion of the effects of disrupting normal oral tactile feedback on the subject's articulatory characteristics. A number of tests for assessment of oral sensation and perception, including those concerned with oral stereognosis, two-point discrimination, tactile sensitivity, tactile acuity, tactile localization ability, and tactile extinction, are described. The relationships between oral tactile perception and articulatory status, stimulability, speech-sound discrimination, and auditory memory, and the general issue of the validity of *functional* articulation disorders and the role of oral tactile perception in such disorders, are discussed. Also included in this section are discussions of the issues of asymmetry and consistency of subjects' two-point limens on several selected oral sites.

This book is not intended to provide a complete coverage of the literature, but rather a representative sampling of relevant articles in each of the four major topics discussed. It is hoped that it will provide the reader with a basic understanding of the topics as well as with an awareness of the issues that exist in each area of investigation.

Norman J. Lass, Ph.D.
West Virginia University
Morgantown, West Virginia

TEMPORAL ASPECTS OF SPEECH

A STUDY OF THE RELATIONSHIP OF DIADOCHOKINETIC RATE, SPEAKING RATE AND READING RATE

ABSTRACT

The purpose of this investigation was to determine the nature of the relationship among three variables: diadochokinetic rate, speaking rate, and reading rate. A group of 40 individuals, 20 males and 20 females, performed three experimental tasks: (1) three repetitions at maximum speed of each of the following: $/p_\Lambda/$, $/t_\Lambda/$, $/k_\Lambda/$, and $/p_\Lambda t_\Lambda k_\Lambda/$; (2) 10 readings of a standard prose passage; and (3) the presentation of a two-minute impromptu speech based on the content of stimulus pictures. Results of subjects' performances indicate that: (1) reading rate is highly related to speaking rate; (2) there is no strong relationship between diadochokinetic rate and speaking rate; and (3) diadochokinetic rate is not highly related to reading rate.

INTRODUCTION

"Diadochokinesis" is the performance of alternating or repetitive movements in rapid succession. The rate of diadochokinesis may be taken as an indication of the relative skill of physiological behavior. Specifically, it indicates the speed of change from inhibition to stimulation of antagonistic sets of muscles. Fletcher believes that diadochokinesis is especially valuable in displaying these physiological skills because of the following reasons:

Free motion in a repetitive activity must be superimposed on balanced equilibrium of muscles. This means that fine balance must be maintained between the muscle tonus necessary for a stable posture in the performing organ and the release of the rapidly moving part or parts of the organ. Thus both integration and segmentation of muscle activity are demanded by alternating movements. Every cycle of movement takes time and time is measurable. Time therefore provides a quantitative reflection of the relative efficiency of normal and pathological performances in complex movement patterns. Since muscle power is distributed around a fulcrum, speed of movement is susceptible to imbalance in muscle force and, since dynamic motion is sustained over time, subtle differences can be accumulated and summated to display their effect.[1]

Diadochokinesis of the speech articulators has received considerable attention from speech pathologists because of the proposed relationship between motor ability and defective speech production.[2] Speech is described as ". . . a highly integrated physiological act characterized by a series of complex movements executed in sequences of kinetic chains."[3] It involves very rapid shifts of muscular excitation and inhibition. A test of diadochokinesis of the speech articulators is ". . . a measure of the maximum rate at which the reciprocal synapses of the central nervous system may function for speech uses."[4]

A relationship between diadochokinetic movements and speech is proposed to exist. West and Ansberry state that, "The person who can negotiate rapid shifts of inhibition of muscle contraction is, generally speaking, possessed of a high speed of diadochokinesis and, correlatively, of the ability to make rapid articulatory movements."[5] Thus, information on the diadochokinetic rate of an individual's articulators may be very useful in determining the status of his physiological mechanism for speech production purposes. This proposed importance of diadochokinesis to speech production has led to the accumulation of a body of research concerned with norms for diadochokinetic movements of the articulators.[6]

Despite this proposed relationship between diadochokinesis and speech pro-

TODAY'S SPEECH, 1971, vol. 19, 49-54.

duction, it has never been systematically shown that diadochokinetic rate of an individual's articulators is in any way related to the rate at which he speaks or reads. Nor has it been shown that there is any relationship between an individual's reading rate and speaking rate. The purpose of the present investigation was to determine if such a relationship exists among an individual's diadochokinetic rate, speaking rate, and reading rate.

METHOD

Subjects

A total of 40 individuals, 20 males and 20 females, served as subjects. All were students at West Virginia University. The subjects ranged in age from 19 to 28 years, with a mean age of 21 years. All had normal voice, articulation, hearing, and neurological status.

Procedure

The following tasks were included in each session: (1) a hearing screening evaluation on a Beltone model 12-D portable audiometer from 500 through 8000 Hz at 20 dB (re:ISO, 1964); (2) the completion of a questionnaire on neurological history and status; (3) an impromptu speech based on the content of stimulus pictures; (4) readings of a standard prose passage; and (5) repetitions at maximum speed of /p$_\Lambda$/ /t$_\Lambda$/, /k$_\Lambda$/, and /p$_\Lambda$ t$_\Lambda$ k$_\Lambda$/.

Speaking rate. Each subject's speaking rate was obtained from a two-minute impromptu speech based on the content of several stimulus pictures. The subject was asked to compose a story about a picture shown to him and to talk about the picture as long as he could. If he stopped talking before the required two minutes, he was shown another picture and was asked to compose another story. This procedure was repeated until each subject completed two minutes of speaking. The stimulus pictures employed were obtained from the Thematic Apperception Test.[7]

Reading rate. The reading rate of each subject was based on ten readings of the first paragraph of Fairbanks' "The Rainbow Passage."[8] The subject was told to read the passage in his normal manner. All readings were required to be errorless.

Diadochokinetic rate. Each subject's diadochokinetic rate was obtained from three trials of /p$_\Lambda$/, /t$_\Lambda$/, /k$_\Lambda$/, and /p$_\Lambda$t k$_\Lambda$/. The subject was allowed one practice trial before attempting each diadochokinetic task. The order of performance of the four diadochokinetic tasks was randomized for each of the 40 subjects.

Recording Equipment

All experimental tasks (reading, speaking, and diadochokinetic) were recorded. Recording equipment consisted of an Ampex model 602 tape recorder and an Altec model 681A condensor microphone. All recordings were made in a sound-treated room at the West Virginia University Medical Center.

Data Analysis

Speaking rate. The impromptu speech of each subject was monitored and transcribed verbatim by two listeners working independently. The two transcriptions were compared, and any differences in transcriptions were resolved by a third listener. The subject's speaking rate was based on the middle one-minute portion of his two-minute speech.

Reading rate. For each of the subject's ten readings, only the middle four sentences of the paragraph, a total of 55 words, were employed for analysis purposes. The first and last sentences were deleted from analysis to avoid any possible effects involved in initiating and terminating reading.[9]

For determination of speaking and reading rates, analysis of all recordings was made by means of a General Radio model 1521-B graphic level recorder. The paper speed of the recorder was 31.75 mm per second, with a writing speed of 100 mm per second and a potentiometer setting of 50 dB. The recorded samples were played from an Apex model 602 tape recorder into the graphic level recorder. Simultaneous aural and visual monitoring of the playback and graphic level tracings allowed the invesigators to place a mark on the tracings at the beginning and end of each reading or speech. A line was drawn perpendicular to the baseline at these marks and the distance between the two points where the drawn line bisected the baseline was measured in millimeters. Since the paper speed of the graphic level recorder was 31.75 mm per second, each millimeter corresponded to .031 second. In the above manner, the millimeter measurements on the tracings were converted to time measurements in seconds.

Diadochokinetic rate. Of the seven seconds allowed for each of the 12 diadochokinetic tasks (three performances of each of the four diadochokinetic syllables), only the middle five seconds were used for analysis purposes. The recordings were played into the graphic level recorder and from the graphic level tracings obtained for each subject's performances, the number of repetitions of each syllable achieved by the subject in the five-second period was determined by counting the number of peaks (corresponding to syllables) on the trancings.

RESULTS

Results of subjects' performances on the diadochokinetic, speaking, and reading tasks are presented in Table 1. The table indicates the following: (1) of the three single-syllable diadochokinetic tasks included in the study, the fastest average syllable per second rate was obtained for $/p_\Lambda t_\Lambda k_\Lambda/$, with the slowest average rate exhibited for $/k_\Lambda/$. However, the differences between the four diadochokinetic tasks appear to be very small; the largest difference between any two tasks is less than one syllable per second (0.64 syllable per second difference); (2) in comparing the performance of male and female subjects for all rate tasks investigated, it appears that there are only slight differences between them. The largest difference between male and female groups is for reading rate, and this difference is only 0.23 syllable per second; and (3) of the six rate tasks included in the study, it appears that the diadochokinetic rates are considerably faster than the reading and speaking rates.

To determine if these observed differences in the tasks were significant, a two-factor analysis of variance (Sex X Rate Tasks) was performed, with the subsequent employment of a Newman-Keuls test to locate the significant differences.[10] Results of the analyses indicate the following: (1) there are no significant differences among the subjects' four diadochokinetic rates ($/p_\Lambda/$, $/t_\Lambda/$, $/k_\Lambda/$, and $/p_\Lambda t_\Lambda k_\Lambda/$); (2) significant differences exist between each of the four diadochokinetic tasks and speaking rate; (3) there are significant differences between $/p_\Lambda/$, $/t_\Lambda/$,

Table 1. Diadochokinetic rates, speaking rate, and reading rate (in syllables per second) for the 20 male subjects, 20 female subjects, and the total group of 40 subjects.

Task	Males X	S. D.	Range	Females X	S. D.	Range	Total X	S. D.	Range
$/p_\Lambda/$	6.27	0.53	5.20-7.40	6.15	0.61	5.00-7.80	6.21	0.57	5.00-7.80
$/t_\Lambda/$	6.14	0.50	5.00-7.80	6.15	0.64	4.40-7.80	6.14	0.57	4.40-7.80
$/k_\Lambda/$	5.78	0.55	4.60-6.80	5.55	0.75	4.00-7.40	5.66	0.66	4.00-7.40
$/p_\Lambda t_\Lambda k/$	6.36	0.42	4.80-7.20	6.27	0.31	4.80-7.20	6.30	0.36	4.80-7.20
Speaking	3.50	0.64	2.71-4.58	3.48	0.61	2.35-5.02	3.49	0.62	2.35-5.02
Reading	4.58	0.37	3.61-5.73	4.34	0.44	3.10-5.39	4.46	0.42	3.10-5.73

/p$_A$t$_A$k$_A$/ and reading rate; (4) there is no significant difference between/k$_A$/ and reading rate; and (5) no significant differences were found between male and female subjects' rates for all six rates investigated in the study.

Four multiple regression analyses, involving both linear and quadratic terms,[11] were employed to determine the relationship of diadochokinetic rate to speaking and reading rates. The analyses were performed on the combined data of the male and female subjects. Each regression analysis involved a different diadochokinetic task as dependent variable, with reading rate and speaking rate as independent variables. The equation employed for the analyses was as follows:

y(/p$_A$/,/t$_A$/,/k$_A$/,/p$_A$t$_A$k$_A$/) = a + b0 + b1 (reading rate) + b2 (reading rate)^2 + b3 (speaking rate) + b4 (speaking rate)^2.

reading rate and its quadratic term were statistically significant at the .05 level, but only accounted for 8% of the total variation.

DISCUSSION

From the results of the multiple regression analyses, it appears that diadochokinetic rate is not strongly related to reading and speaking rates. The production of /p$_A$/ seems most strongly related to reading and speaking rates; however, the fact that only 16% of the variation was accounted for by the regression coefficient for /p$_A$/ indicates that its relationship to the other two variables is very negligible.

A significant relationship between reading and speaking rates was found to exist. This finding allows for the conclusion that the individual who **speaks** at

Table 2 Summary of multiple regression analyses: estimates of regression coefficients in linear and quadratic terms.

Term	/p$_A$/	/t$_A$/	/k$_A$/	/p$_A$t$_A$k$_A$/
Reading Rate	−5.52*	−4.69	−5.74	−3.50*
(Reading Rate)^2	0.65*	0.54	0.65	0.41*
Speaking Rate	2.58*	1.05	1.69	0.49
(Speaking Rate)^2	−0.38*	−0.17	−0.22	−0.07
% Variation Accounted for:	16%	9%	9%	8%

p < .05

A summary of the multiple regression analyses is presented in Table 2. The table contains the estimates of regression co-efficients in quadratic and linear terms. The table indicates the following: (1) for /p$_A$/, reading rate, speaking, and their quadratic terms (i.e., (reading rate)^2 and (speaking rate)^2) were statistically significant at the .05 level, although they accounted for relatively little of the total variation (16%); (2) for the /t$_A$/ and /k$_A$/ tasks, none of the variables (reading rate, speaking rate, and their respective quadratic terms) were statistically significant and accounted for only 9% of the total variation; and (3) for /p$_A$t$_A$k$_A$/,

a faster than average rate will be expected to **read** at a faster than average rate. And, conversely, the slower than average speaker will probably also be a slower than average reader (provided, of course, that the individual's reading rate reflects his true rate and is not the result of his poor reading skills).

Since some of the quadratic terms in the regression analyses were found to be significant, it can be asserted that some of the relationships among diadochokinetic rate, speaking rate, and reading rate are not linear and thus cannot be accurately described by employment of correlation coefficients, since such statistics have as a basic underlying assumption that the relationship between the variables under investigation is linear.[12]

The results of this study have in no way proven that diadochokinetic rates are not useful measures in assessment of an individual's speech mechanism. Information on the diadochokinetic rate of an individual's articulators may be very useful in determining the status of his physiological mechanism for speech production purposes. The present study's findings have not contradicted West and Ansberry's statement that, "The person who can negotiate rapid shifts of inhibition of muscle contraction is, generally speaking, possessed of a high speed of diadochokinesis and, correlatively, of the ability to make rapid articulatory move-

ments."[13] What this study has found is that there is no high relationship between an individual's diadochokinetic rate and his speaking and reading rates. That is, we cannot predict an individual's speaking or reading rate from his performance on a diadochokinetic task. Therefore, an individual who performs a diadochokinetic task at a faster than average rate will not necessarily read or speak at a faster than average rate. However, it should be noted that these statements can only be applied to the four diadochokinetic tasks under investigation in the present study.

NORMAN J. LASS and
JEANNE C. SANDUSKY

Notes

[1] Samuel G. Fletcher, "Measurement of Oral Coordination by Syllable Rate," **Threshold,** III (1968), pp. 12-17.

[2] Robert W. West, "A Neurological Test for Stutterers," **Journal of Neurology and Psychotherapy,** XXXVIII (1929), pp. 114-123; William B. Blackburn, "A Study of Voluntary Movements of Diaphragm, Tongue, Lips and Jaw in Stutterers and Normal Speakers," **Psychological Monographs,** XXXXI (1931), pp. 1-13; H. M. Cross, "The Motor Capacity of Stutterers," **Archives of Speech,** I (1936), pp. 112-132; Isaac W. Karlin, Adella C. Youtz, and Lou Kennedy, "Distorted Speech in Young Children," **American Journal of Diseases of Children,** LIX (1940), pp. 1203-1218; E. William Bilto, "A Comparative Study of Certain Physical Abilities of Children With Speech Defects and Children with Normal Speech, **Journal of Speech Disorders,** VI (1941), pp. 187-203; George J. Harbold, "A Study of the Relationship Between Motor Coordination and the Incidence of Speech Defects Among Selected Individuals With Oral Anomalies" (unpublished M.A. thesis, University of Florida, 1947); Robert W. Albright, "Motor Abilities of Speakers with Good and Poor Articulation," **Speech Monographs,** XV (1948), pp. 164-172; Richard L. Schiefelbusch, "A Developmental Study of Speech Retarded Children" (unpublished Ph.D. dissertation, Northwestern University, 1951); Edna Jenkins and Francis E. Lohr, "Severe Articulation Disorders and Motor Ability," **Journal of Speech and Hearing Disorders,** XXIX (1964), pp. 286-292.

[3] Fletcher, op. cit., p. 12.

[4] Russell L. Jenkins, "The Role of Diadochokinetic Movement of the Jaw at the Ages from Seven to Maturity," **Journal of Speech Disorders,** VI (1941), p. 13.

[5] Robert W. West and Merle Ansberry, **The Rehabilitation of Speech** (New York: Harper and Row, 1968), p. 40.

[6] West, op. cit.; Calvin W. Pettit, "Diadochokinesis of the Musculature of the Jaw During Puberty and Adolescence" (unpublished M.A. thesis, University of Wisconsin, 1939); Bernard Schlanger, "The Rate of Diadochokinetic Jaw Movement

of Young Children in the Age Groups Seven, Eight, and Nine" (unpublished M.A. thesis, University of Wisconsin, 1939); Jenkins, op. cit., pp. 13-22; Charles R. Strother and Lois S. Kriegman, "Diadochokinesis in Stutterers and Non-Stutterers," **Journal of Speech Disorders,** VIII (1943), pp. 323-335; Albright, op. cit.; Betty L. Blomquist, "Diadochokinetic Movements of Nine-, Ten-, and Eleven-Year-Old Children," **Journal of Speech and Hearing Disorders,** XV (1950), pp. 159-164; Dale J. Lundeen, "The Relationship of Diadochokinesis to Various Speech Sounds," **Journal of Speech and Hearing Disorders,** XV (1950), pp. 54-59; Keith L. Maxwell, "A Comparison of Certain Motor Performances of Children with Normal and Children with Defective Consonant Articulation" (unpublished Ph.D. dissertation, University of Michigan, 1953); John V. Irwin and Orville Becklund, "Norms for Maximum Repetitive Rates for Certain Sounds Established with the Sylrater," **Journal of Speech and Hearing Disorders,** XVIII (1953), pp. 149-165.

[7] Henry A. Murray, **Thematic Apperception Test** (Cambridge, Massachusetts: Harvard University Press, 1943).

[8] Grant Fairbanks, **Voice and Articulation Drillbook** (New York: Harper and Row, 1960), p. 127.

[9] Charles L. Hutton, "A Psychophysical Study of Speech Rate" (unpublished Ph.D. dissertation, University of Illinois, 1954).

[10] B. J. Winer, **Statistical Principles in Experimental Design** (New York: McGraw-Hill Book Co., 1962), pp. 298-318.

[11] E. J. Williams, **Regression Analysis** (New York: Wiley, 1959).

[12] J. P. Guilford, **Fundamental Statistics in Psychology and Education** (New York: McGraw-Hill Book Co., 1965), pp. 304-355.

[13] West and Ansberry, op. cit., p. 40.

ACKNOWLEDGEMENT

The authors wish to thank Dr. Edwin C. Townsend, Associate Professor of Statistics, West Virginia University, for his consultation and advice on statistical procedures employed in this study. Sincere appreciation is also extended to the West Virginia University Computer Center for providing the computer services for this research project.

COMPARATIVE STUDY OF TEMPORAL CHARACTERISTICS OF PICTURE-ELICITED AND TOPIC-ELICITED SPEECH

NORMAN J. LASS AND JULIA D. CLEGG

Summary.—The temporal characteristics of picture-elicited and topic-elicited speech were compared in 25 adult *S*s. No significant differences were noted in temporal measures between these two types of speeches. The speech-eliciting technique cannot be validly used to explain differences in prior research on speaking rate.

In studies concerned with speaking rate, several approaches have been employed to elicit speech samples from *S*s. The two most common techniques have employed stimulus pictures (Hahn, 1949; Goldman-Eisler, 1961a, 1961b; Ramsay, 1968; Lass & Noll, 1970; Lass & Sandusky, 1971) and popular topics (Snidecor, 1943; Hanley, 1949; Hahn, 1949; Caraway, 1965; Minifie, 1963; Osser & Peng, 1964; Boomer, 1965; Webb, 1971; Hawkins, 1971).

Stimulus pictures provide the content upon which *S* must speak and thus determine the basic composition of the speech. Topics, on the other hand, allow *S* to draw upon his own experiences and interests and thus allow him more freedom to express his own ideas and views on the chosen topic. However, it is not currently known if these two methods differ in eliciting speech. Since both approaches have been used in prior studies of speaking rate, such information may be very helpful in interpreting differences in previous findings as well as in determining the best approach for future studies.

The purpose of the present investigation was to compare the temporal characteristics, including over-all rate, total time, speech time, pause time, number of pauses, speech-time ratio, and pause-time ratio, of picture-elicited and topic-elicited speech.

METHOD

Subjects

*S*s were 22 females and 3 males, students at West Virginia University. *S*s had normal judged articulation and voice characteristics and none reported hearing difficulty. They ranged in age from 18 to 22 yr. and had a mean age of 20 yr.

Recording Session

Each *S* participated in one recording session. In the session, he presented two 2-min. impromptu speeches; one speech was based on the contents of stimulus

PERCEPTUAL AND MOTOR SKILLS, 1973, vol. 36, 995-998.

pictures (Murray, 1943) and the second speech was based on topics selected from a list of topics provided by the examiner.

For both the picture-elicited and topic-elicited speeches, S was given approximately 1 min. to prepare his speech and was asked to speak for as long as he could. However, if he stopped before the required 2 min., he was shown another picture or asked to choose another topic and to make up another speech. This procedure was repeated until each S completed 2 min. of speaking.

All speeches were recorded using an Ampex Model 602 tape recorder and an Altec Model 681A condensor microphone. Each session, which lasted approximately 20 min., was held in a sound-treated room at the West Virginia University Medical Center.

Data Analysis

Each S's impromptu speeches were aurally monitored and transcribed verbatim onto a sheet of paper. His speaking rate was based on a middle 1-min. portion of each of his two speeches. The middle portion was chosen to represent S's speaking rate in an attempt to avoid any possible rate variation effects associated with the beginning and ending of a speaking task (Hutton, 1954).

For the determination of the temporal speech characteristics of each speaker, all speeches were analyzed by means of a General Radio Model 1521-B graphic level recorder. The recorder had a paper speed of 31.75 mm per second and a writing speed of 100 mm per second. The recorded speech samples were played from an Ampex Model 602 tape recorder into the graphic level recorder. Simultaneous aural and visual monitoring of the playback and graphic level recorder tracings allowed for the placement of marks at the beginning and end of each speech. A line was drawn perpendicular to the baseline at these marks and the distance between them was measured in millimeters. Since the paper speed of the graphic level recorder was 31.75 mm per second, each millimeter corresponded to .031 sec. In the above manner, the millimeter measurements on the tracings were converted to time measurements in seconds.

Temporal Measures

The following temporal measures were obtained for each S's two impromptu speeches: (1) over-all rate (in syllables per second); (2) speech time (in seconds); (3) pause time (in seconds); (4) number of pauses; (5) speech-time ratio; and (6) pause-time ratio.

Over-all rate in syllables per second was determined by dividing total time into the total number of syllables used by S in his speech. Speech time, pause time, and number of pauses were obtained directly from measurements on the graphic level recorder tracings. Speech-time ratio is the ratio of time spent in vocalizing (speech time) to the total time (speech time plus pause time) involved in the speech. It was obtained by dividing total time into speech time. Pause-time ratio is the ratio of pause time to the total time (speech time plus pause time) and was determined by dividing total time into pause time. A minimum pause in this study was defined as one which measured at least one millimeter in length (310 msec. in duration).

RESULTS AND DISCUSSION

Results of Ss' performances on the two tasks are presented in Table 1, which shows a remarkable similarity in temporal measures between picture-elicited and topic-elicited speech. The largest time difference between the two tasks is only 1.12 sec., for speech time. A correlated t test (Guilford, 1965) was computed for over-all rate, and the obtained t of 0.22 ($df = 24$) was not significant, indicating no real differences in rate between the two types of speeches.

These findings indicate that, despite the fact that picture-elicited speeches are limited to the content of the pictures employed while topic-elicited speeches allow more freedom of expression by drawing upon Ss' own experiences and interests, the temporal characteristics of speech do not appear to be affected by such content differences. Therefore, the procedure used to elicit impromptu speeches cannot be used to explain differences in speech rate in prior studies. Furthermore, the present findings suggest that either or both speech-eliciting techniques may be used in future studies to obtain reliable measures of speaking rate.

The present finding of similarity of temporal speech characteristics in topic-elicited and picture-elicited speeches agrees with the work of Goldman-Eisler (1968) and, in fact, is predictable from her findings. She has shown that the temporal characteristics of speech are dependent on the cognitive level of the verbal operation required in a given task and that the description of pictures and interview require the same cognitive level of verbal operation as interpretations of pictures. Since picture-elicited and topic-elicited speeches require the same cognitive level of verbal operation, it is not surprising that there are no real differences in their temporal characteristics.

TABLE 1

MEANS, STANDARD DEVIATIONS, AND RANGES FOR TEMPORAL MEASURES
OF PICTURE- AND TOPIC-ELICITED SPEECHES

Temporal Measures	Picture-elicited Speech			Topic-elicited Speech		
	M	SD	Range	M	SD	Range
Over-all Rate (sps)	3.38	0.45	2.20-4.37	3.41	0.57	2.32-4.60
Speech Time (sec.)	37.37	5.31	26.72-47.01	38.49	5.47	28.52-45.23
Pause Time (sec.)	22.78	4.84	15.76-32.80	21.69	5.23	15.32-30.77
Speech-time Ratio	0.62	0.10	0.45-0.78	0.64	0.50	0.48-0.76
Pause-time Ratio	0.38	0.10	0.29-0.55	0.36	0.10	0.24-0.52
Number of Pauses	30.12	6.67	16-47	33.48	10.57	19-57

REFERENCES

BOOMER, D. S.   Hesitation and grammatical encoding. *Language and Speech*, 1965, 8, 148-158.

CARAWAY, K. E.   Measurements of speaking rates and oral reading rates for boys in grades four through twelve. Unpublished Master's thesis, Univer. of Kansas, 1965.

GOLDMAN-EISLER, F.   Continuity of speech utterance, its determinants and its significance. *Language and Speech*, 1961, 4, 220-231. (a)

GOLDMAN-EISLER, F.   The distribution of pause durations in speech. *Language and Speech*, 1961, 4, 232-237. (b)

GOLDMAN-EISLER, F.   *Psycholinguistics: experiments in spontaneous speech.* New York: Academic Press, 1968.

GUILFORD, J. P.   *Fundamental statistics in psychology and education.* New York: McGraw-Hill, 1965.

HAHN, E.   An analysis of the delivery of the speech of first grade children. *Quarterly Journal of Speech*, 1949, 35, 338-343.

HANLEY, T. D.   Analysis of vocal frequency and duration characteristics of selected samples of speech from three American dialect regions. *Speech Monographs*, 1949, 16, 78-93.

HAWKINS, P. R.   The syntactic location of hesitation pauses. *Language and Speech*, 1971, 14, 277-288.

HUTTON, C. L.   A psychophysical study of speech rate. Unpublished doctoral dissertation, Univer. of Illinois, 1954.

LASS, N. J., & NOLL, J. D.   A comparative study of rate characteristics of cleft palate and noncleft palate speakers. *Cleft Palate Journal*, 1970, 7, 275-283.

LASS, N. J., & SANDUSKY, J. C.   A study of the relationship of diadochokinetic rate, speaking rate, and reading rate. *Today's Speech*, 1971, 19, 49-54.

MINIFIE, F. D.   An analysis of the durational aspects of connected speech by means of an electronic speech-duration analyzer. Unpublished doctoral dissertation, Univer. of Iowa, 1963.

MURRAY, H. A.   *Thematic Apperception Test.* Cambridge, Mass.: Harvard Univer. Press, 1943.

OSSER, H., & PENG, F.   A cross-cultural study of speech rate. *Language and Speech*, 1964, 7, 120-125.

RAMSAY, R. W.   Speech patterns and personality. *Language and Speech*, 1968, 11, 54-63.

SNIDECOR, J. C.   A comparative study of the pitch and duration characteristics of impromptu speaking and oral reading. *Speech Monographs*, 1943, 10, 50-56.

WEBB, J. T.   Subject speech rates as a function of interviewer behaviour. *Language and Speech*, 1971, 14, 54-67.

The Timing of Utterances and Linguistic Boundaries

ILSE LEHISTE

INTRODUCTION

This paper is concerned with the effect of morphological and syntactic boundaries on the temporal structure of spoken utterances. The investigation was prompted by the observation made in a previous study,[1,2] that the duration of a base word may be considerably reduced, if a derivational suffix is added to it. In this earlier study, the base words *stead*, *skid*, and *skit* were compared with the derived words *steady*, *skiddy*, and *skitty*. It might have been expected that the derived set would be longer than the former by the average duration of the derivational suffix. It turned out instead that the duration of the base part of the derived word was considerably shortened, so that even with the addition of a fairly long -*y*, the over-all duration of the derived words was not much longer than the base words.

The purpose of the current study was to explore whether there are any differences in the duration of the base part, depending on whether it is followed by a morpheme boundary within the same word, or by a major syntactic boundary coinciding with the word boundary. Four sets of words were examined, built around the base words *stick*, *sleep*, *shade*, and *speed*. The test material is presented in Table I. Each of the words occurred by itself and in eight additional utterance types. Five derivational suffixes were used, three of them monosyllabic and two disyllabic. The base words were further placed in short sentences in which they were followed by a major syntactic boundary—the boundary between the noun phrase functioning as subject and the verb phrase functioning as predicate. The verb

JOURNAL OF THE ACOUSTICAL SOCIETY OF AMERICA, 1972, vol. 51, no. 6, 2018-2024.

phrase itself either consisted of a stressed monosyllable (in three cases) or started with a stressed syllable (in one case); or it started with one or two unstressed syllables. The sentences thus reproduced the syllabic sequences of the derived words. For example, the words *shading* and *speeding* may be directly compared with the sequences *shade in-* (from the sentence *the shade increased*) and *speed in-* (from the sentence *the speed increased*), where *shade* and *speed* are followed by an unstressed syllable with the same phonemic stucture as in *shading* and *speeding*. Other sequences, while not reproducing the same phonemes, are analogous with regard to syllable structure.

I. METHOD

The test material was recorded by two speakers, R. G. (male) and L. S. (female), both graduate students at the Ohio State University. The recordings were made under standard conditions in an anechoic chamber using high-quality recording equipment. The utterances were produced in two ways, to test the comparability of different contexts and to vary the fairly artificial recording technique of repeating the same word a large number of times. One of the ways was indeed the repetition technique: each word was uttered 10 times under a subjectively established "constant" rate. Then each set, consisting of base word, derived words, and three short sentences, was read 10 times in succession. Each speaker thus produced two sets of 10 tokens of each word, for a total of 720 utterances by each speaker. The recordings were made in a single session, with a 10-min

TABLE I. Test materials used in the study. The symbol - is used to indicate the boundary between stem and derivative suffix. # symbolizes word boundary; ∠ and ⌣ refer to stressed and unstressed syllables.

Base	stick	sleep	shade	speed
-y	sticky	sleepy	shady	speedy
-er	sticker	sleeper	shader	speeder
-ing	sticking	sleeping	shading	speeding
-ily	stickily	sleepily	shadily	speedily
-iness	stickiness	sleepiness	shadiness	speediness
# ∠	the stick fell	sleep heals	the shade lingered	speed kills
# ⌣ ∠	the stick is broken	sleep refreshes	the shade increased	the speed increased
# ⌣ ⌣ ∠	the stick was discarded	my sleep was disturbed	the shade was refreshing	the speed was controlled

21

pause between the two different repetition tasks. The number of productions was monitored by the experimenter, who signaled the speaker when the repetitions had been completed.

The durations of words and segments were measured from oscillograms, produced by processing the recorded tapes through a Frøkjær–Jensen trans-pitch meter and intensity meter, connected to a four-channel Elema–Schönander Mingograph. The measurements were performed according to segmentation principles outlined by Peterson and Lehiste[3] and subsequently elaborated by Naeser.[4] In particular, the duration of a plosive consonant was equated with the duration of the closure; the consonant was considered terminated at the moment of release. The duration data were analyzed statistically, using the IBM 360 model 75 computer available at the Ohio State University Instruction and Research Computer Center.

II. COMPARABILITY OF THE TWO SETS OF DATA

For both sets of data—one from successive productions of single test utterances, the other from successive productions of sequential sets—the following computations were carried out: the mean duration of each segment; the mean duration of each word; the mean duration of the base component of the derived word (e.g., *stick* in *sticky*); and the variances and standard deviations of each segment and word. The differences between the corresponding means for each segment and word were tested for significance according to the standard Z-test. The difference in variability between the two sets was tested by Hartley's and Cochran's tests.[5] It was found that the differences between the two sets of utterances for each speaker were random, and that there was little overlap between the two speakers in the few cases of statistically significant differences. Combining the two sets would tend to increase the extreme ranges for each combined set of utterances and thus increase the variability; but since the difference in variability between the two sets was negligible, it was decided to combine the two sets in future calculations. The resultant increase in variability was actually quite small. It is hoped that the method of producing the test utterances in the two different ways described above will have reduced the artificiality of the situation in which long lists of words are produced out of context, and that the results represent a more natural speech situation.

22

TABLE II. Mean durations (in milliseconds), standard deviations, and B/D ratios for two sets of words and corresponding syllable nuclei produced by speaker R. G.

Utterance	Duration of base	σ	B/D ratio	Duration of syllable nucleus	σ	B/D ratio
stick	401.55	29.45		130.70	6.94	
sticky	312.80	23.68	1.284	93.45	6.53	1.399
sticker	302.50	17.49	1.327	89.45	8.85	1.461
sticking	295.45	16.92	1.359	88.80	7.28	1.472
stickily	291.10	17.90	1.379	84.15	6.75	1.553
stickiness	265.75	15.79	1.511	78.90	5.63	1.657
the stick fell	274.85	14.10	1.461	87.90	7.02	1.487
the stick is broken	248.20	12.65	1.618	81.65	7.57	1.601
the stick was discarded	245.10	13.49	1.638	77.90	5.84	1.678
sleep	409.80	18.96		123.55	14.55	
sleepy	336.80	19.70	1.217	84.15	7.97	1.468
sleeper	341.25	19.83	1.201	83.10	9.21	1.487
sleeping	330.35	18.12	1.241	81.50	10.11	1.516
sleepily	313.35	13.99	1.308	69.60	8.58	1.775
sleepiness	287.05	13.81	1.428	62.05	6.79	1.991
sleep heals	305.95	16.33	1.339	75.95	8.41	1.627
sleep refreshes	299.60	19.90	1.368	61.85	4.67	1.998
my sleep was disturbed	307.45	17.44	1.333	59.65	9.65	2.071

III. EFFECT OF MORPHEME BOUNDARIES

In order to study the effect of morpheme boundaries and word boundaries on the duration of the base to which derivative suffixes were added, B/D ratios were computed. This term refers to the ratio of the durations of the base word (pronounced by itself) and the durations of the same segments occurring in the derived word (e.g., the mean duration of *stick* would be divided by the mean duration of the *stick* part of the word *sticky*). These ratios were calculated for all test words and, separately, for the syllable nuclei (vowel phases) in all test words. The differences between the mean base durations and mean derived durations were highly significant in all instances; the Z-values were always higher than the critical value. The B/D ratios are presented in Tables II through V and graphically in Figs. 1 and 2.

On each figure, the derived word types and sentence types are given on the vertical axis. The horizontal axis is scaled in increasing B/D ratio. Points representing B/D ratios for words are connected with solid lines; points representing B/D ratios for syllable nuclei are connected with dashed lines. The curves start in the left-hand top corner at the B/D value 1: Base/Base

23

TABLE III. Mean durations (in milliseconds), standard deviations, and B/D ratios for two sets of words and corresponding syllable nuclei produced by speaker L. S.

Utterance	Duration of base	σ	B/D ratio	Duration of syllable nucleus	σ	B/D ratio
stick	431.80	43.33		168.90	23.25	
sticky	346.00	34.44	1.248	115.50	15.83	1.462
sticker	331.95	25.88	1.301	109.65	14.75	1.540
sticking	348.30	30.56	1.240	109.20	17.36	1.547
stickily	303.10	17.93	1.425	77.50	6.89	2.192
stickiness	271.60	20.78	1.590	76.50	6.92	2.208
the stick fell	311.15	22.74	1.388	91.35	11.17	1.849
the stick is broken	283.90	19.46	1.521	88.85	10.83	1.901
the stick was discarded	268.15	28.40	1.610	80.75	8.42	2.092
sleep	442.45	39.62		180.30	16.85	
sleepy	363.40	19.64	1.218	131.45	9.24	1.372
sleeper	363.35	22.87	1.218	127.25	8.90	1.417
sleeping	374.45	18.26	1.182	132.45	10.87	1.361
sleepily	342.60	16.72	1.291	114.50	8.72	1.575
sleepiness	307.70	16.39	1.438	96.55	8.45	1.867
sleep heals	325.00	25.33	1.361	113.55	14.77	1.588
sleep refreshes	282.75	18.96	1.565	93.55	9.74	1.927
my sleep was disturbed	314.90	26.82	1.405	99.40	19.27	1.814

TABLE IV. Mean durations (in milliseconds), standard deviations, and B/D ratios for two sets of words and corresponding syllable nuclei produced by speaker R. G.

Utterance	Duration of base	σ	B/D ratio	Duration of syllable nucleus	σ	B/D ratio
speed	511.50	34.95		266.00	28.17	
speedy	359.75	15.09	1.422	150.50	10.25	1.767
speeder	344.75	16.42	1.484	141.50	11.01	1.880
speeding	342.50	13.13	1.493	136.00	9.81	1.956
speedily	322.50	18.03	1.586	120.00	8.27	2.217
speediness	313.25	16.57	1.633	115.50	7.76	2.303
speed kills	344.00	17.06	1.487	125.50	8.87	2.120
the speed increased	301.25	15.12	1.698	110.00	7.61	2.418
the speed was controlled	293.50	20.53	1.743	104.00	8.97	2.558
shade	454.10	28.88		266.15	18.61	
shady	327.20	20.08	1.388	181.85	14.79	1.464
shader	324.20	18.81	1.401	172.40	9.54	1.544
shading	306.95	23.39	1.479	158.00	11.24	1.684
shadily	276.70	10.20	1.641	132.50	8.74	2.016
shadiness	265.20	17.60	1.712	125.35	9.83	2.123
the shade lingered	324.80	18.49	1.398	146.95	16.23	1.811
the shade increased	298.60	18.44	1.521	130.15	12.93	2.045
the shade was refreshing	307.60	26.05	1.476	131.50	18.61	2.024

yields a ratio of 1. Increasing ratios show decrease in the duration of the base component of the derived word or, respectively, of its syllable nucleus.

Several observations are made by referring to the figures. In no case was the duration of the same set of segments greater in a derived word than in the base form. The suffixes -*y*, -*er* and -*ing* seem to be equivalent with respect to their effect on the duration of the stem. It appears that the number of phonemic segments in the suffix has no systematic effect on the duration of the stem. This observation is confirmed by looking at the behavior of stem forms before the suffix -*ily*. This suffix was in fact pronounced with a syllabic /l/ by both speakers in all productions; thus the stems of words like *sticking* and *stickily* were followed by two segments each, but the -*ing* suffix was monosyllabic and the -*ily* suffix was disyllabic. In all cases, the disyllabic -*ily* suffix produced greater reduction in the duration of the stem than the monosyllabic suffix -*ing*, although both consisted of the same number of segments.

The suffix -*iness* constitutes a special case. In each instance, the B/D ratio was greatest under this condition. This is a disyllabic suffix, as is -*ily*; however, its rhythmic structure is considerably different. It seems possible

TABLE V. Mean durations (in milliseconds), standard deviations, and B/D ratios for two sets of words and corresponding syllable nuclei produced by speaker L. S.

Utterance	Duration of base	σ	B/D ratio	Duration of syllable nucleus	σ	B/D ratio
speed	574.25	30.00		297.85	16.25	
speedy	394.85	23.89	1.454	163.30	11.69	1.824
speeder	403.85	18.44	1.422	171.75	13.52	1.734
speeding	396.10	24.54	1.450	158.75	12.86	1.876
speedily	354.50	29.75	1.620	126.25	16.98	2.359
speediness	322.70	23.41	1.780	104.40	6.66	2.853
speed kills	416.55	27.28	1.379	163.05	19.07	1.827
the speed increased	342.85	20.97	1.675	127.30	11.68	2.340
the speed was controlled	305.50	22.00	1.880	96.65	7.92	3.082
shade	454.65			267.70	22.88	
shady	321.65	20.72	1.413	165.25	11.26	1.620
shader	326.75	26.61	1.391	160.50	14.16	1.668
shading	312.95	22.09	1.453	159.30	19.72	1.680
shadily	294.15	26.41	1.546	139.95	21.89	1.913
shadiness	261.65	25.37	1.738	112.55	11.65	2.378
the shade lingered	331.95	36.24	1.370	154.40	23.93	1.734
the shade increased	282.20	22.03	1.611	135.75	16.90	1.972
the shade was refreshing	273.40	23.97	1.633	114.25	15.97	2.343

25

that in the case of the -iness suffix we are dealing with two cycles of derivation—that, for example, *sticky* is derived from *stick* in the first cycle, and *stickiness* from *sticky* in the second cycle. If this is so, then the ratios of *stick/sticky* and *sticky/stickiness* (involving the base forms *stick* and *sticky*, respectively) should be approximately equal. Some support for this assumption is indeed seen in the data of Table VI, which presents the pertinent ratios.

A comparison of the curves for words with the curves for syllable nuclei (vowels) indicates that the reduction in the duration of a stem in the derived form is achieved more at the expense of vowels than at the expense of consonants. The nature of the vowel and the postvocalic consonant seem to play an equally important role. Intrinsically long syllable nuclei (like those in *sleep*, *speed*, and *shade*) are more compressible than intrinsically short syllable nuclei (as in *stick*). But /i/ in *sleep*, when followed by a voiceless plosive, is much less compressible than /i/ in *speed* and /eɪ/ in *shade*. Tendencies for being reduced under a certain condition become accentuated when one looks at the most compressible segment: for both speakers, the greatest effects of the various positions are manifested in the syllable nuclei of *speed* and *shade*.

IV. EFFECT OF SYNTACTIC BOUNDARIES

One of the hypotheses tested in this experiment was the hypothesis that syntactic boundaries would have temporal effects that are clearly distinct from those of morpheme boundaries. However, the results of this study show that, as far as the temporal structure of utterances is concerned, effects of morpheme boundaries and effects of syntactic boundaries cannot be separated from each other. The figures show that, by and large, the ratios are the same for disyllabic words consisting of the base plus suffix, and for disyllabic sequences taken from sentences in which the base word is followed by an unstressed syllable. This applies, mutatis mutandis, to trisyllabic words and analogous sequences: there is no way in which morpheme boundaries and word boundaries could be distinguished on the basis of the associated temporal patterns. Furthermore, it is not certain that the boundaries as such have any effect at all, since the temporal structure of the utterances seems to depend most of all on their syllabic structure, regardless of the nature of the boundaries involved.

In sentences like *speed kills*, we find durations of the

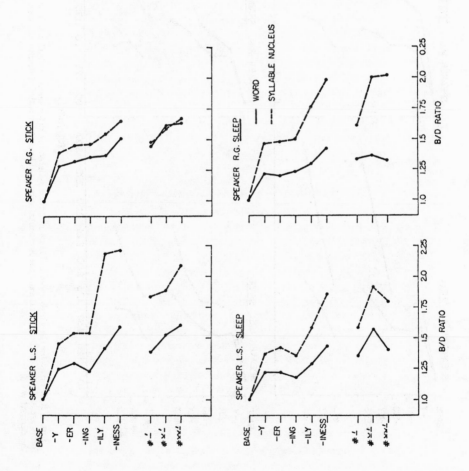

FIG. 1. B/D ratios for the words *stick* and *sleep* and their syllable nuclei for speakers R.G. and L.S. The base word and the derivative forms are indicated on the vertical axis; the horizontal axis is calibrated for ratios of duration of base word/duration of the base part of the derived word.

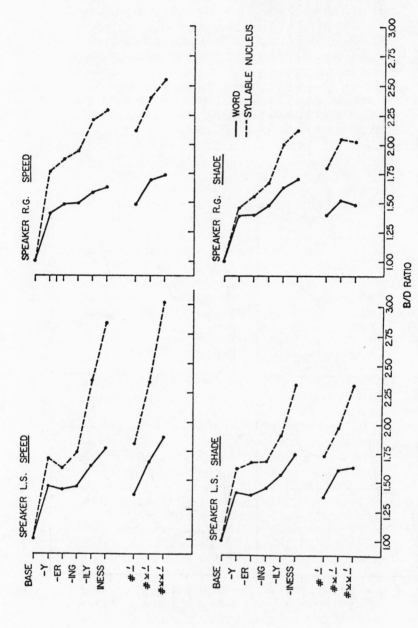

FIG. 2. B/D ratios for the words *speed* and *shade* and their syllable nuclei for speakers R. G. and L. S. The base word and the derivative forms are indicated on the vertical axis; the horizontal axis is calibrated for ratios of duration of base word/duration of the base part of the derived word.

28

test word that are very similar to those of disyllabic bimorphemic words; sentences like *the speed increased* resemble most words like *speediness*, with an unstressed short syllable followed by a relatively long syllable. The addition of another unstressed syllable may have a further reducing effect, but the data are not consistent at this point. The major result here is the absence of any clear differences between the effects of morpheme boundaries and syntactic boundaries; it appears that the durational structure is conditioned by the number of syllables rather than either by the number of segments or by the presence of boundaries.

V. GENERALITY OF THE FINDINGS

One of the ways to test the results would be to form predictions on the basis of these data and then compare the predictions with further observations. I intend to record other sets of words by the same speakers, as well as the same sets of words by different speakers, and calculate the goodness of fit between predicted and observed B/D ratios. The basis for predictions might be the ratio effects in Table VII, which combines words that seem to behave in a similar fashion for the two speakers.

VI. DISCUSSION

The results of this study confirm earlier studies in some respects, but differ from them in certain important aspects.

Bolinger[6] stated that long syllables tend to acquire extra length if followed by another long syllable (long syllables being those that contain a full vowel); if followed by a short syllable, long syllables cannot acquire that extra length and therefore appear shorter. This process tends to ignore morpheme and word boundaries, and may take place across a syntactic boundary.

The present study confirms Bolinger's notion that temporal readjustment processes tend to ignore morpheme and word boundaries. The shortening of a long syllable before a short syllable is likewise confirmed in all the data. However, in sentences of the type *speed kills*, the word *speed* (and words in analogous sentences) certainly did not acquire any extra length, at least in comparison to isolated productions of the same word.

Gaitenby[7] found a common ratio of segment-to-utterance length for all dialects of American English sampled

TABLE VI. Mean durations (in milliseconds), standard deviations, and B/D ratios for words derived with -y and -ness, in which the -ness words are derived by a two-cycle operation from the base.

Utterance	Speaker R. G. Duration of base	σ	B/D ratio	Utterance	Speaker L. S. Duration of base	σ	B/D ratio
stick	401.55	29.45		stick	431.80	43.33	
stick-y	312.80	23.68	1.284	stick-y	346.00	34.44	1.248
sticky	513.25	37.52		sticky	557.45	36.59	
sticky-ness	376.75	17.66	1.362	sticky-ness	388.50	24.34	1.435
sleep	409.80	18.96		sleep	442.45	39.62	
sleep-y	336.80	19.70	1.217	sleep-y	363.40	19.64	1.218
sleepy	517.55	26.58		sleepy	544.20	30.99	
sleepy-ness	369.65	14.15	1.400	sleepy-ness	392.20	18.46	1.388
speed	511.50	34.95		speed	574.25	30.00	
speed-y	359.75	15.09	1.422	speed-y	394.85	23.89	1.454
speedy	529.95	26.23		speedy	597.40	16.94	
speedy-ness	396.35	16.60	1.337	speedy-ness	410.55	31.19	1.455
shade	454.10	28.88		shade	454.65	35.84	
shade-y	327.20	20.08	1.388	shade-y	321.65	20.72	1.413
shady	477.90	25.81		shady	490.60	24.43	
shady-ness	346.30	16.46	1.380	shady-ness	329.70	23.87	1.488

TABLE VII. Average B/D ratios (speakers R. G. and L. S. combined).

| | stick, sleep | | shade, speed | |
	Word	SN	Word	SN
Base	1.00	1.00	1.00	1.00
-y	1.242	1.425	1.420	1.669
-er	1.262	1.476	1.425	1.706
-ing	1.256	1.474	1.469	1.799
-ily	1.351	1.774	1.599	2.126
-iness	1.492	1.931	1.716	2.415
# ´	1.388	1.638	1.409	1.873
# ˘ ´	1.518	1.857	1.626	2.194
# ˘ ˘ ´	1.497	1.914	1.683	2.502

in her study. When segment durations were converted to percentages of total utterance time, it was found that 90% of all the segments varied less than 5.3% for any speaker. The longer the utterance in terms of number of segments, the shorter the absolute duration of any given segment, until an approximate minimum duration was reached beyond which segments could not be compressed any further. She noted also that words immediately preceding a pause tended to expand in utterances of all lengths. According to Gaitenby, it would thus be the word closest to the pause that would acquire extra length, while in longer utterances the preceding parts of the sentence would be produced at a faster rate. This seems to be borne out by the findings: the base word became successively shorter, the farther it was removed from the end of the sentence. Table VIII presents the mean durations of the word (or, respectively, the base part of a morphologically complex word), the mean durations of the utterances in which the word appeared, and the percent the duration of the base word constitutes of the total utterance duration. In almost all instances, the word is shortened, both in absolute and relative terms, when the utterance becomes longer. With the position of the test word remaining constant at the beginning of the utterance, its shortening can well be attributed to its increasing distance from the end of the utterance. A difference between Gaitenby's results and those obtained in this study is the observation that utterance length should be determined with reference to number and type of syllables rather than with reference to the number of segments.

Chomsky and Halle[8] have postulated a hierarchy of boundaries which delimit linguistic units that serve as domains of application of different kinds of phonological rules. Although the authors are careful to state that

TABLE VIII. Mean duration (in milliseconds) of test words and utterances and their ratios (in percent), averaged from productions of speakers R. G. and L. S.

Utterance	Speaker R. G.			Speaker L. S.		
	Duration of word	Duration of utterance	Ratio of word/utterance	Duration of word	Duration of utterance	Ratio of word/utterance
stick	401.55	401.55	100.0	431.80	431.80	100.0
sticky	312.80	513.25	60.9	346.00	557.45	62.1
sticker	302.50	518.05	58.4	331.95	543.35	61.1
sticking	295.45	568.45	52.0	348.30	614.45	56.7
stickily	291.10	612.50	47.5	303.10	637.75	47.5
stickiness	265.75	798.35	33.3	271.60	725.40	37.4
the stick fell	274.85	747.70	36.8	311.15	779.00	39.9
the stick is broken	248.20	922.35	26.9	283.90	935.15	30.4
the stick was discarded	245.10	812.15	30.2	268.15	1084.10	24.7
sleep	409.80	409.80	100.0	442.45	442.45	100.0
sleepy	336.80	517.55	65.1	363.40	544.20	66.8
sleeper	341.25	535.30	63.7	363.35	555.65	65.4
sleeping	330.35	591.70	55.8	374.45	606.25	61.8
sleepily	313.35	602.00	52.1	342.60	645.50	53.1
sleepiness	287.05	739.00	38.8	307.70	705.25	43.6
sleep heals	305.95	836.80	36.6	325.00	777.35	41.8
sleep refreshes	299.60	928.80	32.3	282.75	933.15	30.3
my sleep was disturbed	307.45	1087.50	28.3	314.90	1089.45	28.9

shade	454.10	454.10	100.0	454.65	454.65	100.0
shady	327.20	477.90	68.5	321.65	490.60	65.6
shader	324.20	485.35	66.8	326.75	506.45	64.5
shading	306.95	529.15	58.0	312.95	543.60	57.6
shadily	276.70	552.40	50.1	294.15	613.00	48.0
shadiness	265.20	648.75	40.9	261.65	637.90	41.0
the shade lingered	324.80	799.95	40.6	331.95	746.45	44.5
the shade increased	298.60	938.85	31.8	282.20	823.30	34.3
the shade was refreshing	307.60	1111.40	27.7	273.40	1012.85	27.0
speed	511.50	511.50	100.0	574.25	574.25	100.0
speedy	359.75	529.95	67.9	394.85	597.40	66.1
speeder	344.75	530.50	65.0	403.85	615.50	65.6
speeding	342.50	603.25	56.8	396.10	660.75	59.9
speedily	322.50	631.00	51.1	354.50	711.25	49.8
speediness	313.25	814.25	38.5	322.70	788.95	40.9
speed kills	844.00	990.50	34.7	416.55	999.65	41.7
the speed increased	301.25	968.10	31.1	342.85	999.15	34.3
the speed was controlled	293.50	1142.45	25.7	305.50	1128.55	27.1

phonetic effects need not be associated with (word) boundaries, the postulation of a hierarchy of boundaries naturally prompts a phonetician to look for possibly hierarchical differences in the manifestations of these boundaries. I had previously formulated the hypothesis that phonological units are definable in terms of suprasegmental patterns, while their boundaries are mainly manifested in terms of modifications of segments.[9] Timing patterns are, of course, suprasegmental; therefore it might not be too surprising that few, if any, indications of word boundaries emerged from the present study. (This does not exclude the possibility of boundaries being signaled by other means.) There were a small number of instances in which the duration of the segment preceding a word boundary was greater than the duration of the same segment preceding a morpheme boundary. As far as the over-all temporal organization of the utterances is concerned, no evidence for a hierarchical organization of boundaries was found as a result of this study. The temporal organization of spoken language seems to take place in terms of speech production units which are fairly independent of the morphological or syntactic structure of the utterances.

ACKNOWLEDGMENTS

Grateful acknowledgment is made of the help of Mr. Thomas G. Whitney of the Ohio State University Instruction and Research Computer Center, who wrote the computer programs employed in this study. The work was supported, in part, by Grant GN-534 from the National Science Foundation to the Research Center for Computer and Information Science of The Ohio State University.

[1] I. Lehiste, "The Temporal Organization of Higher-Level Linguistic Units," Paper presented at the April 1970 meeting of the Acoustical Society of America, Atlantic City, N. J. (1970).

[2] I. Lehiste, "Temporal Organization of Spoken Language," in *Form and Substance: Phonetic and Linguistic Papers Presented to Eli Fischer-Jørgensen*, L. L. Hammerich, Roman Jakobson, and Eberhard Zwirner, Eds. (Akademisk Forlag, Copenhagen, 1971), pp. 159–169.

[3] G. E. Peterson and I. Lehiste, "Duration of Syllable Nuclei in English," J. Acoust. Soc. Amer. **32**, 693–703 (1960).

[4] M. A. Naeser, "Criteria for the Segmentation of Vowels on Duplex Oscillograms," Tech. Rep. No. 124, Center for Cognitive Learning, Univ. Wisconsin, Madison, Wisc. (1970).

[5] B. J. Winer, *Statistical Principles in Experimental Design* (McGraw–Hill, New York, 1962), p. 94.

[6] D. Bolinger, "Length, Vowel, Juncture," Linguistics **1**.1, 5–29 (1963) (to be revised).

[7] J. Gaitenby, "The Elastic Word," Paper given at the Tenth Annual National Conference on Linguistics, sponsored by the Linguistic Circle of New York, 13 March 1965. Also, *Status Report on Speech Research* SR-2 (Haskins Laboratories, New York, 1965), pp. 3.1–3.12.

[8] N. Chomsky and M. Halle, *The Sound Pattern of English* (Harper & Row, New York, 1968).

[9] I. Lehiste, *Suprasegmentals* (MIT Press, Cambridge, Mass., 1970).

THE SIGNIFICANCE OF INTRA- AND INTERSENTENCE PAUSE TIMES IN PERCEPTUAL JUDGMENTS OF ORAL READING RATE

NORMAN J. LASS

A total of 31 pause-altered recordings was constructed and played to a group of 78 judges for rate evaluation. Results indicate that pause time is an important variable in perceptual judgments of oral reading rate.

Pauses and duration of pause times are well recognized as important factors in determining speaking and reading rates. Goldman-Eisler (1964) asserts,

> . . . An average of 40 to 50 per cent of utterance time is occupied by pauses. . . . Evidently pausing is as much part of the act of speaking as the vocal utterance of words itself, which suggests that it is essential to the generation of spontaneous speech. . . . Pausing is the main factor accounting for variation in the rate of speech production. (pp. 119-120)

Minifie (1963, p. 62), using an automatic duration analyzer, found, ". . . the changes in reading rate are more a function of the compression and expansion of silence-intervals than a variation in speech-intervals."

Pauses and pause times are also important factors in the perception of reading rate. Franke (1939, p. 19) found overall reading rate and perceptual judgments of rate to be highly correlated (+0.93) and that ". . . pauses were an element in perceived rate."

Agnello (1963) studied the relationship between intra- and interphrasal pauses and the rate of speech as perceived by a group of listeners. He found that duration of intraphrasal pauses related significantly (−0.58) to utterances scaled on a six-point equal-appearing interval scale, while the duration of interphrasal pauses did not (−0.40).

Normally when one attempts to alter his overall reading rate, he exhibits changes in both speech and pause times (Lass and Noll, 1970; Minifie, 1963). However, since a review of the literature indicates that pause time is a very important variable in the perceptual judgment of oral reading rate, it was the purpose of this investigation to experimentally alter only the pause time in an individual's reading of a standard prose passage to determine if perceptual judgments of rate are altered as a result of such changes.

JOURNAL OF SPEECH AND HEARING RESEARCH, 1970, vol. 13, no. 2, 275-283.

Reading Material

The "Rainbow Passage" (Fairbanks, 1960) was used for pause alteration purposes in the study. A 30-year-old male speaker who was judged to have normal voice, articulation, and rate characteristics by a group of 10 graduate students majoring in speech and hearing read the passage.

The reading was recorded in an IAC model 1200 chamber using an Electro-Voice model 664 dynamic cardiod microphone and an Ampex model 602 tape recorder.

Location of Pauses

Alterations within the recording were made only at those points where the reader was found to exhibit pauses in his reading. A group of 20 individuals determined the location of pauses in the reading by listening to the recording and placing pencil marks on copies of the reading where they thought pauses occurred. It was necessary for 15 of the 20 listeners (75%) to agree on a pause point in order for it to be considered and used as a pause in the study. A total of five intrasentence and five intersentence pauses were located in the reading in the above manner.

Pause Alteration Procedure

Duration of intra- and intersentence pause times was determined by an Ampex model 602 tape recorder and a Bruel and Kjaer model 2305 power level recorder. Paper speed of the power level recorder was 30 mm per second, with a pen writing speed of 100 mm per second. The recording was played from the tape recorder through the power level recorder. Simultaneous aural and visual monitoring of the playback and tracing allowed the investigator to place a mark on the power level tracing to delineate each spoken sentence as well as each preestablished pause point. A line was drawn perpendicular to the baseline of the tracing at the beginning and end of each sentence and pause point. The distance between the two points where the drawn line bisected the baseline was measured in millimeters by means of a millimeter ruler. Since the paper speed of the power level recorder was 30 mm per sec, each millimeter corresponded to 0.033 sec. In the above manner, the millimeter measurements on the trace were converted to time measurements in seconds for both intra- and intersentence pauses. It was found that the intrasentence pause time for the entire reading passage was 2.2 secs, while duration of intersentence pause time totaled 3.5 secs.

It was arbitrarily decided to manipulate intra- and intersentence pause times in one of seven ways: (1) no change; (2) 25% increase; (3) 25% decrease; (4) 50% increase; (5) 50% decrease; (6) 75% increase; and (7) 75% decrease. Any changes of pause times involved either increasing both pause types or decreasing them. Increases in one pause type and decreases in the other were not used. Thus, a total of 31 pause alteration conditions were employed. (See Table 1.) Thirty electronic reproductions of the original recording were made. The removal or addition of pause time was accomplished in all cases by the removal or addition of the appropriate percentages of actual tape at each pause point. All pause alterations in a particular recording were distributed approximately equally over the total number of pauses involved. Thus, for ex-

TABLE 1. Mean ratings, pause alteration conditions, and overall reading time (in seconds) for the 31 readings of the "Rainbow Passage."

	Percentages of Pause Alteration		
Mean Rating	Intrasentence	Intersentence	Time (sec)
2.6	+75	+75	31.4
2.6	+50	+75	30.9
2.8	+75	+50	30.8
2.6	+25	+75	30.7
2.8	+50	+50	30.3
2.8	0	+75	30.2
3.1	+75	+25	30.2
3.1	+25	+50	29.8
3.2	+50	+25	29.7
3.1	+75	0	29.6
3.0	0	+50	29.5
3.2	+25	+25	29.2
3.3	+50	0	29.0
3.5	0	+25	28.9
3.5	+25	0	28.8
3.4	0	0	28.2
3.8	−25	0	27.7
4.0	0	−25	27.3
3.9	−50	0	27.2
3.9	−75	0	26.9
4.0	−25	−25	26.7
4.1	0	−50	26.6
4.0	−50	−25	26.4
4.3	−25	−50	26.1
4.5	0	−75	26.0
4.3	−75	−25	25.9
4.4	−50	−50	25.6
5.1	−25	−75	25.4
4.6	−75	−50	25.3
4.9	−50	−75	25.0
5.2	−75	−75	24.7

ample, if a total of 5.0 secs were to be added to (or subtracted from) the intrasentence pause time in a recording, each of the five intrasentence pauses would be increased (or decreased) by 1.0 sec. To control for background noise in all recordings, in those recordings where tape was to be added, tape added was erased on the same recorder used for the original recording.

After all pause alterations were completed, the 30 altered recordings, plus the original unaltered recording, were arranged in random order on a master tape. In addition, five of the 31 recordings (15%) were randomly selected and included at the end of the master tape for intrajudge reliability purposes. Thus, a total of 36 recordings were included on the master experimental tape.

Rating Session

Judges. A total of 78 individuals, 40 males and 38 females, served as judges. All were volunteer subjects from a basic psychology course at the University of Kansas. The group ranged in age from 18 to 28 years, with a mean age of 19 years.

Rating Scale. A six-point equal-appearing interval scale was used for evaluation of reading rate (Agnello, 1963). On the scale, the numbers represented the following rates: 1, very slow; 2, slow; 3, moderate; 4, moderate; 5, fast; and 6, very fast. The judges were asked to listen carefully to the entire reading before circling the number which they thought best represented the reading rate for each reading.

Instructions to Judges. A set of prerecorded instructions was included on the master tape. It contained an explanation of the six-point equal-appearing interval scale, examples of slow, moderate, and fast reading rates, and five readings to be evaluated by the judges for practice purposes. All examples and practice readings involved the same reader and reading passage as was used in the experimental recordings. The examples were obtained from recordings made by the subject in another study (Lass, 1969)[1] in which he was asked to read at moderate, fast, and slow rates. Upon completion of the instructions, all questions of the judges were answered and the experimental readings were played. Playback equipment included an Ampex model 602 tape recorder and an Ampex model 622 speaker-amplifier system.

The rating session, which lasted approximately 60 minutes, was held in a quiet room in one of the buildings on the University of Kansas campus.

RESULTS

Table 1 contains the mean ratings of the judges for each of the 31 pause-altered readings as well as the total time, in seconds, for each reading. The results indicate that changes in perceptual judgments of oral reading rate followed changes in pause times. In addition, the resulting perceptual changes occurred in the expected directions. That is, with increases in pause times, there were corresponding changes toward lower ratings on the scale (slower perceived rates); decreases in pause times produced judgmental changes toward higher ratings (faster perceived rates). Thus, there appears to be a strong inverse relationship between pause time alterations and changes in per-

---

[1]Lass, N. J., Rate alteration patterns in oral reading. Unpublished manuscript, Univ. Kansas (1969).

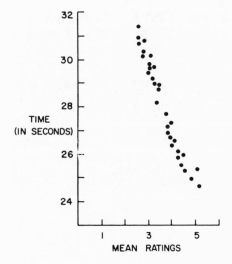

FIGURE 1. Scattergram showing the relationship of overall reading time (in seconds) to mean ratings.

ceptual judgments of reading rate. However, as can be seen from Figure 1, the overall reading time (in seconds) also appears to be related to perceptual judgments of rate ($r = -0.99$). Since it was impossible to alter pause times without also altering overall reading times, it was necessary to determine if the changes in mean ratings were due to changes in overall reading time alone or also to pause time alterations. An analysis of covariance, involving adjustment for a linear dependence of ratings on time (Williams, 1959; Winer, 1962), was used to answer this question. A summary of this analysis is shown in Table 2. An F value of 117.02, significant at the 0.01 level, indicated that pause time alterations had a significant effect on changes in mean ratings.

Intra- vs Intersentence Pauses

Figure 2 shows a comparison of intra- and intersentence pause time alterations and their effect on mean ratings of reading rate. It appears that intersentence pause time alterations affected mean rate ratings more than did alterations of

TABLE 2. Summary of analysis of covariance for determining the effect of pause times on mean ratings of oral reading rate.

Source	SS	df	MS	F
Between Judges	392.84	77	5.10	–
Between Conditions	1323.54	30	44.12	–
Regression	0.06	1	0.06	–
Deviation from Reg.	1323.48	29	45.64	117.02°
Error	902.72	2310	0.39	–
Total	2619.10	2417	–	–

°$F_{0.99}$ (29, 2310) = 2.06

40

intrasentence pause time. The range of mean ratings for intersentence pause time alterations was 2.8 (slow rate) to 4.5 (moderate rate), while intrasentence pause time alterations showed a range of mean ratings of 3.1 (moderate rate) to 3.9 (moderate rate).

In addition, in those pause alteration conditions where both intra- and intersentence pause times are altered by equal percentages, intersentence pause time alterations show greater changes than those of intrasentence pause time. For example, in Table 1, a 75% increase in intrasentence pause time and a 25% increase in intersentence pause time produced a mean rating of 3.1 (moderate rate); while a 25% increase in intrasentence pause time and a 75% increase in intersentence pause time produced a mean rating of 2.6 (slow rate). However,

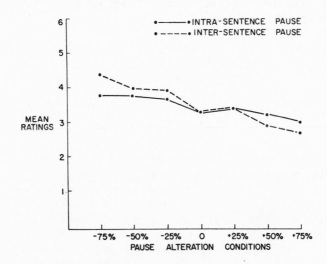

FIGURE 2. The effects of intra- and intersentence pause time alterations on mean ratings of reading rate.

since in the original unaltered recording, total intersentence pause time is greater than total intrasentence pause time, any changes in intersentence pause time will result in longer overall reading time than identical percentage changes in intrasentence pause time. Therefore, from the results of this study it is impossible to make any definitive statement concerning the relative importance of these two types of pauses in influencing perceptual judgments of reading rate.

Intrajudge Reliability

To obtain an estimate of intrajudge reliability, mean discrepancy scores were computed for each of the five repeated readings on the master tape. For each of these readings, the difference between each of the 78 judges' first and second ratings was determined, summed, and divided by the total number of judges, to yield a mean discrepancy score. The grand mean discrepancy, based on the 5 readings, was 0.62 of a scale value, indicating a satisfactorily small dispersion within each of the 78 judges between his first and second ratings of the 5 repeated readings.

Interjudge Reliability

Interjudge reliability was estimated by means of an analysis of variance (Winer, 1962). An r of 0.99 was obtained from this analysis. The interpretation of this finding is as follows: if the experiment were to be repeated with another sample of 78 judges, but with the same readings, the correlation between the mean ratings obtained from the two sets of data on the same readings would be approximately 0.99.

DISCUSSION

Pause time appears to play a definite role in affecting perceptual judgments of oral reading rate. It should be noted that speech time was in no way altered; it remained the same for all of the 31 readings. Moreover, the alterations in pause time were relatively small. A 75% change, the largest amount allowable in the study, involved only a change of approximately 1.7 seconds for intrasentence pause time and 2.6 seconds for intersentence pause time. The largest time change possible for combinations of intra- and intersentence pause time alterations (75% change in both intra- and intersentence pause times) totaled only approximately 4.2 seconds. Nevertheless, such pause changes appear to have affected the listeners' perceptual judgments of reading rate. It is assumed from these findings that larger changes in pause times than the ones used in this study would produce greater changes in perceptual judgments of rate.

The results of this investigation may provide some useful clinical application. Since alterations in pause time, with speech time unaltered, have produced changes in perceptual judgments of rate, perhaps emphasis in speech therapy on pause time alterations, rather than speech time alterations (Fairbanks, 1960; Weiss, 1964), will result in the desired changes in perceptual judgments of rate. In addition, since it has been found that when one attempts to change his reading rate in a given direction (increase or decrease rate), he manifests changes in both speech and pause times (Gilbert and Burk, 1969; Lass and Noll, 1970), there is the possibility that in his attempt to change the duration of his pauses, he will also manifest similar changes in his speech time as well.

However, it should be noted that the results of this investigation pertain to reading rate alone; caution must be exercised in generalizing results from reading to speaking situations. The author is currently involved in the planning stages of a research project concerned with the effect of pause time alterations in impromptu speaking on perceptual judgments of speaking rate. Since there are some basic differences with regard to pause time between reading and speaking (Lass and Noll, 1970; Snidecor, 1943), such a study is necessary before statements concerning pause time alterations in speaking tasks and perceptual judgments of rate can be made.

ACKNOWLEDGMENT

This research was supported by Public Health Service Research Grant No. NB 05362-07 from the National Institute of Neurological Diseases and Blindness to the Bureau of Child Research of the University of Kansas. It was conducted while the author was a postdoctoral research fellow of the Bureau. Papers based on this study were presented at the Second Louisville Conference on Rate and/or Frequency Controlled Speech, University of Louisville, October 22-24, 1969; at the 45th Annual Convention of the American Speech and Hearing Association, Chicago, November 12-15, 1969; and at the 79th Meeting of the Acoustical Society of America, Atlantic City, April 21-24, 1970. Special thanks are extended to Robert Mostellar, Department of Biometry, University of Kansas Medical Center, for his statistical consultation and advice, and to Ralph Shelton, Department of Hearing and Speech, University of Kansas Medical Center, for his helpful comments throughout the research.

REFERENCES

AGNELLO, J. G., A study of intra- and inter-phrasal pauses and their relationship to the rate of speech. Unpublished doctoral dissertation, Ohio State Univ. (1963).

FAIRBANKS, G., *Voice and Articulation Drillbook*. New York: Harper (1960).

FRANKE, P., A preliminary study validating the measurement of oral reading rate in words per minute. Unpublished master's thesis, Univ. Iowa (1939).

GILBERT, J. H., and BURK, K .W., Rate alterations in oral reading. *Lang. Speech*, 12, 192-201 (1969).

GOLDMAN-EISLER, F., Discussion and Further Comments. In Lenneberg, E. H. (Ed.), *New Directions in the Study of Language*. Cambridge, Mass.: M.I.T. Press (1964).

LASS, N. J., and NOLL, J. D., A comparative study of rate characteristics in cleft palate and noncleft palate speakers. *Cleft Palate J.*, 7, 275-283 (1970).

MINIFIE, F. D., An analysis of the durational aspects of connected speech by means of an electronic speech duration analyzer. Unpublished doctoral dissertation, Univ. Iowa (1963).

SNIDECOR, J. C., A comparative study of the pitch and duration characteristics of impromptu speaking and oral reading. *Speech Monographs*, 10, 50-56 (1943).

WEISS, D. A., *Cluttering*. Englewood Cliffs: Prentice-Hall (1964).

WILLIAMS, E. J., *Regression Analysis*. New York: Wiley (1959).

WINER, B. J., *Statistical Principles in Experimental Design*. New York: McGraw-Hill (1962).

A COMPARATIVE STUDY OF RATE EVALUATIONS OF EXPERIENCED AND INEXPERIENCED LISTENERS

Norman J. Lass and Marcia D. Puffenberger

PREVIOUS studies involving perceptual judgments of rate have employed either experienced or inexperienced judges.[1] Although this selection criterion implies that rate evaluations may be affected by the experience of judges, no study has been conducted to assess the effect of this factor on rate evaluations. The present investigation stems directly from the results of a study in which it was found that pause time played a significant role in affecting perceptual judgments of reading rate.[2] Since the judges were college students who had no experience in listening tasks involving the evaluation of speech characteristics, it was not known if the obtained findings were simply the result of the judges' naïveté. The purpose of the present investigation was to resolve this issue: to determine if differences exist between judgments of rate made by experienced and inexperienced observers. In addition, the effect of pause time alterations on rate evaluations by experienced and inexperienced listeners was also explored.

METHOD[3]

Reading material. Fairbanks' "The Rainbow Passage"[4] was read by a 30-year-old male speaker who was judged to have normal voice, articulation, and rate characteristics by a group of ten graduate students majoring in speech and hearing. Recording of the reading was made in an IAC model 1200 chamber using an Electro-Voice model 664 dynamic cardioid microphone and an Ampex model 602 tape recorder.

Location of pauses. Alterations within the recording were made only at those points where the reader was found to exhibit natural pausing in his reading. A group of twenty individuals determined the location of pauses in the reading by listening to the recording and placing pencil marks on copies of the reading where they thought pauses occurred. It was necessary for fifteen of the twenty listeners (75%) to agree on a pause point in order for it to be considered and used as a pause in the study. A total of five intrasentence and five intersen-

[1] Phyllis E. Franke, "A Preliminary Study Validating the Measurement of Oral Reading Rate in Words Per Minute" (unpublished M.A. thesis, University of Iowa, 1939), p. 7; J. C. Kelly and M. D. Steer, "Revised Concept of Rate," *Journal of Speech and Hearing Disorders*, XIV (September 1949), 222-226; Charles L. Hutton, Jr., "A Psychophysical Study of Speech Rate" (unpublished Ph.D. dissertation, University of Illinois, 1954); Joseph G. Agnello, "A Study of Intra- and Inter-Phrasal Pauses and Their Relationship to the Rate of Speech" (unpublished Ph.D. dissertation, Ohio State University, 1963); and Norman J. Lass, "The Significance of Intra and Inter Sentence Pause Times in Perceptual Judgments of Oral Reading Rate," *Journal of Speech and Hearing Research* (in press).

[2] Lass.

[3] The method described below is identical to the one used in *ibid*.

[4] Grant Fairbanks, *Voice and Articulation Drillbook*, 2nd ed. (New York, 1960), p. 127.

QUARTERLY JOURNAL OF SPEECH, 1971, vol. 57, no. 1, 89-93.

tence pauses were located in the above manner.

Pause alteration procedure. Duration of intrasentence and intersentence pause times was determined by means of a Bruel and Kjaer model 2305 high-speed power level recorder. Simultaneous aural and visual monitoring of the playback and tracing allowed the investigators to mark the beginning and ending of each sentence as well as each preestablished pause. The distance between such marks on the tracings were measured (in millimeters) and converted to duration (in seconds) for intrasentence and intersentence pauses. Since the paper speed of the power level recorder was 30 mm per second, each millimeter corresponded to .033 seconds.

It was arbitrarily decided to manipulate intrasentence and intersentence pause times in one of seven ways: (1) no change; (2) 25% increase; (3) 25% decrease; (4) 50% increase; (5) 50% decrease; (6) 75% increase; and (7) 75% decrease. Any changes of pause times involved either increasing or decreasing both pause types. Increases in one pause type and decreases in the other were not allowed. Thus, a total of 31 pause alteration conditions were employed. (See Table I.) Thirty electronic reproductions of the original recording were made. The removal or addition of pause time was accomplished in all cases by the removal or addition of the appropriate percentages of actual tape at each pause point. All pause alterations in a particular recording were distributed approximately equally over the total number of pauses involved.

After all pause alterations were completed, the 30 altered recordings, plus the original unaltered recording, were arranged in random order on a master tape. In addition, 5 of the 31 recordings (15%) were randomly selected and included at the end of the master tape for intrajudge reliability estimations. Thus, a total of 36 recordings were included on the master tape.

Rating sessions: judges. The group of inexperienced listeners consisted of 78 individuals, 40 males and 38 females. All were volunteer subjects from a basic psychology course at the University of Kansas. The group of experienced listeners consisted of 30 persons, 28 females and 2 males. Members of this group were seniors and graduate students in the speech pathology-audiology program at West Virginia University. All had training and experience in listening to, and evaluating, the speech characteristics of speakers. In addition, all were currently involved in speech therapy work at the University Speech and Hearing Clinic. The average number of clock hours of therapy for the group was 172 hours. In view of the geographical locations of the two universities employed, the two groups of judges differed not only in experience but in dialect region as well.

Rating scale. A six-point equal-appearing intervals scale was employed for evaluation of reading rate.[5] On the scale, the numbers represented the following rates:

1 = very slow
2 = slow
3 = moderate
4 = moderate
5 = fast
6 = very fast

The judges were asked to listen carefully to the entire reading before circling the number which they thought best represented the reading rate for each reading.

Instructions to judges. A set of prerecorded instructions was included on the master tape. The instructions were as follows:

5 See Agnello.

45

You will hear the same reader read a standard prose passage a total of 36 times. Please listen carefully to each reading and then make a decision about his oral reading rate. Base your decision on the entire passage and not merely on the first few sentences. Therefore, do not make any final decisions until the reader has completed the entire passage.

Your task will be to assign a numerical value to represent the rate for each reading. Numbers "1" and "2" on the scale represent a slow reading rate, numbers "3" and "4" are considered moderate rate, and "5" and "6" represent a fast reading rate.

You will now hear a sample of the reading rates. The following is an example of a slow reading rate (play reading). Most likely you would have circled the "1" or "2" on the scale, depending on how slow you thought it was. "1" is a rating for a very slow reading. The following is an example of a moderate reading rate (play reading). Most likely you would have circled the "3" or "4" on the scale, depending on whether it was closer to being slow, "3," or closer to being fast, "4." The following is an example of a fast reading rate (play reading). Most likely you would have circled the "5" or "6" on the scale, depending on whether you thought it was closer to the moderate rate, "5," or extremely fast, "6."

To allow you to become familiar with the rating task, you will judge the reading rate of five practice readings. Circle the number which you feel best represents the rate for each reading (play five readings).

You will now hear the same reader read the same passage a total of 36 times. Judge the rate of each reading in the same manner as you did for the practice evaluations.

The concept of rate is an important one in many areas of communication. The judgments obtained from you in this study will be important factors in future research in this area. Therefore, it is important that you do a good, honest job. Are there any questions?

Upon completion of the instructions, all questions of the judges were answered and the experimental readings were played. Playback equipment included an Ampex model 602 tape recorder and an Ampex model 622 speaker-amplifier system. Two rating sessions were held in quiet rooms on the University of Kansas and West Virginia University campuses for the inexperienced and experienced groups, respectively. Each session lasted approximately 60 minutes.

RESULTS[6]

Table I contains the mean ratings of the experienced and inexperienced judges for each of the 31 pause-altered readings as well as the total time (in seconds) for each reading. The results indicate that for both groups of listeners, changes in perceptual judgments of oral reading rate accompanied changes in pause times. In addition, the resulting perceptual changes were in the expected directions. That is, with increases in pause times, there were corresponding changes toward lower ratings on the scale (slower perceived rates); decreases in pause times produced judgmental changes toward higher ratings on the scale (faster perceived rates). Thus, a strong inverse relationship appears to exist between pause time alterations and changes in perceptual judgments of oral reading rate for both groups of judges.

Two three-factor analyses of variance (judge groups X intrasentence pause time alterations X intersentence pause time alterations), one for increases in pause times and one for decreases in pause times, were performed. The analyses involved a least squares solution technique to account for the unequal sizes of the two groups of judges (78 inexperienced; 30 experienced).[7] The analyses indicate the following: (1) there are no significant differences in rate evaluations between the experienced and inexperienced judges when pause times are increased; (2) there are significant differences in rate evaluations between the two groups of judges when pause times

6 The results reported for the inexperienced group of judges were obtained from the study of Lass.

7 B. J. Winer, *Statistical Principles in Experimental Design* (New York, 1962), pp. 374-378.

TABLE I

OVERALL READING TIME (IN SECONDS), PAUSE ALTERATION CONDITIONS, AND MEAN RATINGS OF
EXPERIENCED AND INEXPERIENCED JUDGES FOR THE 31 READINGS

Time (sec.)	Pause Alterations		Mean Ratings	
	Intra-Sent.	Inter-Sent.	Inexperienced	Experienced
31.4	+75%	+75%	2.6	2.7
30.9	+50%	+75%	2.6	2.8
30.8	+75%	+50%	2.8	2.9
30.7	+25%	+75%	2.6	2.7
30.3	+50%	+50%	2.8	3.1
30.2	0	+75%	2.8	2.8
30.2	+75%	+25%	3.1	3.3
29.8	+25%	+50%	3.1	3.4
29.7	+50%	+25%	3.2	3.3
29.6	+75%	0	3.1	3.0
29.5	0	+50%	3.0	3.1
29.2	+25%	+25%	3.2	3.4
29.0	+50%	0	3.3	3.5
28.9	0	+25%	3.5	3.6
28.8	+25%	0	3.5	3.5
28.2	0	0	3.4	3.6
27.7	−25%	0	3.8	3.9
27.3	0	−25%	4.0	4.4
27.2	−50%	0	3.9	4.2
26.9	−75%	0	3.9	4.2
26.7	−25%	−25%	4.0	4.4
26.6	0	−50%	4.1	4.5
26.4	−50%	−25%	4.0	4.3
26.1	−25%	−50%	4.3	4.5
26.0	0	−75%	4.5	4.5
25.9	−75%	−25%	4.3	4.5
25.6	−50%	−50%	4.4	4.8
25.4	−25%	−75%	5.1	5.2
25.3	−75%	−50%	4.6	4.8
25.0	−50%	−75%	4.9	5.5
24.7	−75%	−75%	5.2	5.3

are decreased; (3) intrasentence and intersentence pause time alterations significantly influence the perceptual rate judgments of both experienced and inexperienced listeners; and (4) there is a significant interaction between the two pause types.

Descriptively, for both increases and decreases in pause times, the experienced judges consistently assigned higher scale values (i.e., faster perceived rates) in their evaluations of the readings than did the inexperienced judges. The mean difference between the two groups' overall evaluations for the 31 readings was 0.2 of a scale value. In addition, it appears that there were larger differences in ratings between the two groups of judges for the readings involving decreases in pause times (mean difference of 0.3 of a scale value) than for those involving increases in pause times (mean difference of 0.1 of a scale value).

Intrajudge reliability. To obtain an estimate of intrajudge reliability for each of the two groups of judges, mean discrepancy scores were computed for each of the five repeated readings on the master tape. Grand mean discrepancy scores of 0.62 and 0.54 of a scale value were obtained for the inexperienced and experienced listeners, respectively. These mean discrepancy scores indicate a satisfactorily small dispersion within each of the judges between his first and second ratings of the five repeated readings.

Interjudge reliability. Interjudge reliability for the judges in each of the two groups was estimated by means of two analyses of variance.[8] The obtained *r* values of .99 and .98 for the inexperi-

8 *Ibid.,* pp. 124-132.

47

enced and experienced listeners, respectively, should be interpreted as follows: if the experiment were to be repeated with another sample of judges in each group, but with the same readings, the correlation between the mean ratings obtained from the two sets of data on the same readings would be approximately .98 for the experienced group and .99 for the inexperienced group.

DISCUSSION

The results of this investigation indicate that for both experienced and inexperienced listeners, pause time is an important variable in influencing perceptual judgments of oral reading rate. In the experimental procedure, speech time was in no way altered; it remained the same for all readings. Moreover, the alterations in pause times were relatively small. A 75% change, the largest amount allowable in the study, involved only approximately 1.7 seconds and 2.6 seconds for intrasentence and intersentence pause times, respectively. The largest time change possible for combinations of both pause types (75% change for intrasentence and intersentence pause times) totalled only approximately 4.2 seconds. Nevertheless, both experienced and inexperienced listeners appear to be sensitive to such small pause time alterations.

In addition, the finding of no significant interaction between the judge groups and pause type alterations indicates that, except for differences in initial points of reference, both groups of judges appear to be influenced by pause time alterations in the same manner.

48

DURATION OF SILENT INTERVAL AS A
PERCEPTUAL CUE OF SPEECH PAUSES[1]

KENNETH F. RUDER

Summary.—The effect of duration of silent interval on the perception of pauses in speech was investigated. The stimuli consisted of 5 recorded sentences within which the words "lost" and "contact" were manipulated so that their syntactic relation to one another varied in complexity from sentence to sentence. *Ss,* working individually, mechanically adjusted the silent interval duration between the words "lost" and "contact" within each sentence in order to make judgments of (1) the pause-detection threshold, (2) the optimal fluent pause, and (3) the minimal hesitation pause. Across the 5 sentences, the mean durations were 23 msec., 186 msec., and 505 msec. for the three types of pause, respectively. Statistical analysis, however, showed that durations of silent interval for these three types of pause differed significantly only when occurring between phrases. This was not true of within-phrase pauses. Thus, contrary to usual assumptions in the literature, these results suggest that for within-phrase pauses, at least, duration of silent interval is an insufficient perceptual cue for differentiation of fluent and hesitation pauses.

Most of the research literature on speech pauses (the unfilled variety) has been concerned with an examination of hesitation pauses. The resultant tendency has been to infer the existence of other types of pauses therefrom. This is especially true of Goldman-Eisler's (1968) research. Boomer and Dittman (1962), on the other hand, did examine juncture pauses in relationship to hesitation pause perception but on the basis of an implicit assumption that a pause, if other than a hesitation, served a grammatical function. An implicit attitude is held in the literature, therefore, that there are two types of pauses—those which interrupt the "smooth flow of speech" (hesitation pauses), and those which do not (fluent pauses if you will). Thus, more direct examination of the question of dichotomous (hesitation versus fluent) types of pause seemed in order. Such an examination, if done in relation to what might be termed minimal pause perception (or pause-detection threshold), might even be more helpful in clarifying the general nature of perception of pauses.

An equally important consideration motivated the study reported here. When one compares the various studies in which duration of the silent interval has served as the primary parameter underlying the perceptual distinction among types of pause, it is evident that considerable disagreement exists concerning their durational characteristics. Lounsbury (1954) reports that pauses of durations

[1]This research was supported by NSF Grant GS-2337 and by Grant NB-06459 of the National Institute of Neurological Diseases and Stroke granted to the University of Florida and by PHS Training Grant NS-05362 from NINDS to the Bureau of Child Research, University of Kansas. The data were reported in part at the 78th and 79th meetings of the Acoustical Society of America.

PERCEPTUAL AND MOTOR SKILLS, 1973, vol. 36, 47-57.

greater than 100 msec. are perceived as hesitations, while Goldman-Eisler (1961) sets 250 msec. as the lower bound of hesitation pauses. Hargreaves and Starkweather (1959), on the other hand, state that perceptual identification of hesitation pauses is consistent only for durations of silent intervals greater than 1 sec., although acceptable reliability was obtained for pause judgments down to 500 msec. Boomer and Dittman dispute this finding and indicate that Ss discriminate hesitation pauses reliably at durations down to 200 msec. Thus, it is evident that the durational specification of silent intervals perceived as hesitation pauses needs clarification.

The lack of consistent data is even more acute in regard to fluent pauses due to the largely inferential basis of their durational characteristics. It is natural to assume that the durational domain of the fluent pauses ranges from the point at which a silent interval is just perceived, to that point where the silent interval is perceived as being a hesitation. However, in view of the contradictory evidence on duration of hesitation pauses, any measures of fluent pauses derived from hesitation-pause thresholds are likely to be equally inconsistent. A further shortcoming of the inferred durational basis of fluent pauses is that their lower bound, the threshold of pause detection in speech, has yet to be established. In any case, the study of the durational specifications of those silent intervals perceived as fluent pauses cannot profitably proceed until more reliable data about the threshold of hesitation pauses and pause detection are obtained.

As a result of the implicit nature of presently available information on the existence of various perceptual types of speech pauses and the contradictory reports of their underlying durational characteristics, the present study was directed toward investigating duration of silent interval as it affects the perception of pauses in speech.

PROCEDURE

The psychophysical method of adjustment was employed to obtain the perceptual judgment of pause types on the basis of duration of silent intervals. Judgments were obtained within identical phonetic environments for each of five recorded sentences. The sequence "lost contact" was embedded in each sentence in such a manner that the syntactic relations between "lost" and "contact" varied from sentence to sentence. These syntactic relations were specified both through use of a structural complexity index (Miller & Chomsky, 1963) and Ss' rankings of the complexity of these relations. The rank order of complexity thus obtained ranged from sentence one being least complex to sentence five being most complex. The stimulus sentences, listed in order of complexity of the syntactic relations between "lost" and "contact," were as follows:

1. He lost contact with reality.
2. The lost contact lens case was finally found.
3. The team that lost contacted the authorities.

4. If you're lost, contact the nearest policeman.

5. Even though the battle was lost, contact had been established with the rear guard.

Pause adjustment was accomplished in the following manner: Four adult male speakers were recorded reading the five stimulus sentences. No special instructions were given to the speakers except to read the sentences as naturally as possible. The four recordings of each sentence were presented together to 15 students in an advanced speech pathology class for ranking of the speakers with respect to the following attributes: (1) rate, (2) quality, (3) fluency, (4) naturalness, (5) precision and (6) over-all effectiveness. In ranking the speakers on rate, for example, Ss were told to give the highest ranking to the individual who attained the best rate for the given sentence; that is, the rate was neither too fast nor too slow. In like manner, the highest ranking went to the speaker who had the best quality, was most fluent, most natural, etc. The speaker ultimately selected from this original pool of four, attained the highest mean ranking on all attributes for each sentence (87% of the judges ranked this speaker best on all sentences). The speaker's recorded sentences were then dubbed onto a two-track tape such that the portion of the sentence up to and including the word "lost" was recorded on Track A, while the remainder of the sentence (beginning with the word "contact") was recorded on Track B.

A modified two-track playback head system (Ruder, Jensen, & Brandt, 1970) was constructed so that adjustment of pause duration could be accomplished through delaying, to a greater or lesser degree, the playback of the Track B signal (that part of the sentence beginning with the word "contact"). To provide for such a variable delay, a tape guide attached to a worm gear assembly, as shown in Fig. 1, was mounted between the fixed Track A and Track B playback heads. Since the tape guide was attached to the worm gear, its position, relative to the horizontal plane of the playback heads, could be varied up and down the worm gear, thereby increasing or decreasing the effective distance between the playback heads. Pause duration between "lost" and "contact" could be increased, then, by moving the tape guide away from the playback heads and decreased by moving the tape guide toward the playback heads, since this movable guide altered the time of onset of the Track B signal relative to that on Track A by changing the distance the tape must travel to reach the "B" playback head. The outputs from Tracks A and B were combined so that the signals from both tracks were received in both ears.

The young adults (26 males and 4 females, aged 21 to 35 yr.), working individually, were asked to adjust the duration of the pause between "lost" and "contact" to that point at which they just detected a pause; that is, if the duration had been any shorter, a pause would not have been perceived between those two words. Twelve of these Ss (all males) also were asked to adjust the duration of the pause between the words "lost" and "contact" so that (1) the duration of

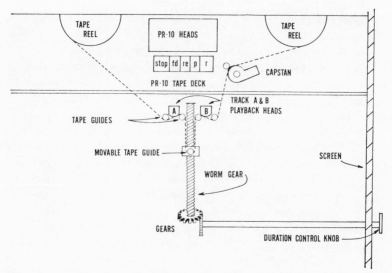

FIG. 1. Apparatus to provide variable pause adjustment. The screen shields the instrumentation from *S*'s view (from Ruder, *et al.* (1970), © 1970 by the Society for the Experimental Analysis of Behavior, Inc.).

the pause was considered optimal for "fluent" presentation of the sentence and (2) the pause was just perceived as a hesitation. Each pause adjustment within each task was repeated three times to obtain an estimate of within-subject variability. *S*s were given as much time and as many trials as necessary to make each adjustment. The interval of the sentence containing the adjusted pause was displayed on an oscilloscope screen and photographed.

The adjusted durations of pause were measured from the oscilloscope photographs in the following manner. A straight-edge ruler was placed along the top of the Channel A baseline on the extreme right-hand corner of the photo display so that it was parallel to the horizontal scale division. This procedure is depicted as line AB in Fig. 2. Moving right to left along line AB, the point at which the speech signal first departed from this baseline reference was identified (indicated by point X in Fig. 2). A perpendicular (line EF) was erected at this point. In similar fashion, point Y was located by moving along the Channel B baseline from left to right and a perpendicular (line GH) erected at this point also. The distance between lines EF and GH is depicted in Fig. 2 as line IJ. This distance represents the time between the end of the Channel A signal and the beginning of the Channel B signal. This distance was converted to pause time in milliseconds by multiplying this distance by the time scale value used for that particular oscillographic display.

RESULTS AND DISCUSSION

The mean durations for the three pause types—pause-detection threshold,

52

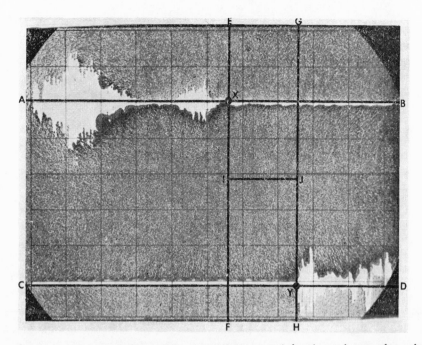

FIG. 2. Reference points used in the measurement of durations of pause from the oscillographic photographs: line AB, the top of the Channel A baseline; line EF, a perpendicular erected through AB at point X (point where the speech signal drops to the baseline); line GH, a perpendicular erected at point Y (point at which the Channel B signal drops to the baseline); line IJ, the distance in centimeters from the end of Channel A signal to the beginning of Channel B signal

fluent pause, and hesitation pause are shown in Fig. 3. From this figure, it can be seen that the mean duration of hesitation pause (505 msec.) differs considerably from the mean duration of fluent pause (186 msec.) and that both of these pause types differ in duration from the mean pause-detection threshold (23 msec.). To determine whether these differences were statistically significant, a treatment by subjects analysis of variance was performed. Results indicated that pause durations for hesitation pause, fluent pause, and pause-detection threshold did differ significantly from each other ($F = 43.63$, $df = 2/22$, $p < .01$). However, there was also a significant interaction between type of pause and syntactic complexity ($F = 8.97$, $df = 8/88$, $p < .01$). In order to more meaningfully interpret the effects of pause type, then, this significant interaction was analyzed further by computing the simple main effects of pause-type at each level of syntactic complexity. The outcome, summarized in the table below, indicates no significant differences among the durations of pause-detection threshold, fluent pause, and hesitation pause at the two lowest levels of syntactic complexity; there are significant differences, however, at the other three levels.

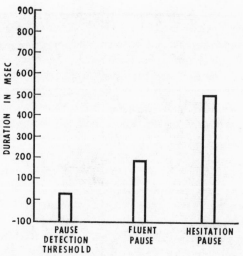

FIG. 3. Comparison of mean durations of pause-detection threshold, fluent pause, and hesitation pause

The differences between the two lowest levels of complexity and the other three sentences were further clarified by examination of the raw data. While Fig. 3 indicates that durations of hesitation pause were greater than durations of fluent pause, and durations of fluent pause were greater than pause-detection thresholds, this held true only for the three highest levels of syntactic complexity. Numerous reversals of this order occurred at the two lowest levels of complexity. Since the syntactic boundaries at these two lowest levels of complexity represent within-phrase relations and those at the higher levels of complexity represent between-phrase relations the effects of pause duration on perceived pause types will be discussed, in turn, with respect to this within-phrase, between-phrase distinction.

Within-phrase Durations of Pause

The lack of significance among pause-detection threshold, fluent pause and durations of hesitation pause at the within-phrase pause boundaries in sentences

TABLE 1

SIMPLE MAIN EFFECTS FOR FACTOR A (PAUSE TYPE) AT EACH LEVEL OF FACTOR B (SYNTACTIC COMPLEXITY)

Source	SS	df	MS	F	p
A at B_1	648,627	2	324,314	1.23	
A at B_2	1,019,351	2	509,675	1.94	
A at B_3	3,960,353	2	1,980,177	7.53	.01
A at B_4	10,029,195	2	5,014,598	19.08	.01
A at B_5	14,112,191	2	7,056,095	26.85	.01
Error (A at B_j)	5,782,012	22	262,819		

one and two suggest that within-phrase pauses are functionally distinct from between-phrase pauses. Goldman-Eisler (1968), as well as Boomer and Dittman (1962), make a similar distinction between juncture (grammatical) pauses and hesitation pauses in which the former are limited to between-phrase and the latter to within-phrase occurrences. It is clearly implied in their works that duration of the silent interval is the only significant cue for within-phrase hesitation pauses; the present study, however, indicates that duration, in itself, is not a sufficient cue for such pauses. An alternative is that allophonic changes, such as prepausal phoneme lengthening, combine with duration of silent interval in providing for the perception of within-phrase hesitation pauses. Such a viewpoint would be supported by the work of Martin (1970), however, the extent to which such cues might interact in the perception of pauses remains to be investigated.

The discrepancy that has been cited relative to the parameters cueing perception of hesitation pause might relate as well to definitional considerations. In the present study, hesitation pauses were defined with reference to durations of fluent pause; it is not clear that this was the case in the earlier investigations. Although Goldman-Eisler (1968, pp. 11-79), Lounsbury (1954), and Maclay and Osgood (1959) define hesitation pauses as silent intervals of "unusual" duration, they fail to state an explicit reference for the concept "unusual." Their conception of "unusual" duration may not be referenced to duration of fluent pause, but rather, to some internalized standard of the listener. The large degree of variability in Ss' mean durations of hesitation pause suggests that this is plausible.

Between-phrase Pause Durations

To determine which of the pause types accounted for the over-all significance of the simple main effect in the between-phrase durations, the Newman-Keuls test of treatment differences (Winer, 1962, pp. 80-85), following an over-all significant F ratio was applied to this portion of the data. The results of this test indicated that pause durations for pause-detection threshold, fluent pause, and hesitation pause differed significantly from each other at all three between-phrase syntactic boundaries.

Essentially, then, the data for between-phrase pauses can be viewed as support for the notion that pause-detection threshold, fluent pause, and hesitation pause are perceptually differentiated on the basis of duration of the silent interval. However, it should be noted that in many previous investigations, between-phrase pauses have been systematically excluded. This has been particularly true in the study of hesitation pauses (Goldman-Eisler, 1968) although the rationale for the exclusion of such between-phrase pauses was never made clear. While the present data do suggest that within-phrase pauses are functionally distinct from between-phrase pauses, they would also argue against any such exclusion. For instance, if the present study had been confined to either within- or between-phrase pauses, the answer to the question concerning the role of duration of silent interval in the perception of pauses would have been answered quite differently.

55

It is apparent, therefore, that an understanding of the perceptual nature of speech pauses *per se* must take into account both within-phrase and between-phrase environments if further investigation is to be considered at all valid and meaningful.

The question initially posed as to the extent to which duration of pause is used to differentiate pause-detection thresholds, fluent pauses, and hesitation pauses may, therefore, be answered briefly as follows. Pause duration was found to be an insufficient perceptual cue, in and of itself, in differentiating between these pause types when such pauses occurred within phrases. However, with regard to between-phrase pauses, duration of the silent interval was a significant perceptual cue. In light of the differences found in the perception of within- and between-phrase pauses, further explication of the perceptual nature of speech pauses will have to take this within-between phrase distinction into account. Therefore, these results suggest that for within-phrase pauses, at least, other perceptual cues, as well as duration of the silent intervals, should be considered in any study of the differences between fluent and hesitation pauses.

Pause Detection as a Function of Syntactic Complexity

Inspection of the pause-detection threshold raw data for sentences two through five showed numerous negative pause durations (that is, the point at which S indicated he just detected a pause was in reality an overlap of the words "lost" and "contact"). For sentence one, however, only one of 90 judgments resulted in a negative pause-detection threshold.

Comparison of the acoustic signals of the five stimulus sentences did show a possible explanation for these negative values. In sentences two through five, the word "lost" was terminated by a plosive burst which was perceptible both in the auditory and visual (oscilloscope) signal. Sentence one contained no such plosive burst. Thus, it was hypothesized that Ss were disregarding, or were perceptually unaware of, the overlapping of this plosive burst with the word "contact." This overlap may well have not been perceived since the plosive burst is often redundant information for the identification of plosive stops (Cooper, Delattre, Liberman, Borst, & Gerstman, 1952) and was also, presumably, masked by the onset of "contact." Therefore, the silent interval corresponding to the period of closure for the stop consonant may well have been taken to be part of the pause interval.

If it were assumed that Ss did indeed disregard the plosive burst in the pause-detection task, then a pause-duration remeasurement which also ignored this plosive burst should eliminate the negative pause-detection thresholds. Fig. 4 shows the results of the remeasurement procedure compared with the original pause-detection thresholds and mean durations of fluent pause. As can be seen from this figure, not only did the remeasurement eliminate most of the negative pause-detection thresholds, but it also made the pause-detection curve resemble

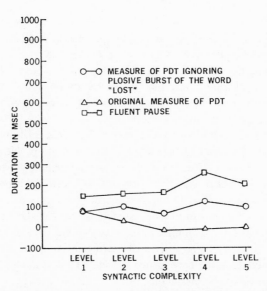

FIG. 4. A comparison of fluent pause durations with pause-detection thresholds obtained from measures in which the plosive burst terminating the word "lost" was included as part of the speech signal and pause-detection thresholds obtained from measures in which this plosive burst was ignored

the curve for fluent pauses. The striking similarity between these two curves suggests, then, that fluent-pause duration at a particular boundary may well be a function of the pause-detection threshold at that same boundary. This, however, needs verification by further research.

The remeasurement of the pause-detection thresholds also had the effect of increasing the over-all mean pause-detection threshold from 23 msec. to 95 msec. This value, however, is still far short of the minimum detected duration of pause of 190 msec. reported by Agnello (1963). There are, however, several important procedural differences which might account for this discrepancy. First of all, the present study directed Ss specifically to locate the duration at which the silent interval was just detected as a pause. Agnello assumed *a priori* that pauses shorter than 150 msec. were not perceived. Furthermore, the pause-detection thresholds reported in the present study are the result of direct measures, whereas Agnello's minimum duration of pause is merely an estimate based on comparison of the total number of perceived pauses with the total number of pauses measured by machine. Agnello's data cannot, therefore, really be taken as an indication of the pause-detection threshold in speech nor can they really be compared to the results of the present study. It should be pointed out as well that the present data provide but an indication of the speech pause-detection threshold. Considerably more data, obtained from more Ss and more phonetic environments, are needed before any substantial statements about such thresholds can be made.

Subject Variability

To provide an estimate of within-subject variability in making duration judgments of pause types, each S was asked to replicate each pause adjustment three times. The treatments by Ss analysis of variance indicated that there was no statistically significant effect due to replications ($F = 2.65$, $df = 2/22$, $p > .05$). This suggests that, within themselves, Ss were performing consistently from one replication to the next.

Since the replications effect was shown to be non-significant in the over-all analysis of variance, the replication scores were pooled to provide an estimate of within-cell variance to be used in a test of these apparent between-subject differences. The results of this analysis showed that Ss differed significantly among themselves ($F = 22.38$, $df = 11/24$, $p < .01$).

These subject differences in pause perception parallel the situation found in the production aspect. Goldman-Eisler (1968) and Scholes (1971) report considerable variation among individuals in the use of pauses in speech. The subject differences reported here in this perceptual study, as well as the reported individual variation in the production studies, thus point out one important fact. Any study of pauses, be it perceptual or production, should take care to use a relatively large group of randomly selected Ss since the outcome could well reflect the bias of a small group of Ss and not be representative of the population as a whole. Although the present study was restricted to a selected group of Ss (undergraduate college students), this was done to control for possible unwanted sources of variation due to age, socioeconomic, and/or educational differences. While there is no *a priori* reason to assume that these factors would affect the perception of pauses in speech, they do need to be considered for further study.

The fact that considerable individual differences exist both in the production and perceptual aspects of pausal behavior leads to the obvious conclusion that these individual differences may be related. More specifically, the question could be asked whether or not a person who habitually produces longer pauses at a particular pause boundary would also use a longer adjusted duration of pause at this boundary in a perceptual study such as this one. An experiment to test this aspect is currently in progress.

REFERENCES

AGNELLO, J. A study of intra- and inter-phrasal pauses and their relationship to the rate of speech. Unpublished dissertation, Ohio State Univer., 1963.

BOOMER, D., & DITTMAN, A. Hesitation pauses and juncture pauses in speech. *Language and Speech*, 1962, 5, 215-226.

COOPER, F. S., DELATTRE, P., LIBERMAN, A., BORST, J., & GERSTMAN, L. Some experiments on the perception of synthetic speech sounds. *Journal of the Acoustical Society of America*, 1952, 24, 597-606.

GOLDMAN-EISLER, F. A comparative study of two hesitation phenomena. *Language and Speech*, 1961, 4, 232-237.

GOLDMAN-EISLER, F. *Psycholinguistics: experiments in spontaneous speech.* New York: Academic Press, 1968.

HARGREAVES, W. A., & STARKWEATHER, J. Collection of temporal data with the duration tabulator. *Journal of the Experimental Analysis of Behavior,* 1959, 2, 179-183.

LOUNSBURY, F. Sequential psycholinguistics. In C. Osgood & T. Sebeok (Eds.), *Psycholinguistics, a survey of theory and research problems.* Baltimore: Waverly, 1954. Pp. 93-125.

MACLAY, H., & OSGOOD, C. Hesitation phenomena in spontaneous English speech. *Word,* 1959, 15, 19-44.

MARTIN, J. G. On judging pauses in spontaneous speech. *Journal of Verbal Learning and Verbal Behavior,* 1970, 9, 75-78.

MILLER, G., & CHOMSKY, N. Finitary models of language users. In R. Luce, R. Bush, & E. GALANTER (Eds.), *Handbook of mathematical psychology.* Vol. 2. New York: Wiley, 1963. Pp. 419-492.

RUDER, K., JENSEN, P., & BRANDT, J. An apparatus and procedure for the perceptual study of speech pauses. *Journal of the Experimental Analysis of Behavior,* 1970, 14, 287-289.

SCHOLES, R. *Acoustic cues for constituent structure: Janua Linguarum, No. 121.* The Hague: Mouton, 1971.

WINER, B. J. *Statistical principles in experimental design.* New York: McGraw-Hill, 1962.

PERCEPTION OF READING RATE BY SPEAKERS AND LISTENERS

HARLAN LANE   FRANÇOIS GROSJEAN

The generalization that sensation grows more rapidly for the speaker than for his listener is supported by scaling autophonic and extraphonic reading rate, using the methods of magnitude production and estimation respectively. The obtained exponents of the two power functions 2.6 and 1.5, show that when a speaker doubles his reading rate he perceives a sixfold increase, whereas a listener perceives less than a threefold increase. This disparity, about the same size as that for voice level, indicates that the speaker's judgments of rate, like his judgments of level, are not based solely on the sound of his voice. When a speaker varies his rate of reading a known passage in order to produce a desired apparent rate, he primarily adds or subtracts pauses at strategic syntactic locations. It is the number of pauses, much more than the rate of articulation or the duration of the pauses, that determines the changes in overall rate.

When a speaker judges the characteristics of his own speech, the cues available include tactile and proprioceptive feedback, as well as bone-and-air-conducted sidetone. When he stops speaking and judges someone else's speech, he is deprived of all of these cues save the last and, as a listener, must found his judgments differently. Since the sensory characteristics of speaking and listening are so different structurally, it is not surprising to learn, from the accumulated experimental evidence, that they are quite different functionally (Lane, 1971b). As a rule, the speaker's perception of the properties of his own speech, his autophonic output, grows more rapidly than the corresponding physical magnitudes and more rapidly than his perception

of these properties in the speech of another. The autophonic functions for voice level, vowel duration, and voice pitch are all steeper than the corresponding extraphonic functions (Lane, 1962).

In the present study, we turn to examine the speaker's perception of his own rate of reading against this background. Does apparent rate, like apparent level, grow as a power of physical rate and, if so, with what exponent? Does this autophonic scale have a slope greater than 1.0 (log–log coordinates), and is it steeper than the corresponding extraphonic scale? One more question helps to set the stage for this attempt to determine the autophonic scale of speech rate: To what extent does the speaker change his articulation rate and

JOURNAL OF EXPERIMENTAL PSYCHOLOGY, 1973, vol. 97, no. 2, 141-147.

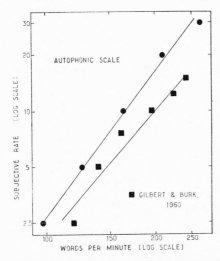

FIG. 1. Autophonic scale of reading rate. (Each circle represents the geometric mean of 96 magnitude productions, 8 by each of 12 speakers. The squares represent the arithmetic means of 288 fractionations or multiplications of reading rate, 24 by each of 12 speakers, in an experiment by Gilbert and Burk, 1969.)

to what extent the frequency and duration of his pauses, in order to produce an overall change in apparent rate of reading?

METHOD

Subjects. Twelve graduate students, native speakers of English with no reported speech or hearing defects, served for about an hour in the experiment on autophonic rate. Four of them, plus four additional classmates, served in the subsequent experiment on extraphonic rate, lasting about a half hour.

Procedure. The method of magnitude production was used to determine the autophonic scale (Lane, Catania, & Stevens, 1961). The *S* was asked to read the experimental passage at normal rate. To the apparent rate of this reading, *E* assigned the numerical value 10. A series of values (2.5, 5, 10, 20, 30) was then named in irregular order, eight times each in all, and the speaker responded to each value by reading the passage with a proportionate apparent rate.

The method of magnitude estimation was used to measure extraphonic perception of speech rate. The *E* played a recording of the experimental passage read at moderate rate (162 wpm); to this standard he assigned the numerical value 10. Next he played 40 recordings of the passage, and the listener

assigned to each a number proportional to its apparent rate. In all, five rates of reading by the same speaker were presented eight times in irregular order: 92, 131, 162, 255, and 360 wpm.

Materials. The experimental passage contained 51 words of text (including contractions), comprising 75 syllables: AS FAR AS I KNOW, I'M A FAIRLY NORMAL FIFTEEN YEAR OLD, NEITHER A COMPLETE PSYCHOLOGICAL CASE, NOR A CUT ABOVE THE OTHERS. I LISTEN TO RADIO LUXEMBOURG, MY HAIR FALLS FORWARD IN THE FASHIONABLE STYLE, AND I WEAR POLO NECK SWEATERS, BUT I DON'T CONSIDER MYSELF A GREAT POP FAN.

The magnitude productions were tape recorded (Uher 4000L) in an audiometric room. The tapes were played back into an oscillographic recorder (Mingograph EM 34) and the tracings measured with dividers to an accuracy of ± .02 sec. (paper speed, 25 mm/sec). These measures yielded, for each passage, the number and duration of the pauses and the runs (the stretches of speech between the pauses), with a pause defined as an interruption of the sound wave lasting more than .24 sec. The magnitude estimations were obtained from *S*s in the same audiometric room, listening to the tape recordings at comfortable level, with parallel headsets (Opelem-Socapex) supplied by an Opelem tape recorder (2M70).

RESULTS AND DISCUSSION

Autophonic perception of rate. The speaker's perception of his own reading rate is plotted in Figure 1 as a function of the rate actually produced. The results are well represented by a straight line in log–log coordinates. Consequently, the relation between perceived and actual rate can be considered a power function whose exponent is given by the slope of best fit to the geometric means of the data. The subjective scale of autophonic rate has a slope of 2.58 when determined by the method of magnitude production. Thus, autophonic rate joins the list of several dozen other continua on which psychological magnitude has been shown to be a power function of the stimulus (Stevens, 1962); and, more specifically, it joins the other autophonic scales indicating that the sensory mechanisms mediating the speaker's perception of his own speech amplify constant stimulus ratios into much larger constant subjective ratios. If we estimate the slope of the autophonic scale of reading rate to a first approximation at 2.6, then a subjective ratio of $\frac{1}{2}$ corresponds to a physical ratio of rate of $\frac{3}{4}$.

The most thoroughly studied of the other autophonic scales is certainly that for voice level, with exponent 1.2 (Lane, 1962, 1963; Lane et al., 1961; Lane, Tranel, & Sisson, 1970). The variability of magnitude productions of speech rate is compared to that for voice level in Table 1. Three sources of variability should be distinguished in both cases: (*a*) variability due to *S*'s choice of the standard 10, that is, his modulus; (*b*) variability due to *S*'s conception of a subjective ratio; and (*c*) variability due to different sense-organ operating characteristics. The first component of the total variance was removed to obtain the "corrected" estimates of population standard deviations shown in the table in the following way: A grand mean of the log vocal rates of the group was first computed. The mean of all of the log rates of a given *S* was then subtracted from the grand mean and the difference was added to each one of that *S*'s log rates. This operation left unchanged the slope of each *S*'s autophonic rate function, but it minimized the sum of the squared deviations of his productions around the regression line for the group. On the other hand, it should be noted that these standard deviations are unaffected by changes in the unit of measurement. Table 1 shows that almost half of the total variability obtained with the method of magnitude production is accounted for by differences among *S*s in their choice of modulus and that the productions of rate were less variable than those of level.

When the autophonic scale of speech rate is constructed from fractionations and multiplications of reading rate, the results are reasonably consistent with those obtained by magnitude production in this study. Gilbert and Burk (1969) had 12 *S*s read a 55-word passage at speeds $\frac{1}{4}$, $\frac{1}{2}$, and $\frac{3}{4}$ normal, and $\frac{1}{4}$ and $\frac{1}{2}$ greater than normal. When their results are plotted in log–log coordinates (Figure 1), the straight line of best fit has a slope of 2.3. On the one hand, the use of fractionation below the standard and multiplication above is expected to steepen the psychophysical function (cf. the results for halving and doubling of loudness, Poulton & Stevens, 1955). On

TABLE 1

Standard Deviations (in db.) of Vocal Levels[a] and Reading Rates Obtained by Magnitude Production

Criterion value	Vocal level ($n = 72$)[b]		Reading rate ($n = 96$)[c]	
	Uncorrected	Corrected	Uncorrected	Corrected
2.5	5.2	3.4	2.6	1.9
5	6.3	3.3	1.9	1.3
10	6.6	2.6	1.2	.5
20	6.9	2.8	1.2	1.1
30	6.7	4.0	1.7	1.6

Note. The *SD*s were corrected for the component of variability due to *S*'s choice of modulus and for bias due to sample size. The *SD*s are expressed in db. to facilitate comparison.
[a] The *SD*s of vocal levels were taken from Lane, Catania, and Stevens (1961).
[b] 72 = 24 *S*s × 3 Magnitude Productions/*S*.
[c] 96 = 12 *S*s × 8 Magnitude Productions/*S*.

the other hand, curiously enough, these *E*s played *S*'s standard back to him after each production, which may have encouraged him to found his judgments of rate more heavily on auditory impressions than he would otherwise have done; that is, the rate of growth of autophonic changes may have been attenuated by the more moderate growth of extraphonic changes. The fractionation data are probably more in line with the autophonic scale of speech rate than it already appears for yet another reason. The lowest reading rates are associated with the largest variance (Table 1) and the greatest skewness. Since Gilbert and Burk used the arithmetic mean as a measure of central tendency, the rates at the lowest fractionation values and therefore the slope of the psychophysical function may be underestimated. In fact, if the arithmetic mean had been used in the present study instead of the geometric mean, a slope of 2.50 and not 2.58 would have been obtained for the autophonic scale.

Extraphonic perception of rate. The extraphonic perception of reading rate is described in Figure 2. The magnitude estimates are well fit by a straight line in log–log coordinates, with slope 1.5 (the mean and *SD* of the eight individual slopes are 1.5 and .37). The figure also shows the transformed category estimates of reading rate from an experiment in which a 55-word passage recorded at eight differ-

62

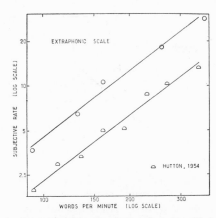

FIG. 2. Extraphonic scale of reading rate. (Each circle represents the geometric mean of 40 magnitude estimations, 5 by each of 8 listeners. Also plotted are transformed average category estimates of rate assigned by 10 listeners [Hutton, 1954].)

ent rates was presented to 10 listeners. Hutton (1954) reported that $G = 11.97 \log R - .46$, where G is a category estimate from 1 to 9, and R is the rate in words per minute. Schneider and Lane (1963) have shown that when a category scale is a simple logarithmic function of a physical continuum, as in this case, then it is related to the ratio estimation scale of the same continuum by: $\log M = n/b(G - a)$, where M is a magnitude estimate, a and b the intercept and slope, respectively, of the category scale, and n the exponent of the ratio scale. The excellent fit of the transformed category estimates of rate to the extraphonic function obtained in the present study confirms that the category scale of rate is concave downward when plotted against the ratio scale, as is expected for a prothetic continuum (Stevens & Galanter, 1957).

The disparity between the slopes of the autophonic and extraphonic functions (Figures 1 and 2), which was displayed by each of the four Ss who served in both experiments as well as by the groups, is quite instructive. It means that when a speaker doubles his reading rate he perceives a sixfold increase, whereas a listener perceives less than a threefold increase.

It is noteworthy that this ratio, approximately 2:1, between the sensory dynamics of speaking and listening is similar to that obtained for voice level (Lane et al., 1970). The generalization that sensation grows more rapidly for the speaker than for the listener seems to be borne out.

The disparity between the perception of spoken rate and heard rate also shows that the speaker does not rely exclusively on his hearing in judging his rate. This was expected. It is clear that, as far as judging his voice level is concerned, the speaker does not rely on his hearing. The autophonic scale of voice level is the same for normal speakers, for those who are experimentally deafened with intense masking noise, and for those who are deaf from birth (Lane, 1963). All three populations claim they are judging vocal effort when judging their own voice level, and indeed, the autophonic level of a speech sound and the work done on the air in producing it are proportional; they both grow as the 1.2 power of sound pressure (Ladefoged & McKinney, 1963). Further evidence that autophonic judgments are not loudness judgments is obtained whenever speakers vary their levels in order to match changes in the loudness of a criterion stimulus, to compensate for changes in sidetone loudness, or to maintain intelligibility despite increasing noise (Lane et al., 1970). All of these tasks confirm the 2:1 disparity in the operating characteristics of the underlying sensory mechanisms. Finally, the finding that judgments of one's own reading rate must depend more on interoceptive cues than on hearing was expected in the light of the evidence that it is these cues and not sidetone that are critically involved in the servomechanism control of speech (Lane, 1971a).

Rate as a complex variable. The autophonic scale plotted in Figure 1 shows the changes in the speaker's perception of his rate associated with changes in the rate of reading a passage. These latter changes, however, are the sum of changes in the time spent articulating and in the time spent pausing, and it is natural to wonder about the relative contribution of these two vari-

63

ables to the autophonic perception of rate. Since the exponent of a power function $y = x^m$ is unchanged under the similarity group transformation, $x' = cx$, the slope of the autophonic scale will not change whether it is plotted against articulation time, pause time, or their sum (or words per minute) *if* articulation time is a constant fraction of the total time. Figure 3 shows, however, that the articulation time ratio (= phonation time ratio) is not a constant. The percentage of the time spent articulating seems to grow about linearly with the rate, reaching nearly 100% in the present experiment. The whole picture does not agree with that painted by Gilbert and Burk (1969) who thought that "the results for w.p.m. rate indicate a significant serial increase as subjects progress from the slowest to the fastest rates studied, p.t.r. [phonation time ratio] on the other hand being altered only for establishing a difference between the

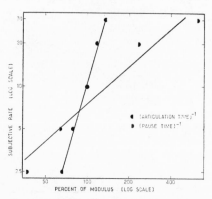

Fig. 4. Autophonic judgments of reading rate as a function of articulation time and pause time that comprise the physical rate. (For convenience, the reciprocals of these two components of the measures plotted in Figure 1 are shown, expressed as a percentage of their average values at the modulus.)

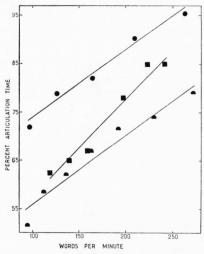

Fig. 3. Percentage of time spent articulating as a function of the overall rate. (Each circle represents the articulation–time ratio [×100] averaged across the 12 speakers. The squares represent the articulation-time ratios for the fractionations and multiplications of reading rate obtained by Gilbert and Burk, 1969. The half circles show articulation-time ratios of category productions by 1 speaker [Hutton, 1954].)

faster and slower rates [p. 201]." Average articulation time ratios are less in the latter experiment and in Hutton's (1954) experiment (data reported for one S), but then the passage employed had four sentences compared to two here, and hence two more places for "full stops." Another factor probably contributing to reduced articulation–time ratios in these two experiments is the duration criterion for a pause; reported in neither study, it was probably shorter than in the present experiment.

The speaker in fact changes articulation time much less than pause time to achieve a given increase in apparent rate. When autophonic judgments are plotted against these two component variables of physical rate in log–log coordinates, the slopes of the straight lines of best fit are − 3.4 and − 0.9, respectively. For convenience, Figure 4 shows the reciprocals of these two functions, with articulation time and pause time expressed as a percentage of their average values at the average modulus (165 wpm), specifically, 15.4 and 3.4 sec. (82% articulation time). In terms of articulation rates, the modulus, 4.8 syllables/sec, was bracketed by a range of only 3.4 syllables/sec. Apparently, the speaker who wishes to double his apparent

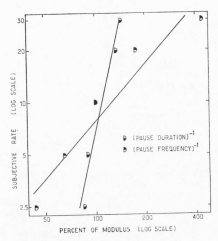

Fig. 5. Autophonic judgments of reading rate as a function of pause duration and pause frequency, which comprise total pause time (Figure 4). (For convenience, the reciprocals of these two components of the measures plotted in Figure 4 are shown, expressed as a percentage of their average values at the modulus.)

rate simply spends half as much time pausing.

Does he do this by pausing half as often or by cutting the durations of his pauses in half—or both? The former, according to Figure 5, is correct. On the average, twice the apparent rate was associated with about half the number of pauses but 85% of the average pause duration. The

slopes of the straight lines of best fit in log–log coordinates are, respectively, $- 1.1$ and $- 4.3$. Incidentally, the slope relating autophonic rate to total pause time (Figure 4) follows necessarily from the slopes reported in Figure 5 for pause frequency and duration and the fact that pause time is their product. In general, if $y = x^a$ and $y = z^b$, then $y = (xz)^{ab/a+b}$.

The nearly linear reduction in pause frequency with increasing autophonic rate (Figure 5) is not accomplished, of course, by indiscriminate suppression of pauses. Goldman-Eisler (1968) states that, with passages read aloud, pauses should be found after phrases, clauses, and at the end of sentences. Table 2 shows the percentage of all pause slots filled, as a function of the nature of the grammatical juncture and the rate of reading. At the modulus rate (165 wpm), her prediction is indeed confirmed, with the addition of two pauses after content words not located at clause boundaries: GREAT and POP. These exceptions are most likely caused by the particular stress distribution over the expression A GREAT POP FAN. At the next highest speed, the pause after GREAT is dropped, while all the others are retained. At the very highest speed, only the sentence-final and three of the clause-final pauses are retained, namely those before the constructions beginning NEITHER . . . NOR, AND, and BUT. When the reader gives magnitude productions of rate below his modulus, he prefers to add pauses after content words, inserting them after function words and after syllables within a word only as a last resort. Two content words are never followed by pauses: YEAR in FIFTEEN YEAR OLD, and POLO in POLO NECK SWEATERS. Clearly, stress is the conditioning factor, as it may have been in creating an occasional pause after A in I'M A FAIRLY NORMAL FIFTEEN YEAR OLD; the other occurrences of A are never followed by pauses, nor are those of THE and TO.

The results for pause frequency taken together with those for pause location (Figure 5 and Table 2) lead to the following conclusion. Although rate in wpm is a

TABLE 2

PERCENTAGE OF PAUSE SLOTS FILLED BY TWO OR MORE SPEAKERS AS A FUNCTION OF RATE OF READING THE EXPERIMENTAL PASSAGE AND NATURE OF THE GRAMMATICAL JUNCTURE

Pause slot following	No. of pause slots[a]	Speech rate (wpm)				
		97	126	165	210	263
Sentence[b]	1	100	100	100	100	100
Clause	6	100	100	100	100	50
Content word	23	91	65	13	9	0
Function word	20	60	10	0	0	0
Internal syllable	24	8	4	0	0	0
Overall	74	57	34	14	12	5

[a] All but the last of the categories are mutually exclusive.
[b] There is no pause slot after the last word of the passage.

convenient variable for comparisons across studies carried out with diverse materials and methods, it turns out that a particular component of rate accounts for most of the variance in magnitude productions; this rate component is the number of pauses. When the speaker varies his rate of reading a known passage, he primarily adds or subtracts pauses of largely the same duration at strategic syntactic locations; he alters articulation rate and pause duration much less. In so doing, the speaker seems to be guided not only by autophonic sensation but also by several other variables that remain to be disentangled: the volume of air in his lungs, mechanical limits on the rate of articulator displacement, the punctuation of the passage, its stress distribution, and the demands of intelligible communication (Grosjean, 1971; Lane, 1971a; Lane, Grosjean, LeBerre, & Lewin, in press).

REFERENCES

GILBERT, J. H., & BURK, K. W. Rate alterations in oral reading. *Language and Speech*, 1969, **12**, 192–201.

GOLDMAN-EISLER, F. *Psycholinguistics: Experiments in spontaneous speech.* London: Academic Press, 1968.

GROSJEAN, F. Le rôle joué par trois variables temporelles dans la compréhension orale de l'anglais, étudié comme seconde langue. Unpublished doctoral dissertation, Université de Paris VIII, 1971.

HUTTON, C. L. A psychophysical study of speech rate. Unpublished doctoral dissertation, University of Illinois, 1954.

LADEFOGED, P., & McKINNEY, N. P. Loudness, sound pressure, and subglottal pressure in speech. *Journal of the Acoustical Society of America*, 1963, **35**, 454–460.

LANE, H. L. Psychophysical parameters of vowel perception. *Psychological Monographs*, 1962, **76** (44, Whole No. 563).

LANE, H. L. The autophonic scale of voice level for congenitally deaf subjects. *Journal of Experimental Psychology*, 1963, **66**, 328–331.

LANE, H. L. The Lombard Sign and the role of hearing in speech. *Journal of Speech and Hearing Research*, 1971, **14**, 677–709. (a)

LANE, H. L. Production et perception de la parole: Rapports et différences. *Phonetica*, 1971, **23**, 94–125. (b)

LANE, H. L., CATANIA, A. C., & STEVENS, S. S. Voice level: Autophonic scale, perceived loudness, and effects of sidetone. *Journal of the Acoustical Society of America*, 1961, **33**, 160–167.

LANE, H. L., GROSJEAN, F., LEBERRE, J., & LEWIN, K. Properties of foreign language utterances that control their comprehension. *International Journal of Psycholinguistics*, in press.

LANE, H. L., TRANEL, B., & SISSON, C. Regulation of voice communication by sensory dynamics. *Journal of the Acoustical Society of America*, 1970, **47**, 618–624.

POULTON, F. C., & STEVENS, S. S. On the halving and doubling of the loudness of white noise. *Journal of the Acoustical Society of America*, 1955, **27**, 329–331.

SCHNEIDER, B., & LANE, H. L. Ratio scales, category scales, and variability in the production of loudness and softness. *Journal of the Acoustical Society of America*, 1963, **35**, 1953–1961.

STEVENS, S. S. The surprising simplicity of sensory metrics. *American Psychologist*, 1962, **17**, 29–39.

STEVENS, S. S., & GALANTER, E. H. Ratio scales and category scales for a dozen perceptual continua. *Journal of Experimental Psychology*, 1957, **54**, 377–411.

TIME-COMPRESSED SPEECH

Methods of Controlling the Word Rate of Recorded Speech

EMERSON FOULKE

Abstract

Six methods for increasing speech rate are presented. They are as follows. 1. Speech at a rate that is faster than normal may be obtained by pacing an oral reader at a rate that is faster than his normal reading rate. 2. The word rate of recorded speech may be increased by reproducing a tape or record at a speed that is faster than the speed used during recording. 3. The word rate of recorded speech may be increased by an electromechanical device that reproduces consecutive samples of a recorded tape. 4. Consecutive sampling may also be accomplished by a computer. 5. The word rate of synthesized speech may be manipulated by instructions in the program followed by a speech synthesizer. 6. The harmonic compressor increases word rate by a method of frequency division without temporal alteration, and frequency restoration with temporal alteration.

There are several methods for increasing the word rate of recorded speech. Each of these methods imposes its own characteristic distortion. By now, a good deal of research has been accomplished in which one or more methods have been evaluated with respect to their effect on word intelligibility and/or listening comprehension. Though a review of such research is not within the scope of this article, summary statements of research findings will be made where appropriate, and pertinent references will be cited.

Before turning to the description of the various methods, a few remarks are in order regarding confusion in the terminology used in talking about recorded speech, the word rate of which has been increased. Any recorded speech that is reproduced in less time than the time required for its original production can be regarded as having been compressed in time. Hence, such speech is often called time-compressed speech, or simply compressed speech. Since reproducing recorded speech in less time than the time required for its original production results in an increase in word rate, it is often called accelerated speech. Such speech has also been described as rapid speech or speeded speech. There has been an attempt on the part of some writers to employ these terms selec-

JOURNAL OF COMMUNICATION, 1970, vol. 20, no. 3, 305-314.

tively in describing the products of the various methods. However, there has been no general agreement about which term should be used for the product of which method. In the present article, there is no need for such terminological differentiation, since the discussion will be primarily of the methods themselves, and not of their products. An attempt to secure agreement among researchers regarding the appropriate term for the product of each of the several methods might be a useful undertaking. In the absence of such agreement, it will continue to be necessary for writers to avoid referring to recorded speech, the word rate of which has been increased, without specifying the method by which this has been accomplished.

Speaking Rapidly

Increasing word rate by speaking rapidly is the only method presented in this paper that does not operate upon recorded speech. Its discussion is included here for the sake of completeness, and because the comparison of this method with other methods exhibits a class of variables that may have to be taken into account in producing comprehensible speech at an increased word rate.

Within limits, word rate is under the control of the speaker [2, 4, 5, 19, 24]. This method requires no exotic apparatus. However, if the increased word rate that results from speaking rapidly is to be well controlled, the speaker must be trained, and he must be provided with feedback to regulate his speaking rate. This method has a distinct disadvantage. When a speaker attempts to operate his speech machinery at a rate that is much faster than normal, it begins to malfunction. That is, when the muscles involved in the articulation of speech sounds are made to respond too rapidly, the coordination of their action begins to deteriorate, with resulting errors in articulation. Furthermore, even below this critical limit, it is doubtful that a speaker can maintain a speaking rate that is faster than his normal rate for very long at a time.

As a speaker produces connected speech, he varies vocal pitch, vocal intensity, and the amount and distribution of pause time. Although there is, at present, an insufficient amount of research regarding the contribution of these variables to the comprehensibility of spoken language, it is a fair hypothesis that, in addition to the information contained in the words the speaker uses and in the order in which he arranges them, he specifies something about his message by the way in which he jointly manages pitch, intensity, and pause time. Goldman-Eisler [18], for instance, has introduced the concept of cognitive rhythm, which she believes to be an essential feature of spoken language, and which is the result of the way in which a speaker distributes pause time in his speech production.

The structure of a spoken message is determined, in part, by factors such as pitch, timbre, intensity, and pause time. When an effort is made to compress the time required for a spoken message by speaking more rapidly, all of these factors may be affected. When compression is accomplished by reproducing a tape or record at a faster speed than the speed at which it was recorded, the patterns of variation in vocal pitch and intensity and the apportionment of pause time are preserved, but the absolute amount of pause time is reduced, overall pitch is elevated, and timbre is altered. When recorded speech is compressed in time by reproducing a succession of time-abutted samples of the original recording, as in the case with compression by the Fairbanks method or by computer, or when it is accomplished by harmonic compression, timbre, patterns of variation in pitch and intensity, and the apportionment of pause time are preserved, but the absolute amount of pause time is reduced. The representation of these factors in the synthetic speech signal is determined by the program that controls the operation of the speech synthesizer. What is preserved and what is not preserved, as speech is compressed in time, may prove to be an important consideration in evaluating the various methods of compression.

THE SPEED CHANGING METHOD

The word rate of recorded speech may be changed simply by reproducing a tape or record at a different speed than the one used during recording. If the playback speed is slower than the recording speed, word rate is decreased and the speech is expanded in time. If the playback speed is increased, the word rate is increased, and the speech is compressed in time. When speech is accelerated in this manner, there is a change in the

70

frequencies that constitute the voice signal. This change is proportional to the change in tape or record speed. If playback speed is doubled, the component frequencies will be doubled, and vocal pitch will be raised one octave. Speech compressed by the speed changing method has been examined in several experiments [9, 17, 20]. These experiments indicate that both the intelligibility of single words and the comprehension of connected discourse withstand only moderate compression in time before losses set in.

The Sampling Method

In 1950, Miller and Licklider [23] demonstrated the signal redundancy in spoken words by deleting brief segments of the speech signal. This was accomplished by a switching arrangement which permitted a recorded speech signal to be turned off periodically during its reproduction. They found that as long as these interruptions occurred at a frequency of ten times per second or more, the interrupted speech was easily understood. The intelligibility of monosyllabic words did not drop below 90% until 50% of the speech signal had been discarded. Thus, it appeared that a large portion of the speech signal could be discarded without serious disruption of communication.

Garvey [17], taking cognizance of these results, reasoned that if the samples of a speech signal remaining after periodic interruption could be abutted in time, the result should be time-compressed intelligible speech without distortion in vocal pitch. To test this notion, he prepared a tape on which speech had been recorded by periodically cutting out short segments of tape and by splicing the ends of the retained segments of tape together again. Reproduction of this tape achieved the desired effect. Garvey's method was, of course, too cumbersome for any but research purposes. However, the success of the general approach having been shown, an efficient technique for accomplishing it was not long to follow.

In 1954, Fairbanks, Everitt, and Jaeger [6] published a description of an electromechanical apparatus for the time compression or expansion of recorded speech, which embodies a principle adumbrated by Gabor [15, 16]. In the Fairbanks apparatus, a continuous tape loop passes over a record head, used to place on this storage loop the signal that is to be compressed. Next, the tape passes over the sampling wheel, which reproduces samples of the

71

signal that has just been recorded. Finally, it passes over an erase head that removes the signal from the storage loop so that it can be re-recorded on the next cycle. The sampling wheel is a cylinder, with four playback heads embedded in it, flush with its curved surface, and equally spaced around the curved surface. The tape, in passing over the curved surface of the sampling wheel, makes contact with approximately one-quarter of its surface. When the sampling wheel is stationary and one of its heads is contacted by the moving tape, the signal on the tape is reproduced as recorded. However, when the apparatus is adjusted for some amount of compression, the sampling wheel begins to rotate in the direction of tape motion. Under these conditions, each of the four heads, in turn, makes and then loses contact with the tape. Each head reproduces the signal on the portion of the tape with which is makes contact. When, as it rotates, the sampling wheel has arrived at a position at which one head is just losing contact with the tape, while the preceding head is just making contact, the segment of tape that is wrapped around the sampling wheel between these two heads never makes contact with a reproducing head, and is therefore not reproduced. The segment of tape that is eliminated from the reproduction in this manner is always the same length, one-quarter of the circumference of the sampling wheel. The amount of speech compression depends upon the frequency with which these tape segments are eliminated, and this frequency depends, in turn, upon the rotational speed of the sampling wheel. The temporal value of the segments of tape that are not reproduced depends upon the speed of the storage loop, since this determines the amount of tape that will pass over a tape head during a given time interval. Since the sampling wheel rotates in the direction of tape motion, the speed of the storage loop, relative to the surface of the sampling wheel, is reduced, with the result that the frequencies in the retained samples of the original signal are lowered. The output of the compressor is recorded on tape, and this tape is reproduced at a speed that is enough faster than the recording speed to restore the lowered frequencies to their original values. The increase in the playback speed of this tape results in its reproduction in less than the original production time, and the result is time-compressed speech that is not altered with respect to vocal pitch. In an alternate mode of operation, the tape or record player which supplies the signal to the record head that transfers it to the compressor's storage loop may be speeded up enough to produce an elevation in the frequencies constituting the signal that is exactly compensated for by the lowering of frequencies which takes place during the sampling process. In this case, the output signal of the compressor is compressed in time without frequency distortion.

Speech may be expanded in time by reversing this process. The sampling wheel is rotated in a direction opposite to that of the storage loop, so that samples of the signal recorded on it are periodically repeated.

The speech compressor now manufactured by Wayne Graham is based upon the Fairbanks design. Like the Fairbanks compressor, it makes use of a storage loop. The temporal value of the samples that are discarded during compression can be varied by changing speed of the storage loop. Operation of the Graham compressor requires two tape recorders—one to provide its input, and one to receive its output. One of these recorders must be continuously variable in speed.

Mr. Anton Springer, relying upon the same basic principle, developed a compressor with a modified mode of operation. In the Springer approach, the storage loop, the record head, and the erase head have been eliminated. Previously recorded tape passes from a supply reel over the surface of the sampling wheel to a take up reel. The tape is sampled in the manner just described. However, as the sampling wheel rotates in the direction of tape motion, the speed of the tape is increased by an amount sufficient to hold tape speed constant in relation to the surface of the sampling wheel over which it passes. Thus, the output of the Springer device is compressed in time, without distortion in vocal pitch. The temporal value of the samples discarded during compression by the Springer device is determined by the distance, along the curved surface of the sampling wheel, separating adjacent playback heads, and is not variable. Operation of a compressor of the Springer type requires a tape recorder to receive its output. In addition, another tape recorder is required to provide the tape transport function, since the commercially available compressors based on the Springer approach have not incorporated provisions for handling tape.

73

A computer may also be used for compressing speech by the sampling method [27]. In this approach, speech that has been transduced to electrical form, for example, the output of a microphone or tape reproducing head, is temporally segmented by an analog-to-digital converter, and these segments are stored in the computer. The computer samples these segments according to a sampling rule for which it has been programmed, for example, discard every third segment. The durations of both retained and discarded samples can be varied over a wide range. The retained samples are abutted in time, and fed to the input of a digital-to-analog converter, and the signal at the output of this converter, compressed in time, is appropriate for transduction to acoustical form again.

Electromechanical compressors of the Fairbanks or Springer type are unselective with respect to the portions of a recorded signal that are discarded. Portions are discarded on a periodic basis, and may be deleted anywhere within or between words. It is quite unlikely that a given signal would be sampled in exactly the same way on two consecutive passes through such a device. With the computer, it is feasible to employ a variety of sampling rules. For instance, a computer might be programmed to dispose of empty time intervals between words, and to sample the time intervals occupied by words differentially, discarding larger fractions of those speech sounds with higher signal redundancy. From what has just been said, it would appear that the computer, because of its greater flexibility, offers the most satisfactory approach for the time compression of speech. This may ultimately prove to be the case. However, at present, computer time is too expensive to justify the employment of a computer in this capacity for any but research purposes. Furthermore, although researchers are working on the problem of writing programs for the differential samplings of speech signals, satisfactory programs have not yet been written.

Speech compressed by the sampling method has been evaluated with respect to word intelligibility [8, 13, 17, 21] and listening comprehension [7, 14, 26]. In general, results have shown that whereas word intelligibility is relatively resistive to the effects of compression by the sampling method, listening comprehension begins to decline after moderate compression. Several investigators have tested training experiences intended to improve the comprehension of time-compressed connected discourse [10, 25]. Although the successful training experience has not yet been devised, Orr, *et al.* [25] have reported encouraging results.

OTHER METHODS FOR THE TIME COMPRESSION OF SPEECH

The technique of speech synthesis suggests another possibility for the production of accelerated speech without distortion in vocal pitch [3, 22]. The speech synthesizer generates an electrical analog of the acoustical materials needed for the construction of speech sounds. A program of rules is provided for generating these analogs for the proper durations, at the proper intensities, and in proper conjunction or sequence. These rules may be varied to produce speech at any desired rate. Speech synthesis is still in the developmental stage, and the method employed in its production is not widely known and available. Nevertheless, it may ultimately prove to be the most satisfactory method for the time compression of speech, because it permits flexible control over all of the parameters of the speech signal. By means of speech synthesis, it should, in principle, be possible to produce a speech signal of any desired description.

Another method for the compression of speech in time is harmonic compression, an outgrowth of research conducted at Bell Laboratories. A description of a device embodying this method was made available by Bell Laboratories to the American Foundation for the Blind, where a working prototype has been developed [1]. By means of a bank of Bessel band-pass filters, energy in the speech signal is distributed among 36 contiguous frequency bands. The width of each band is somewhat less than 100 Hz. The output of each filter is supplied to a frequency divider, which preserves its amplitude and phase relationships, while reducing its frequency by one-half. The outputs of the 36 filters are then combined by means of a summing amplifier. This combined signal may be directly transduced to acoustical form, or recorded on tape or disc for subsequent reproduction. When a record or tape containing recorded speech is reproduced at twice the recording speed, the time required for its reproduction is halved, and the component frequencies of the signal recorded on it are doubled. When this time-compressed, frequency-distorted signal is passed through the Harmonic Compressor, the proper values of these component frequencies are restored, and the result is speech, undistorted with respect to pitch and timbre, that is reproduced at twice the original word rate, and in one-half the original time.

The prototype of the Harmonic Compressor is now in operation at the American Foundation for the Blind, and samples of its output have been prepared for demonstration and evaluation. There is general agreement among those with experience in listening to speech compressed by various methods that the signal quality of the Harmonic Compressor is exceptionally good. However, since it permits only the doubling of word rate, and since doubling the average oral reading rate [12] results in a word rate that is not comprehended very well by most listeners [11], its product may not be as generally useful as the product of compressors which can be adjusted for any desired word rate.

REFERENCES

1. Breuel, J. W. and L. M. Levens. "The A. F. B. Harmonic Compressor." In *Proceedings of the Second Louisville Conference on Rate and/or Frequency Controlled Speech*. Louisville, Ky.: University of Louisville, 1970.
2. Calearo, C. and A. Lazzaroni. "Speech Intelligibility in Relation to the Speed of the Message." *Laryngoscope* 67:410–19, 1957.
3. Campanella, S. J. "Signal Analysis of Speech Time-Compression Techniques." *Proceedings of the Louisville Conference on Time-Compressed Speech*. Louisville, Ky.: University of Louisville, 1967, 108–14.
4. deQuiros, J. B. "Accelerated Speech Audiometry, an Examination of Test Results." *Translations of the Beltone Institute for Hearing Research*, No. 17, 1964.
5. Enc, M. E. and L. M. Stolurow. "A Comparison of the Effects of Two Recording Speeds on Learning and Retention." *The New Outlook for the Blind* 54:39–48, 1960.
6. Fairbanks, G., W. L. Everitt, and R. P. Jaeger. "Method for Time or Frequency Compression-Expansion of Speech." *Transactions of the Institute of Radio Engineers Professional Group on Audio*, AU 2, 7–12, 1954.
7. Fairbanks, G., N. Guttman, and M. S. Miron. "Auditory Comprehension in Relation to Listening Rate and Selective Verbal Redundancy." *Journal of Speech and Hearing Disorders* 22:23–32, 1957.
8. Fairbanks, G. and F. Kodman, Jr. "Word Intelligibility as a Function of Time Compression." *Journal of the Acoustical Society of America* 29: 636–41, 1957.
9. Fletcher, H. *Speech & Hearing*. New York: Van Nostrand, 1929, 293–94.

10. Foulke, E. *The Comprehension of Rapid Speech by the Blind—Part II.* Cooperative Research Project #1370, Office of Education, Washington, D.C.: U. S. Department of Health, Education, and Welfare, 1964.

11. ————. "Listening Comprehension as a Function of Word Rate." *The Journal of Communication* 18:198–206, 1968.

12. ————. *The Comprehension of Rapid Speech by the Blind: Part III.* Final Progress Report Project No. 2430, Grant No. OE-4-10-127. Washington, D.C.: United States Department of Health, Education, and Welfare, Office of Education, 1969.

13. Foulke, E. and T. G. Sticht. "The Intelligibility and Comprehension of Time-Compressed Speech." *Proceedings of the Louisville Conference on Time-Compressed Speech.* Louisville, Ky.: University of Louisville, 1967, 21–28.

14. Foulke, E. and others. "The Comprehension of Rapid Speech by the Blind." *Exceptional Children* 29:134–41, 1962.

15. Gabor, D. "Theory of Communication." *The Journal of the Institution of Electrical Engineers* 93(Part III):429–57, 1946.

16. ————. "New Possibilities in Speech Transmission." *The Journal of the Institution of Electrical Engineers* 94(Part III):369–87, 1947.

17. Garvey, W. D. "The Intelligibility of Speeded Speech." *Journal of Experimental Psychology* 45:102–08, 1953.

18. Goldman-Eisler, F. "The Determinants of the Rate of Speech Output and Their Mutual Relations." *Journal of Psychosomatic Research* 1:137–43, 1956.

19. Goldstein, H. "Reading and Listening Comprehension at Various Controlled Rates." Teachers College, *Columbia University Contributions to Education,* No. 821. New York: Bureau of Publications Teachers College, 1940.

20. Klumpp, R. G. and J. C. Webster. "Intelligibility of Time-Compressed Speech." *Journal of the Acoustical Society of America* 31:265–67, 1961.

21. Kurtzrock, G. H. "The Effects of Time and Frequency Distortion Upon Word Intelligibility." *Speech Monographs* 24: 94, 1957.

22. Mattingly, I. G. "Speech Synthesis by Rule as a Research Technique." *Journal of the Acoustical Society of America* 41:1588, 1967.

23. Miller, G. A. and J. C. R. Licklider. "The Intelligibility of Interrupted Speech." *Journal of the Acoustical Society of America* 22:167–73, 1950.

24. Nelson, H. E. "The Effect of Variations of Rates on the Recall by Radio Listeners of Straight Newscasts." *Speech Monographs* 15:173–80, 1948.

25. Orr, D. B., H. L. Friedman and J. C. C. Williams. "Trainability of Listening Comprehension of Speeded Discourse." *Journal of Educational Psychology* 56(3):148–56, 1965.

26. Reid, R. H. "Grammatical Complexity and Comprehension of Compressed Speech." *The Journal of Communication* 18(3):236–42, 1968.

27. Scott, R. J. "Temporal Effects in Speech Analysis and Synthesis." Doctoral dissertation. Ann Arbor: University of Michigan, 1965.

REVIEW OF RESEARCH ON THE INTELLIGIBILITY AND COMPREHENSION OF ACCELERATED SPEECH[1]

EMERSON FOULKE   AND   THOMAS G. STICHT

Time-compressed or accelerated speech is speech which has been reproduced in less than the original production time. Such speech may prove to be useful in a variety of situations in which people must rely upon listening to obtain the information specified by language. It may also prove to be a useful tool in studying the temporal requirements of the listener as he processes spoken language. Methods for the generation of time-compressed speech are reviewed. Methods for the assessment of the effect of compression on word intelligibility and listening comprehension are discussed. Experiments dealing with the effect of time compression upon word intelligibility and upon the comprehensibility of connected discourse, and experiments concerned with the influence of stimulus variables, such as signal distortion, and organismic variables, such as intelligence, are reviewed. The general finding that compression in time has a different effect upon the comprehensibility of connected discourse than upon word intelligibility is discussed, and a tentative explanation of this difference is offered.

Accelerated speech is speech in which the word rate has been increased. Increasing the word rate reduces communication time for a given message. Hence, accelerated speech is often referred to as time-compressed or simply compressed speech.

Since the announcement by Fairbanks (Fairbanks, Everitt, & Jaeger, 1954) of a practical means for the time compression of recorded speech, there has been an interest in its use to enable blind people to read by listening at a rate that compares favorably with the silent visual reading rate (Foulke, Amster, Nolan, & Bixler, 1962; Iverson, 1956). More recently, time-compressed speech has been considered for use as an audio aid in general education (Friedman, Orr, Freedle, & Norris, 1966; Orr & Friedman, 1964) and as a research tool for studying the auditory perception of language (Foulke & Sticht, 1967).

The present paper is concerned with the communication problems produced by the time compression of speech. Various techniques for the acceleration of speech are described, methods for its evaluation are reviewed, and characteristics of the listener that may affect his perception of time-compressed speech are discussed.

METHODS FOR THE ACCELERATION OF SPEECH

Speaking Rapidly

Within limits, word rate is under the control of the speaker, and this method has been used by several investigators (Calearo & Lazzaroni, 1957; deQuiros, 1964; Enc & Stolurow, 1960; Fergen, 1955; Goldstein, 1940; Harwood, 1955; Nelson, 1948). This method has the virtue of simplicity and requires no special equipment. However, it is limited by the fact that only a moderate increase in the rate of articulation of speech sounds is possible. When the speaker increases his word rate by talking faster, there are changes in vocal inflection and intensity, and in the relative duration of consonants, vowels, and pauses (Kozhevnikov & Chistovich, 1965). When word rate is increased by methods that alter the rate of reproduction of recorded speech, these changes do not take place. The significance of this fact, with respect to word intelligibility or listening comprehension, has not yet been determined.

[1] The work described in the present paper was performed at the University of Louisville as part of Project 7-1254, Cooperative Research Branch, Office of Education, Department of Health, Education, and Welfare.

PSYCHOLOGICAL BULLETIN, 1969, vol. 72, no. 1, 50-62.

The Speed-Changing Method

The word rate of a recorded message may be changed, simply by reproducing it at a different tape or record speed than the one used during recording. If the playback speed is slower than the recording speed, word rate is decreased, and the speech is expanded in time. If playback speed is increased, word rate is increased, and the speech is compressed in time. When word rate is compressed in this manner, there is a shift in the frequencies that constitute the voice signal, which is proportional to the change in tape or record speed. If the speed is doubled, the component frequencies will be doubled, and vocal pitch will be raised one octave. Speech compressed by the speed-changing method has been examined in several experiments (Fletcher, 1929, pp. 292–294; Foulke, 1966a; Garvey, 1953b; Klumpp & Webster, 1961; Kurtzrock, 1957; McLain, 1962).

The Sampling Method

In 1950, Miller and Licklider demonstrated the signal redundancy in spoken words, by deleting brief segments of the speech signal. This was accomplished by a switching arrangement that permitted a recorded speech signal to be turned off periodically during its reproduction. They found that as long as these interruptions occurred at a frequency of 10 times per second, or more, the interrupted speech was easily understood. The intelligibility of monosyllabic words did not drop below 90% until 50% of the speech signal had been discarded. Thus, it appeared that a large portion of the speech signal could be discarded without a serious disruption of communication. Garvey (1953b), taking cognizance of these results, reasoned that if the samples of a speech signal remaining after periodic interruption could be abutted in time, the result should be time-compressed, intelligible speech, without distortion in vocal pitch. To test this notion, he prepared a tape on which speech had been recorded by periodically cutting out short segments of tape, and by splicing the ends of the retained tape together again. Reproduction of this tape achieved the desired effect. Garvey's method was, of course, too cumbersome for any but research pur-

poses. However, once the success of the general approach was shown, an efficient technique for accomplishing it was not long to follow.

In 1954, Fairbanks et al. published a description of an electromechanical apparatus for the time compression or expansion of recorded speech, which embodies a principle adumbrated by Gabor (1946, 1947). The Fairbanks apparatus reproduces periodic samples of a recorded tape. The unreproduced samples are brief enough so that a discarded sample cannot contain an entire speech sound, and the retained samples are abutted in time. Under these condtions, every speech sound in the original recording is sampled, and the result is a time-compressed reproduction without alteration in vocal pitch. With this apparatus, speech can be expanded in time by periodically repeating samples of a recorded tape. A computer may also be used for the time compression or expansion of speech by the sampling method (Scott, 1965). Whereas speech compressors of the Fairbanks type sample periodically and unselectively, a computer permits a variety of sampling rules. For instance, a computer might be programmed to dispose of empty time intervals between words, and to sample the time intervals occupied by words differentially, discarding larger fractions of those speech sounds with higher signal redundancy. Though, because of its flexibility, the computer may provide the most satisfactory method for the time compression or expansion of speech, at present, computer time is too expensive to justify the employment of a computer in this capacity for any but research purposes.

The time compression of speech may be accomplished by the shortening or the elimination of the natural pauses occurring in speech (Diehl, White, & Burk, 1959; Miron & Brown, 1968). This may be done manually, by removal of blank segments of a recorded tape, or by means of a computer, and the remaining speech may be compressed or uncompressed.

The technique of speech synthesis offers another possibility for the compression of speech in time (Campanella, 1967). The harmonic compressor, a device for the time compression of speech based on research performed at Bell Laboratories, is now under construction at the American Foundation for the Blind.

METHODS FOR THE EVALUATION OF ACCELERATED SPEECH

Some Procedural Problems

There is no common practice in specifying the amount of compression to which a listening selection has been subjected. This lack of uniformity can result in confusion, especially when the results of different studies are compared (Bellamy, 1966). The amount of compression may be specified by the percentage of the original recording time that is saved by reproducing the message at a faster word rate. Thirty percent compression means that 30% of the production time has been saved. Conversely, the fraction of original production time remaining after compression may be specified.

Alternatively, specification may be in terms of the acceleration of the original word rate, tape speed, or record speed. An acceleration of 1.5 means that the word rate after compression is 1.5 times the word rate before compression. In comparing these indices, it must be remembered that the relationship between them is not linear. For instance, whereas an increase in acceleration from 1.1 to 1.2 corresponds to an increase in compression from 9% to 17%, an increase in acceleration from 1.9 to 2.0 corresponds to a change in compression from 47% to 50%.

A problem common to both indices is that they do not indicate directly the word rate of compressed speech. The final word rates of two listening selections, compressed or accelerated by the same amount, depend upon the rates of speaking before compression. There is considerable variability in the published estimates of word rate. Part of this variability is undoubtedly due to the difference between spontaneous, conversational word rate and the word rate of oral reading. Nichols and Stevens (1957) found a conversational speaking rate of 125 words per minute (wpm), while Johnson, Darley, and Spriestersbach (1963, p. 220) found a median oral reading rate of 176.5 wpm, and Foulke (1967) found a mean oral reading rate of

174 wpm. The oral reading rate is the rate that is relevant to the process under discussion since, in most cases, the speech that is compressed is recorded oral reading. However, the usefulness of average oral reading rates is limited. The rate of oral reading depends upon the nature of the material being read, and this kind of variability can be reduced by reporting syllable rate, rather than word rate (Carroll, 1967). The oral reading rate also depends upon the style of the individual reader. It varies considerably from reader to reader and from sample to sample of the production of a given reader (Foulke, 1967).

There are reasons for believing that speech rate is the dimension of which listeners are aware. Johnson et al. (1963, pp. 202–203) summarized research supporting the conclusion that perception of the rate of speaking corresponds to the oral reading rate. Hutton (1954) found a logarithmic growth in perceived word rate as measured word rate was increased linearly.

A variety of initial or uncompressed word rates have been used in studies of the effect of time compression on listening comprehension (Fairbanks, Guttman, & Miron, 1957c; Foulke et al., 1962; Goldstein, 1940). These studies indicated that a rapid decline in comprehension commences beyond a word rate of approximately 275 wpm regardless of the compression which may have been required to achieve that word rate. Thus, it seems advisable to describe compressed speech not only in terms of the amount of compression but also in terms of word rate.

For certain purposes, such as the measurement of intelligibility, single words are compressed, and it is, of course, meaningless to speak of the word rate of a single word. In these cases, specification must be made in terms of compression or acceleration ratio.

The Measurement of Intelligibility

The ability to repeat a word, phrase, or short sentence accurately is often taken as an index of the intelligibility of time-compressed speech. A procedure typical of this approach is one in which words are compressed in time by some amount and presented, one at a time, to a listener. The listener's task is to reproduce them orally, or in writing, and his score is the correctly identified fraction of those words. This procedure is sometimes referred to as an articulation test (Miller, 1954, p. 60).

Disjunctive reaction time (RT) may also be taken as an index of intelligibility (Foulke, 1965). The underlying rationale, in this case, is that reduced discriminability means reduced intelligibility. It has been shown that if stimuli are made more similar, and hence less discriminable, choice RT is increased (Woodworth & Schlosberg, 1954, p. 33). The procedure for testing intelligibility, under this approach, is to acquaint the subject with a list of response words. The words are then presented to the subject, one at a time, in random order, for identification. The subject indicates his choice with a discriminative response, for instance, pressing an appropriate response key. He can then be scored for speed and accuracy of reaction. The experiment is performed using words that have been compressed in time by several amounts, and changes in RT and/or accuracy are regarded as indicative of changes in intelligibility. The RT method may be more sensitive than other methods, since a change in the amount of compression may produce a change in RT to words which are discriminated without error.

Calearo and Lazzaroni (1957) reported the use of a method for testing intelligibility, familiar to those in clinical audiology, in order to detect the effects of compression. The minimum intensity required for words to be intelligible is determined for words at several compressions. Threshold intelligibility is defined as that intensity at which some percentage (usually 50%) of a list of words is correctly identified. If the threshold for intelligibility changes as the amount of compression is changed, it is concluded that compression has affected intelligibility.

Tests of Comprehension

In this approach to the evaluation of the effects of compression, the listener first hears a listening selection, compressed in time by some amount, and is then tested for comprehension of that selection. Any kind of test may be used, but researchers have, in most cases, preferred objective tests of specifiable reliability.

Wood (1965) dealt with the problems inherent in assessing the listening comprehension of young children by determining their ability to follow brief, verbal instructions, compressed in time. Instructions consisted of imperative statements, such as "buzz like a bee."

Some tests of listening comprehension may detect differences not detected by others, but this increased sensitivity may have been purchased at the cost of a loss in reliability, or in ease of test administration and scoring. Bellamy (1966) used both a multiple-choice test and an interview technique to determine the listening comprehension of a group of blind subjects and a comparable group of sighted subjects. She reported that the interview technique revealed a difference in favor of the blind subjects not detected by the multiple-choice test. Friedman et al. (1966) used short answer and essay tests to assess the comprehension of accelerated speech and found no discernable trend in performance as a function of practice in listening to such speech. On the other hand, a multiple-choice test revealed considerable improvement. They also found a lack of correlation between the results of short answer and essay tests.

THE INTELLIGIBILITY OF TIME-COMPRESSED SPEECH

Characteristics of the Signal

1. The method of compression. The intelligibility of time-compressed words depends, in part, upon the method used for compression. When a recording is played back at a speed that is enough faster than the recording speed to result in the compressed reproduction of a list of words in two-thirds of their original production time, there is a loss in intelligibility of 40% or more (Fletcher, 1929; Garvey, 1953b; Klumpp & Webster, 1961; Kurtzrock, 1957). On the other hand, Garvey (1953b) found only a 10% loss in the intelligibility of a list of words, each of which was reproduced in 40% of its original production time by means of his manual sampling method and a 50% loss in intelligibility for words reproduced in 25% of their original production times. Kurtzrock (1957), using the electromechanical sampling

method of Fairbanks, obtained an intelligibility score of 50% for a group of words reproduced in 15% of their original production times. Using the same method and similar materials, Fairbanks and Kodman (1957) obtained an intelligibility score of 57% for a group of words reproduced in only 13% of their original production times.

Compression by either the sampling or the speed-changing method increases the rate at which the discriminable elements of speech occur. However, whereas the overall spectrum, the location of formants within that spectrum, and vocal pitch are unaffected by the sampling method, they are altered by the speed-changing method, and these alterations are probably responsible for the difference in intelligibility between the two methods (Nixon, Mabson, Trimboli, Endicott, & Welch, 1968; Nixon & Sommer, 1968).

2. Intelligibility and the sampling rule. The message to be compressed may be conceived as consisting of a succession of temporal segments, called sampling periods. When speech is compressed by the sampling method, compression is accomplished by discarding a fraction of each sampling period and by abutting in time the remainders of sampling periods. It is the retained fraction of the sampling period that determines the amount of compression. If 10 milliseconds (msec.) of a 20-msec. sampling period or 30 msec. of a 60-msec. sampling period are retained, the result is the same—50% compression. For any given sampling period, changing the fraction of the sampling period that is retained changes the amount of compression.

When the sampling method is used, the effect that a given amount of compression has upon the intelligibility of words depends upon the duration of the discarded portion of the sampling period and hence upon the duration of the sampling period itself. The duration of the discarded portion of the sampling period must be short relative to the duration of the speech sounds to be sampled. If it is not, a speech sound may fall entirely within the discarded portion of a sampling period, in which case, it is not sampled at all. Garvey (1953b) used discard intervals of 40, 60, 80, and 100 msec. to compress spondaic words to 50% of their original durations. He obtained

corresponding intelligibility scores of 95, 96, 95, and 86%. In a two-factor experiment in which five discard intervals and eight compressions were represented, Fairbanks and Kodman (1957) also found a substantial loss in intelligibility when the duration of the discard interval exceeded 80 msec. This was true at all eight compressions.

Cramer (1965) reported that when subjects use earphones to listen to speech that has been compressed in time by the sampling method, delaying the signal to one earphone by 7.5 msec. improves intelligibility. This delay provides what Cramer has called "binaural redundancy." If, as Garvey (1953a) suggested, it is the briefness of highly compressed speech sounds that makes them unintelligible, binaural redundancy may restore some intelligibility by increasing the effective duration of speech sounds.

Scott (1965) reported a favorable result when subjects use one earphone to listen to the normally retained samples of compressed speech, and the other earphone to listen, at the same time, to the normally discarded samples of the same compressed speech. He refers to such speech as "dichotic speech."

3. The rate of occurrence of speech sounds. Garvey (1953b) compared the intelligibility of words compressed in time by the sampling method with the intelligibility, reported by Miller and Licklider (1950), of words that had been interrupted periodically. Garvey's words and Miller and Licklider's words were treated alike in that portions of sampling periods were discarded. However, the retained samples of Garvey's words were abutted to produce time-compressed speech, while the retained samples of Miller and Licklider's words were not abutted, and the resulting speech, though interrupted, was not compressed in time. There was no difference between the intelligibility of time-compressed words and interrupted words when 50% of each word was discarded. However, when 62% of each word was discarded, interrupted words were 40% more intelligible than time-compressed words. Since the two groups of words were alike with respect to the amount of speech information that had been discarded, the poorer intelligibility of the time-compressed words, when 62% of the speech

information was discarded, was probably due to the increased rate of occurrence of speech sounds. Garvey used spondaic words, whereas Miller and Licklider used monosyllabic words. Results obtained by Henry (1966) suggest that if Garvey had used monosyllabic words, or if Miller and Licklider had used spondaic words, the difference in favor of interrupted speech would have been even more pronounced.

4. Intelligibility and linguistic factors. Kurtzrock (1957) found that compression by the speed-changing method degraded the intelligibility of vowel sounds more than consonantal sounds and that compression by the sampling method degraded the intelligibility of consonantal sounds more than vowel sounds. Garvey's (1953a) subjects rated the vowel sounds in words that had been compressed in time by the sampling method as higher in "goodness" than consonantal sounds. In a study in which the number of phonemes per word was varied from three to nine, Henry (1966) found that increasing the number of phonemes improved the intelligibility of words that had been compressed in time by the sampling method. In a similar vein, Klumpp and Webster (1961) found short phrases, compressed in time by the speed-changing method, to be more intelligible than single words. The findings of Henry, and of Klumpp and Webster, are probably explained by the increased number of cues available to subjects because of the redundancy in polyphonemic words and short phrases, and could have been predicted from the finding of French and Steinberg (1947) that speech is understandable when composed of syllables that are only 67% intelligible.

Characteristics of the Listener

1. Intelligibility and prior experience. Fairbanks and Kodman (1957) found a group of words compressed by several amounts to be more intelligible than a similar group of words in which the same amounts of speech information had been discarded by interrupting them in the manner of Miller and Licklider. However, the subjects of Fairbanks and Kodman had received extensive familiarization with the words to be identified before the tests were made, whereas the subjects of Miller and Licklider were relatively naïve.

Miller and Licklider (1950), using interrupted words, and Garvey (1953a), using words compressed in time by the sampling method, found that repeated exposure to such words improves their intelligibility.

If a group of listeners agree that a particular speech sound in a word that has been compressed in time by the sampling method is unrecognizable, it may be concluded fairly that the difficulty lies with the signal itself. However, Garvey found that subjects disagreed about the speech sounds that were rendered unintelligible by compression of the words in which they occurred. Garvey explained this finding in terms of the differential exposure of subjects to the words in question. In this connection, Henry (1966) found a positive relationship between word frequency in general language, as revealed in the Thorndike and Lorge (1944) word count, and word intelligibility.

2. Intelligibility and hearing loss. There appear to be no differential effects of time compression upon the intelligibility scores of normal hearing subjects and patients having conductive or sensorineural hearing losses (Bocca & Calearo, 1963; Calearo & Lazzaroni, 1957; deQuiros, 1964; Luterman, Welsh, & Melrose, 1966; Sticht & Gray, in press). However, aged patients, some with diffuse cerebral pathology (Calearo & Lazzaroni, 1957; Sticht & Gray, in press), and patients with temporal lobe lesions (Bocca & Calearo, 1963; deQuiros, 1964) required greater intensity for threshold intelligibility and showed a higher error rate with suprathreshold words when compression was increased. The latter was true for aged subjects having normal hearing or sensorineural hearing losses (Sticht & Gray, in press). Apparently, the changes accompanying aging reduce the rate at which speech information can be processed.

FACTORS AFFECTING THE COMPREHENSION OF TIME-COMPRESSED SPEECH

Stimulus Variables

1. Comprehension and word rate. Within the range extending from 126 to 272 wpm.

Diehl et al. (1959) found listening comprehension to be unaffected by changes in word rate. In the range bounded by 125 and 225 wpm, Nelson (1948) and Harwood (1955) found a slight but insignificant loss in listening comprehension as word rate was increased. Fairbanks et al. (1957c) found little difference in the comprehension of listening selections presented at 141, 201, and 282 wpm. Thereafter, comprehension, as indicated by percentage of test questions correctly answered, declined from 58% at 282 wpm to 26% at 470 wpm, a level of performance near chance. Foulke et al. (1962), using both literary and technical listening selections, found listening comprehension to be only slightly affected by increasing word rate in the range bounded by 175 and 275 wpm. However, in the range extending from 275 to 375 wpm, they found an accelerating loss in listening comprehension as word rate was increased. Foulke and Sticht (1967) found a 6% loss in comprehension between 225 and 325 wpm and a loss of 14% between 325 and 425 wpm. The three studies just cited are in agreement regarding the finding that as word rate is increased beyond a normal word rate, there is initially a moderate linear decline in comprehension, followed by an accelerating decline.

Simple comprehension scores do not take into account the learning time that is saved when speech is presented at an increased word rate. Such an allowance may be made by dividing the comprehension score by the time required to present the listening selection. This index of learning efficiency expresses the amount of learning per unit time. Using such an index, Fairbanks et al. (1957c), Enc and Stolurow (1960), and Foulke et al. (1962) found that learning efficiency increased as word rate was increased until a word rate of approximately 280 wpm was reached. In a similar approach, Enc and Stolurow (1960) computed an index of the efficiency of retention.

The word rate at which a listening selection is presented apparently has no special effect on the rate at which forgetting occurs. Enc and Stolurow (1960), Friedman et al. (1966), and Foulke (1966b) performed studies in which tests of the comprehension of listening selections presented at several word rates were made after several retention intervals. In general, these studies support the conclusion that differences in the course of forgetting are due to differences in original learning. Of course, as has already been shown, the amount of original learning is, in part, a function of the word rate at which a listening selection is presented.

2. Comprehension and the method of compression. McLain (1962) and Foulke (1962), using subjects who were naïve with respect to compressed speech and unaccustomed to reading by listening, compared the comprehension of a listening selection compressed by the sampling method to a rate of 275 wpm with the comprehension of the same selection compressed to the same word rate by the speed-changing method. In both instances, a slight but statistically significant advantage was found for the sampling method. However, in a similar experiment in which blind children, who were accustomed to reading by listening, served as subjects, Foulke (1966a) found no statistically significant difference in favor of either method.

The finding that the obvious superiority of the sampling method when the comparison is based upon a test of the intelligibility of single words is not observed when the comparison is based upon a test of the comprehension of connected discourse is of considerable interest. It suggests that some other factor, such as the rate at which words occur, is also involved in determining the comprehension of accelerated speech. A satisfactory explanation of such comprehension must, therefore, take into account the perceptual and cognitive processes of the listener.

3. Comprehension and the difficulty of the compressed material. The extent to which the comprehension of a listening selection is affected by compression in time may depend upon its difficulty. However, before this question can be examined satisfactorily, a method must be developed for determining the difficulty of a listening selection.

Using one normal and four accelerated word rates, Foulke et al. (1962) measured the comprehension of a scientific selection and a literary selection. In each case, performance on a test containing multiple-choice items covering the listening selection constituted the evi-

84

dence for listening comprehension. Comprehension of the scientific selection was poorer than comprehension of the literary selection at a normal word rate, suggesting that it was relatively more difficult. As word rate was increased, comprehension of the scientific selection did not decline as rapidly as comprehension of the literary selection. Although this interaction was significant, it was probably due to the fact that since comprehension scores for the scientific selection were lower at a normal word rate, the range in which they could vary was relatively smaller. Furthermore, the apparent difference in difficulty of the two selections may have been due, at least in part, to differences in the tests of listening comprehension employed. Certainly, the apparent difficulty of a selection can be manipulated by the choice of items used in testing for its comprehension.

In an investigation of the effect of time compression on message units varying in difficulty, Fairbanks et al. (1957c) distributed the 60 multiple-choice items of a test of listening comprehension equally among five categories of item difficulty. The listening selections covered by the test of comprehension were administered to several groups of subjects, each group experiencing a different accelerated word rate. Each subject received five scores, determined by his responses to the items in each of the five test-item categories. The mean score for each test-item category decreased as the amount of compression in time was increased. They concluded that, assuming item difficulty to be a reflection of the difficulty of the message unit to which it pertained, the effect of time compression on listening comprehension, within the range explored, did not depend upon the difficulty of the listening material.

There are formulas for estimating what might be called the "absolute difficulty" of a selection. These formulas have generally been developed for material that is to be read visually (Dale & Chall, 1948; Flesch, 1948). However, it has often been assumed that the listening difficulty of a selection is the same as its reading difficulty. The results of the experiment by Foulke et al. (1962) suggest that this assumption may not be tenable. In this experiment, although comprehension test scores suggested that the scientific selection was relatively more difficult than the literary selection, they were estimated to be equal in difficulty by the Dale-Chall formula for readability. Similar evidence is presented in a study reported by Enc and Stolurow (1960). They found considerable variability in the mean comprehension test scores of ten listening selections, presented at a normal word rate and a slightly accelerated word rate, in spite of the fact that the selections were rated as equal in difficulty by the Dale-Chall formula. Of course, the formula may have failed to detect differences in listening difficulty because of a relatively large variance in the estimates of reading difficulty.

However, if the difficulty of an aurally received selection is not the same as the difficulty of that selection when visually received, the explanation may be that differences between the oral and the print display make it necessary for the reader to process them differently. The printed page is primarily a spatial display. It permits the kind of scanning that helps in understanding long, complex sentences. On the other hand, when information is specified by spoken language, it is displayed in a temporal dimension. The only sensory information available to the listener at any given instant is the information specified by the display at that instant. Unlike the visual reader, the listener must depend upon memory alone for the availability of speech that has already occurred. Furthermore, unlike the visual reader, he can exert no control over the order in which he encounters the syntactic and semantic components of sentences. The syntactical difference between two selections might be inconsequential when they are received visually, yet quite significant when they are received aurally. The formulas used for estimating reading difficulty (Dale & Chall, 1948; Flesch, 1948; Rodgers, 1962) are based on different considerations, and the estimates of difficulty yielded by these formulas may be expected to vary. However, there has been no comparative study of the extent to which the effect of word rate on listening comprehension depends upon the formula used to estimate difficulty. The finding of a systematic interaction between word rate and listening difficulty, as estimated by a particular formula, would seem to provide a kind of face validity for that formula.

4. Comprehension and the oral reader. Oral readers differ considerably with respect to vocal timbre, and, of course, there are conspicuous sex differences in vocal pitch. Oral readers also differ with respect to such factors as average word rate and variability in word rate, pitch, and loudness. Such factors combine to define the personal, oral reading style. In a preliminary experiment, Foulke (1964) explored the extent to which oral reading style interacts with word rate in determining listening comprehension. Three renditions of a listening selection, each read by a different reader (two males and one female), were presented to three groups of college students at a normal word rate, and to three comparable groups at a word rate that was increased to 275 wpm by the sampling method. After exposure to the listening selection, all subjects took a test of listening comprehension. Significant differences in listening comprehension were associated with the reader variable and with the word-rate variable, but the reader's effect on listening comprehension did not depend upon the word rate at which the selection was presented.

Listener Variables That Affect Listening Comprehension

Foulke (1964) called attention to the considerable variation in the ability of listeners to comprehend accelerated speech. Several experiments have been reported in which there has been an effort to determine those characteristics of the listener that may contribute to the ability to comprehend accelerated speech.

1. The sex of the listener. Comparisons of male and female listeners have revealed no sex-related differences in listening comprehension for word rates ranging from 174 to 475 wpm (Foulke & Sticht, 1967; Orr & Friedman, 1964).

2. The listener's age and educational experience. Fergen (1955) and Wood (1965) found a positive relationship between the age-grade level of school children and their ability to comprehend accelerated speech. Together,

their experiments included Grades 1, 3, 4, 5, and 6.

3. The intelligence of the listener. In the case of children, the evidence presently available is not sufficient to permit a conclusion regarding the effect of intelligence on the comprehension of accelerated speech. Fergen (1955) found no relationship between the IQs of grade school children and their ability to comprehend accelerated listening selections. However, 230 wpm was the fastest word rate represented in her experiment. Wood (1965) found no relationship between the IQs of children in the primary grades and their ability to follow the instructions conveyed by short, imperative, time-compressed statements. However, his procedures resemble more closely those used in testing for intelligibility. A more definite conclusion is possible in the case of adults. Fairbanks et al. (1957b, 1957c), Goldstein (1940), and Nelson (1948) have all found a positive relationship between intelligence and the ability to comprehend accelerated speech. The data of Fairbanks et al. (1957c) and Goldstein (1940) concur in showing a positive relationship between the intelligence of the listener and the magnitude of the decline in listening comprehension as word rate is increased. This relationship may be due, at least in part, to the fact that intelligent subjects earn higher scores than less intelligent subjects on comprehension tests of listening selections presented at normal word rates. Therefore, the scores they earn on tests of the comprehension of materials presented at accelerated word rates have a larger range within which to vary.

4. The visual status of the listener. There are a priori grounds for expecting blind listeners to show better comprehension than sighted listeners. However, the research related to this question is meager and inconclusive. In an experiment performed by Hartlage (1963), blind and sighted subjects did not differ with respect to their comprehension of listening selections presented at a normal word rate. Foulke (1964) presented evidence that blind listeners comprehend time-compressed listening selections better than sighted listeners.

5. Reading rate and listening rate. Those perceptual and cognitive processes that are responsible for individual differences in read-

ing rate may also contribute to individual differences in the ability to comprehend accelerated speech. If this is true, fast readers should be able to comprehend speech at a faster word rate than slow readers. This hypothesis has been tested by Goldstein (1940) and by Orr, Friedman, and Williams (1965). In both experiments, a significant positive correlation was found between reading rate and the ability to comprehend accelerated speech. Of course, in all likelihood, a significant positive correlation would also have been found between reading rate and reading comprehension. In both experiments, it was also found that practice in listening to accelerated speech resulted in an improvement in reading rate.

Goldstein (1940) and Jester and Travers (1965) compared the comprehension resulting from listening to selections presented at several word rates with the comprehension resulting from reading the same selections at the same word rates. In both cases, comprehension declined as word rate was increased. Listening comprehension was superior to reading comprehension up to approximately 200 wpm but inferior to reading comprehension thereafter. Simultaneous reading and listening at 350 wpm resulted in better comprehension than could be demonstrated with either mode of presentation alone.

6. Improving the comprehension of time-compressed speech. In an experiment performed by Fairbanks et al (1957b), a mean comprehension score of 63.8% was obtained by subjects who listened to a selection presented at an uncompressed word rate at 141 wpm. Subjects who listened to the same selection, compressed by 50% to a word rate of 282 wpm, earned a mean comprehension score of 58%. A third group of subjects, who listened to two consecutive reproductions of the listening selection at 282 wpm, earned a mean comprehension score of 65.4% which was slightly, but probably not significantly, higher than the mean comprehension score resulting from a single exposure to the uncompressed selection. In a second study by the same investigators (1957a), augmentations were written for selected facts in a listening selection. The recorded version of the augmented selection was then compressed enough by the sampling method to produce a playback time

equal to the playback time of the uncompressed and unaugmented selection. The objective was to determine whether or not comprehension could be improved by trading the temporal redundancy in the uncompressed version for the verbal redundancy in the augmented version. Analysis of the results revealed better comprehension only for the augmented sections of the listening selection. There was a decline in comprehension of the unaugmented sections. The explanation of this finding may be that subjects associated verbal redundancy with importance and distributed their attention accordingly.

Several investigators have explored the possibility of improving the comprehension of accelerated speech by training. The simplest and least sophisticated training experience that has been evaluated is mere exposure. Voor and Miller (1965) exposed a group of subjects to five listening selections presented at 380 wpm. Total listening time was 17.5 minutes. At the end of each selection, subjects were tested for listening comprehension. Mean comprehension scores increased from the first to the third selection but did not change significantly thereafter. These results probably reflect a simple adjustment to the initially unfamiliar task of listening to accelerated speech.

Orr et al. (1965) found a 29.3% increase in the comprehension of materials presented at 475 wpm, following several weeks of training in which subjects listened to selections, the word rates of which were increased in steps of 25 wpm from 325 to 475 wpm. However, since there was no control group that received training in listening for comprehension at a normal word rate, it is not possible to attribute their results unequivocally to practice in listening to accelerated speech. The improvement may have been due simply to practice in listening for comprehension.

In this regard, Foulke (1964), using blind subjects who can safely be presumed to have had years of experience in listening for comprehension, measured comprehension of speech presented at 350 wpm, before and after training. Training consisted of approximately 25 hours of exposure to (a) speech at a constant rate of 350 wpm, (b) speech that was gradually increased from a normal word rate to a final word rate of 350 wpm, (c) the same as a but with frequent pauses for questioning about the material just heard, and (d) the same as b but with frequent pauses for questioning about the material just heard. There were no significant differences between pre- and posttraining test scores for any of the treatment groups.

Friedman et al. (1966) compared the comprehension test scores of subjects given 35 hours of massed practice in listening to accelerated speech with the comprehension test scores of subjects who received from 12 to 14 hours of distributed practice in listening to accelerated speech. They concluded that the comprehension demonstrated by the distributed-practice group was as good as, or better than, the comprehension demonstrated by the massed-practice group.

From the research reviewed in the present paper, it is clear that an adequate training experience for improving the comprehension of accelerated speech has yet to be found. Simple exposure, at least in the amounts so far tested, is not adequate.

CONCLUSION

It is possible to provide a fairly accurate description of the relationship between word rate and listening comprehension on the basis of the experimental results that have been reviewed. There are two general classes of results which, when taken together, suggest that the relationship between word rate and listening comprehension is structured by more than one underlying process. First, there are those studies in which listening comprehension has been measured at various word rates (see Stimulus Variables). When these studies are considered collectively, the relationship that emerges is one in which listening comprehension declines at a slow rate as word rate is increased, until a rate of approximately 275 wpm is reached, and at a faster rate thereafter.

In the second class of studies, intelligibility has been determined for words compressed by various amounts (see Characteristics of the Signal). These studies are in general agreement regarding the finding that, when compression is accomplished by the sampling method, word intelligibility is not seriously degraded until a relatively large amount of signal information has been discarded. The finding that increasing the amount of compression has a different effect upon listening comprehension than upon word intelligibility suggests that decreased intelligibility is not, in itself, an adequate explanation for the loss in comprehension that is observed at faster word rates. One might expect decreased intelligibility to interfere with comprehension to some extent. However, the listener's uncertainty regarding imminent speech is reduced because of his ability to estimate the sequential dependencies in meaningfully connected words and syllables, and there is a further substantial reduction in uncertainty when he has heard enough of a message to form a valid hypothesis about its contents. The reduction in message uncertainty should significantly counteract losses in word intelligibility, and the finding by French and Steinberg (1947), that listeners can understand messages composed with words whose syllables are only 67% intelligible, suggests that this is the case.

The increase in the rate at which comprehension declines beyond 275 wpm suggests that when a certain critical word rate is reached, a factor in addition to signal degradation begins to determine the loss in comprehension. The understanding of spoken language implies the continuous registration, encoding, and storage of speech information, and these operations require time. When the word rate is too high, words cannot be processed as fast as they are received, with the result that some speech information is lost. To put it another way, when channel capacity is exceeded, some of the input cannot be recovered at the ouput (Miller, 1953, 1956).

The explanation just suggested is, of course, tentative. A good deal of research on sentence, word, and syllable rate, and upon the amount of distribution of processing time in connected discourse, will be required in order to provide a more substantial basis for the hypothesis.

REFERENCES

BELLAMY, M. J. An experimental study to compare the comprehension of speeded speech by blind and sighted children. Unpublished master's thesis, University of Texas, 1966.

88

BOCCA, E., & CALEARO, C. Central hearing processes. In J. Jerger (Ed.), *Modern developments in audiology*. New York: Academic Press, 1963.

CALEARO, C., & LAZZARONI, A. Speech intelligibility in relation to the speed of the message. *Laryngoscope*, 1957, 67, 410–419.

CAMPANELLA, S. J. Signal analysis of speech time-compression techniques. In, *Proceedings of the Louisville conference on time compressed speech*. Louisville: University of Louisville, 1967.

CARROLL, J. B. Problems of measuring speech rate. In, *Proceedings of the Louisville conference on time compressed speech*. Louisville: University of Louisville, 1967.

CRAMER, H. L. Intelligibility of compressed speech as a function of degree and direction of delay of presentation from one ear to the other. Paper presented at the meeting of the American Psychological Association, Chicago, September 1965.

DALE, E., & CHALL, J. S. A formula for predicting readability. *Educational Research Bulletin*, 1948, 27, 11–20, 28.

DEQUIROS, J. B. Accelerated speech audiometry, an examination of test results. *Translations of the Beltone Institute for Hearing Research*, 1964, No. 17.

DIEHL, C. F., WHITE, R. C., & BURK, K. Rate and communication. *Speech Monographs*, 1959, 26, 229–232.

ENC, M. E., & STOLUROW, L. M. A comparison of the effects of two recording speeds on learning and retention. *The New Outlook for the Blind*, 1960, 54, 39–48.

FAIRBANKS, G., EVERITT, W. L., & JAEGER, R. P. Method for time or frequency compression-expansion of speech. *Transactions of the Institute of Radio Engineers Professional Group on Audio*, 1954, AU 2, 7–12.

FAIRBANKS, G., GUTTMAN, N., & MIRON, M. S. Auditory comprehension in relation to listening rate and selective verbal redundancy. *Journal of Speech and Hearing Disorders*, 1957, 22, 23–32. (a)

FAIRBANKS, G., GUTTMAN, N., & MIRON, M. S. Auditory comprehension of repeated high speed messages. *Journal of Speech and Hearing Disorders*, 1957, 22, 20–22. (b)

FAIRBANKS, G., GUTTMAN, N., & MIRON, M. S. Effects of time compression upon the comprehension of connected speech. *Journal of Speech and Hearing Disorders*, 1957, 22, 10–19. (c)

FAIRBANKS, G., & KODMAN, F., JR. Word intelligibility as a function of time compression. *Journal of the Acoustical Society of America*, 1957, 29, 636–641.

FERGEN, G. K. Listening comprehension at controlled rates for children in grades IV, V, VI. (Unpublished doctoral dissertation, University of Missouri, 1954) *Dissertation Abstracts*, 1955, 15, 89.

FLESCH, R. A new readability yardstick. *Journal of Applied Psychology*, 1948, 32, 231–233.

FLETCHER, H. *Speech and hearing*. New York: Van Nostrand, 1929.

FOULKE, E. A comparison of two methods of compressing speech. In R. H. Bixler (Chm.), Speech compression. Symposium presented at the Southeastern Psychological Association, Louisville, March 1962.

FOULKE, E. The comprehension of rapid speech by the blind—Part II. (Cooperative Research Project No. 1370) Washington, D. C.: United States Department of Health, Education, and Welfare, Office of Education, 1964.

FOULKE, E. The comprehension of rapid speech by the blind—Part III. (Semi-annual Progress Report, Cooperative Research Project No. 2430) Washington, D. C.: United States Department of Health, Education, and Welfare, Office of Education, 1965.

FOULKE, E. Comparison of comprehension of two forms of compressed speech. *Exceptional Children*, 1966, 33, 169–173. (a)

FOULKE, E. The retention of information presented at an accelerated word rate. *International Journal for the Education of the Blind*, 1966, 14, 11–15. (b)

FOULKE, E. The comprehension of rapid speech by the blind—Part III. (Interim Progress Report, Cooperative Research Project No. 2430) Washington, D. C.: United States Department of Health, Education, and Welfare, Office of Education, 1967.

FOULKE, E., AMSTER, C. H., NOLAN, C. Y., & BIXLER, R. H. The comprehension of rapid speech by the blind. *Exceptional Children*, 1962, 29, 134–141.

FOULKE, E., & STICHT, T. The intelligibility and comprehension of accelerated speech. In, *Proceedings of the Louisville conference on time compressed speech*. Louisville: University of Louisville, 1967.

FRENCH, N. R., & STEINBERG, J. C. Factors governing the intelligibility of speech sounds. *Journal of the Acoustical Society of America*, 1947, 19, 90–119.

FRIEDMAN, H. L., ORR, D. B., FREEDLE, R. O., & NORRIS, C. M. Further research on speeded speech as an educational medium. (Progress Report No. 2, Grant No. 7-48-7670-267) Washington, D. C.: United States Department of Health, Education, and Welfare, Office of Education, 1966.

GABOR, D. Theory of communication. *Journal of the Institution of Electrical Engineers*, 1946, 93, Part III, 429–457.

GABOR, D. New possibilities in speech transmission. *Journal of the Institution of Electrical Engineers*, 1947, 94, Part III, 369–387.

GARVEY, W. D. The intelligibility of abbreviated speech patterns. *Quarterly Journal of Speech*, 1953, 39, 296–306. (a)

GARVEY, W. D. The intelligibility of speeded speech. *Journal of Experimental Psychology*, 1953, 45, 102–108. (b)

GOLDSTEIN, H. Reading and listening comprehension at various controlled rates. *Teachers College Contributions to Education*, 1940, No. 821.

HARTLAGE, L. Differences in listening comprehension between blind and sighted subjects. *International Journal for the Education of the Blind*, 1963, 13, 1–6.

HARWOOD, K. A. Listenability and rate of presentation. *Speech Monographs*, 1955, 22, 57–59.

89

HENRY, W. G., JR. Recognition of time compressed speech as a function of word length and frequency of usage. Unpublished doctoral dissertation, Indiana University, 1966.

HUTTON, C. L., JR. A psychophysical study of speech rate. (Doctoral dissertation, University of Illinois) Ann Arbor, Mich.: University Microfilms, 1954, No. 10-494.

IVERSON, L. Time compression. *International Journal for the Education of the Blind*, 1956, 5, 78–79.

JESTER, R., & TRAVERS, R. M. Comprehension as a function of rate and modality of presentation. Paper presented at the meeting of the American Psychological Association, Chicago, September 1965.

JOHNSON, W., DARLEY, F., & SPRIESTERBACH, D. C. *Diagnostic methods in speech pathology*. New York: Harper & Row, 1963.

KLUMPP, R. G., & WEBSTER, J. C. Intelligibility of time-compressed speech. *Journal of the Acoustical Society of America*, 1961, 31, 265–267.

KOZHEVNIKOV, V. A., & CHISTOVICH, L. A. *Speech: Articulation and perception*. (Trans. No. JPRS 30, 543, 1965) Washington, D. C.: United States Department of Commerce, Joint Publications Research Service, 1966.

KURTZROCK, G. H. The effects of time and frequency distortion upon word intelligibility. *Speech Monographs*, 1957, 24, 94.

LUTERMAN, D. M., WELSH, O. L., & MELROSE, J. Responses of aged males to time-altered speech stimuli. *Journal of Speech and Hearing Research*, 1966, 9, 226–230.

McLAIN, J. A comparison of two methods of producing rapid speech. *International Journal for the Education of the Blind*, 1962, 12, 40–43.

MILLER, E. C. Effects of learning of variations in oral presentation. Unpublished doctoral dissertation, University of Denver, 1954.

MILLER, G. A. What is information measurement? *American Psychologist*, 1953, 8, 3–11.

MILLER, G. A. The magical number seven, plus or minus two: Some limits on our capacity for processing information. *Psychological Review*, 1956, 63, 81–97.

MILLER, G. A., & LICKLIDER, J. C. R. The intelligibility of interrupted speech. *Journal of the Acoustical Society of America*, 1950, 22, 167–173.

MIRON, M. S., & BROWN, E. R. Stimulus parameters in speech compression. *Journal of Communication*, 1968, 18, 219–235.

NELSON, H. E. The effect of variations of rates on the recall by radio listeners of straight newscasts. *Speech Monographs*, 1948, 15, 173–180.

NICHOLS, P. G., & STEVENS, L. A. *Are you listening?* New York: McGraw Hill, 1957.

NIXON, C. W., MABSON, W. E., TRIMBOLL, F., ENDICOTT, J. E., & WELCH, B. E. Observations on man in an oxygen-helium environment at 380 mm. Hg total pressure: IV. Communications. *Aerospace Medicine*, 1968, 39, 1–9.

NIXON, C. W., & SOMMER, H. C. Subjective analysis of speech in helium environments. *Aerospace Medicine*, 1968, 39, 139–144.

ORR, D. B., & FRIEDMAN, H. L. Research on speeded speech as an educational medium. (Progress Report, Grant No. 7-48-7670-203) Washington, D. C.: United States Department of Health, Education, and Welfare, Office of Education, 1964.

ORR, D. B., FRIEDMAN, H. L., & WILLIAMS, J. C. C. Trainability of listening comprehension of speeded discourse. *Journal of Educational Psychology*, 1965, 56, 148–156.

RODGERS, J. R. A formula for predicting the comprehension level of material to be presented orally. *Journal of Educational Research*, 1962, 56, 218–220.

SCOTT, R. J. Temporal effects in speech analysis and synthesis. Unpublished doctoral dissertation, University of Michigan, 1965.

STICHT, T. G., & GRAY, B. B. The intelligibility of time compressed words as a function of age and hearing loss. *Journal of Speech and Hearing Research*, in press.

THORNDIKE, E. L., & LORGE, I. *The teacher's word book of 30,000 words*. New York: Columbia University Press, 1944.

VOOR, J. B., & MILLER, J. M. The effect of practice on the comprehension of worded speech. *Speech Monographs*, 1965, 32, 452–455.

WOOD, C. D. Comprehension of compressed speech by elementary school children. (Final Progress Report, Grant No. 7-24-0210-263) Washington, D. C.: United States Department of Health, Education, and Welfare, Office of Education, 1965.

WOODWORTH, R. S., & SCHLOSBERG, H. *Experimental psychology*. New York: Holt, 1954.

THE DIFFICULTY OF LISTENING TO TIME-COMPRESSED SPEECH

WILLARD R. ZEMLIN, RAYMOND G. DANILOFF, and THOMAS H. SHRINER

Forty normal college students rated the difficulty of listening to samples of speech subjected to 20, 30, 40, and 50% time compression compared with a standard consisting of normal speech. A male and female speaker were used. Results indicate that difficulty commences to increase and accelerate beyond 20% time compression to reach a value of about five times as difficult at 50% time compression. The male's speech was increasingly less difficult to listen to than the female's speech as the degree of time compression increased.

Investigations of the comprehension of time-compressed speech by Fairbanks, Guttman, and Miron (1957) and Foulke et al. (1962) indicate that comprehension of speech is relatively unaffected by up to 50% time compression (or rates of 275-282 words per minute). However, the "difficulty of listening" to 50% time-compressed speech increases markedly. Foulke and Sticht (1966) permitted normal college students to select a preferred degree of time compression of speech spoken at an original rate of 175 words per minute. The mean preferred rate was 28% or a word rate of 212 words per minute. For blind subjects, Iverson (1956) and Foulke (1966) observed that 35-40% time compression and word rates of 236-275 words per minute were the preferred rates for listening to speech. These data indicate that blind subjects will trade increased difficulty or effort in listening to speech for increased information rate and time savings.

The quality of the speaker's voice may well affect comprehension of time-compressed speech. Evidence of this is Foulke's (1967) observation of significant differences in comprehension by blind subjects of different speakers (two males and a female) speaking the same material. Using a questionnaire, Foulke (1966) found that a majority (64%) of blind listeners preferred to listen to time-compressed male speech; however, in response to another question, a majority (55%) considered time-compressed female speech to be easier to understand. Foulke did not offer a readily investigable explanation to account for this seeming discrepancy.

In order to explore the relationship between degree of time compression and difficulty of listening, a study was designed in which normal college students rated the difficulty of time-compressed speech relative to recorded normal

JOURNAL OF SPEECH AND HEARING RESEARCH, 1968, vol. 11, no. 4, 875-881.

speech. In addition, both a male and female speaker were used in order to detect possible differences in the difficulty of listening to their speech.

METHODS

Experimental Materials

The speech materials used were those prepared and described by Fairbanks et al. (1957). They consisted of straightforward, factual material on aviation meteorology in essay form, prepared so that there was little prior listener knowledge demanded for comprehension.

Both speakers, a mature male with a 98 Hz fundamental speaking frequency and a mature female phonetician with a 190 Hz fundamental speaking frequency, produced their speech with minimum inflection at a conversational level in a sound treated room. A steadily flashing light was used in both cases to aid in pacing their speech. Analysis revealed an average speaking rate of 140 and 141 words per minute for male and female, respectively.

Master tape recordings were made on Magnecord PT-6 and M-90 equipment at 15 ips with an Altec M-11 microphone. The master tapes were then time compressed on the compression apparatus (now modified) described by Fairbanks, Everitt, and Jaeger (1954) to 0, 20, 30, 40, and 50% time compression using a 20 msec interval of discard. The compressor acts so that the spectrum of the speech wave is not frequency shifted. The device effectively records and discards alternate segments of a signal, rejoining the recorded segments into a continuous output signal. For a given interval of speech (I_a), the relationship between the recorded (I_r) and discarded (I_d) intervals is $I_a = I_r + I_d$, and the percent time compression (TC) of interval I_a is

$$TC\% = \frac{I_d}{I_r + I_d} \times 100$$

The size of both I_d and I_r are independently manipulable. Each tape was high-pass filtered (300 Hz, 36 dB per octave) to remove low frequency noise generated by the compression system.

Each of 6 master tapes representing minimally inflected, monotone speech and 0, 20, 30, 40, and 50% time-compressed filtered speech were segmented into 20 sec ($\pm$ 2 sec) segments. Ten segments for each of the 6 conditions were selected, randomized in order, and spliced into an experimental tape, with a 4 sec silence between each sample. In addition, 10 segments of normal speech were placed as standard segments at every 10-segment interval.[1] Two experi-

---

[1] The standard used in this study anchored the lower end of the rating scale. The uncompressed speech standard was used because preliminary work indicated that subjects had difficulty forming stable judgments using a sample of compressed speech as the standard. As is well known (Stevens, 1956), the location and stated size of the standard along the scale of samples to be scaled affects the size of the rated values. In this case, the rated values of difficulty may be somewhat larger and the growth of difficulty slower than with a standard in the middle or upper ranges of scaled values (Beck and Shaw, 1965).

mental tapes, one for the male and one for the female speaker, were made, as well as two practice tapes of 18 segments each.

Subjects

Subjects consisted of 40 students enrolled in an introductory University Speech course, each with declared normal hearing. They were divided into 2 groups of 20 subjects, and each group was assigned to listen to one of the two experimental tapes.

Experimental Procedures

Subjects were seated in individual carrels in a sound treated room at the center of which was placed a high quality 15″ speaker and enclosure connected to a Magnecord M-90 tape recorder and amplifier. Ambient noise levels with subjects in place were 38 and 50 dB as measured on the A and B bands of a B & K Type 2203 sound level meter and Type 4131 condenser microphone. The speech material presented averaged 70 dB as measured on the B band, indicating satisfactory sound pressure level and signal-to-noise ratio for the speech.

The method of direct-magnitude estimation was used for the scaling procedures. Subjects were instructed to listen to the standard speech and to consider it to have a difficulty of 10. They were to rate the difficulty of the various time compressed speech samples relative to the standard sample. *Difficulty* was defined as follows: (1) the degree of strain needed to listen to the speech, (2) the troublesomeness of listening, (3) the annoyance caused by the speech, (4) the ease of understanding the speech, (5) the degree of effort needed for listening to the speech, and (6) the unpleasantness of the speech.

A practice tape consisting of 18 items was presented after written instructions were read aloud. After a short period for questions and restatement of the task, subjects judged the experimental tapes in one sitting. There were 4 judgment sessions, each involving 10 subjects.

RESULTS

The mean and median scaled values as well as standard deviations and semi-interquartile ranges of the scaled values which are divided by 10 are reported in Table 1.

As a check upon the reliability of the ratings of each speaker, intraclass correlations for average scores were computed (Ebel, 1951). The correlations were both high and identical for each speaker ($r_k = 0.98$). The reliabilities for individual scores were $r_i = 0.87$ and $r_i = 0.86$ for male and female respectively, indicating satisfactory reliability for both average (r_k) and individual (r_i) scores.

Each datum point in Figure 1 represents the mean score divided by 10 for 10 judgments by each rater averaged over 20 raters. In Table 1, it can be seen that the variability of the ratings for the female was slightly higher than for the male; the divergence between mean and median scale values at 40 and 50% time compression indicates a skewing of judgments toward high values at high degrees of compression.

The data indicate that for both the male speaker and female speaker, rated difficulty accelerated to a high, almost linear growth of difficulty, with the female voice showing both more rated difficulty and a faster growth of difficulty for 20 to 50% time compression. At 20% time compression, both male and female voices were rated about equally difficult, only to diverge steadily at high values of compression.

TABLE 1. Mean values, standard deviation (SD), median values, and semi-interquartile ranges (Q) of scaled difficulty for listening to both male and female speech subjected to various degrees of time compression.

		Amount of Time Compression				
	Normal	0	20	30	40	50
Mean (male)	0.98	1.15	1.33	2.05	3.38	4.42
Mean (female)	1.08	0.92	1.40	2.37	4.55	6.31
SD (male)	0.73	1.20	2.60	2.10	4.70	6.30
SD (female)	1.00	1.00	1.74	3.10	6.00	8.40
MdN (male)	1.00	1.18	1.32	2.08	3.10	3.90
MdN (female)	1.00	0.91	1.34	2.25	4.20	5.60
Q (male)	0.05	0.25	0.20	0.19	0.54	0.50
Q (female)	0.12	0.13	0.24	0.50	1.00	1.24

The data show that at 50% time compression, the difficulty ratings of listening to speech has grown to be between 4.4 and 6.3 times the ratings for normal speech, while at 40% compression, this ratio is between 3.4 and 4.5 times. At 30% compression, difficulty ratings are twice normal, while a 20% speed-up shows a difficulty little different from normal speech. The data indicate that ratings for female speech are 1.51, 1.35, and 1.45 times as large as the difficulty ratings for the male's going from 30 to 50% compression, suggesting that the

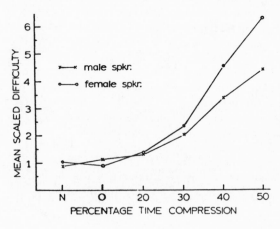

FIGURE 1. Mean scaled difficulty (divided by 10) of male and female speech for various degrees of time compression. Each datum point is the mean for 20 raters.

general preference of blind listeners for male speakers may be related to the increased difficulty of listening to the female at 30% or more time compression.

DISCUSSION

The results of this study agree only in part with those of the Foulke 1966 study. Assuming that the less difficult speech is most preferable, then both studies agree in concluding that time-compressed male speech is preferable to time-compressed female speech. However, our findings disagree with Foulke's observation that time-compressed female speech is more easily understood than the male speech. The Foulke study separated preference for speakers of one sex from the question as to which speaker, male or female, was most easily understood. The present investigators made ease of understanding one of the six subcriteria for difficulty of listening. Because time-compressed male speech was the less difficult, it can be assumed that the male speech is also the easier to understand. These conflicting results may reflect differences in listeners (blind vs. normal), or experimental conditions (questionnaire vs. scaling procedure, speech materials, readers, etc.), or may indicate that ease of understanding is too vague a construct when used alone to permit generalization between studies. Interestingly enough, recent work by Daniloff, Shriner, and Zemlin (1968) indicates that vowels produced by a female (same speaker as this study) are generally more intelligible under all degrees of time compression (0 to 80%) and bandwidth compression than a comparable male's. From this evidence, we conclude that time compressed vowel intelligibility can not be very closely connected with difficulty of listening to time-compressed speech except at extreme (greater than 50%) levels of time compression.

Normal listeners prefer speech at about 30% time compression, speech not more than twice rated difficulty relative to normal speech. As Foulke (1966) indicates, blind listeners prefer 35 to 40% time compression. If the generalization is made that both the normal-sighted and the blind have an initially similar conception of the difficulty of speech, then it is clear that the blind tolerate speech at conditions rated 3 to 4 times higher in difficulty relative to normal in exchange for increased rate of flow of information. With repeated hearings of compressed speech, the apparent difficulty might well decrease because of familiarization. However, if familiarization were to occur, speech at more than 50% time compression, even if intelligible, would still be prohibitively difficult to listen to. Extrapolating the function for the male to 60% compression indicates speech 5 times as difficult to listen to as normal speech, probably a prohibitively difficult condition for listening. The difficulty of listening would probably interact with the decline in speech intelligibility above 50% time compression, rendering measurement of difficulty impracticable.

Speech intelligibility and comprehension do not appreciably decline in the 0 to 50% time compression region (Fairbanks et al., 1957). The increased difficulty, aside from novelty removable with listener training, lies in the decrease of temporal redundancy and in degradation of phonetic quality of the speech.

The data indicate that nearly 30% time compression can be effected before difficulty increases appreciably; the acceleration in difficulty occurs at about 30% time compression. On this basis then, it may be ventured that the first 25 to 30% of the time segments removed in compression are redundant, but since difficulty of listening begins to accelerate at that point, the next 20 to 30% of the speech time discarded is redundant only insofar as information is concerned, but not in regard to the extra attention, strain, and effort demanded to monitor such speech.

The second result of interest is the fact that for 30% or more time compression, there is a difference in difficulty between listening to male and female speakers, a difference which grows so that the ratio of the difficulty ratings increases from 1 to 1.43 at 50% compression. Provided that the male-female differences in this study are related to the differences in voice quality between the sexes and not to some artifact unique to these two speakers, the differential difficulty probably contributes to the preference for male readers of time-compressed speech. Listeners may well tolerate additional time compression provided that the readers are male. Of course, the lack of a difference in difficulty between the male and female speaker at normal rates and at 20% compression indicate that causative factors are not operative except at higher rates of time compression. The source of this difference in difficulty may not be attributed to a differential decline in intelligibility with increasing time compression, but perhaps to the alteration of the phonetic quality or prosodic elements of speech.[2] The verbal reaction of subjects to the female voice at high compression rates indicates that they feel a "pseudo" Donald Duck effect is operating, that is, the pitch is abnormally high, compared to that of uncompressed female speech. At present, vowel and consonant differences in male and female speaker intelligibility for various degrees of time and bandwidth compression are being investigated in an attempt to account for this difference.

ACKNOWLEDGMENT

This work was supported in part by Public Health Research Grant No. NB-07346 from the National Institute of Mental Health. The authors are grateful to Elaine Paden and Dan Beasley for their assistance.

REFERENCES

BECK, J., and SHAW, W. A., Magnitude of the standard, numerical value of the standard, and stimulus spacing in the estimation of loudness. *Percept. motor Skills*, 21, 151-153 (1965).
DANILOFF, R., SHRINER, T. H., and ZEMLIN, W. R., The intelligibility of time and bandwidth altered vowels. Champaign: Univ. Illinois (1968).

[2]We would predict more difficulty in listening and poorer intelligibility for female speech than for the male because the 20 msec discard interval would remove about two pitch periods of the male voice as compared to four for the female. Recent research by Daniloff, Shriner, and Zemlin (1968) shows, however, that vowels produced by a female voice (same speaker as this study) are more intelligible than a male's for nearly all conditions (0 to 80%) of time compression and bandwidth compression (with and without time distortion) examined.

EBEL, R. L., Estimation of the reliability of ratings. *Psychometrika*, 16, 407-425 (1951).

FAIRBANKS, G., EVERITT, W. L., and JAEGER, R. P., Methods for time or frequency compression-expansion of speech. *Trans. I.R.E.-P.G.A.*, AU-2, 7-11 (1954).

FAIRBANKS, G., GUTTMAN, N., and MIRON, M., Effects of time compression upon the comprehension of connected speech. *J. Speech Hearing Dis.*, 22, 10-19 (1957).

FOULKE, E., A survey of the acceptability of rapid speech. *New Outlook Blind*, 60, 261-265 (1966).

FOULKE, E., The influence of a reader's voice and style of reading on comprehension of time-compressed speech. *New Outlook Blind*, 61, 65-68 (1967).

FOULKE, E., AMSTER, C. H., NOLAN, C. Y., and BIXLER, R. H., The comprehension of rapid speech by the blind. *Except. Child.*, 29, 134-141 (1962).

FOULKE, E., and STICHT, T. G., Listening rate preferences of college students for literary material of moderate difficulty. *J. auditory Res.*, 6, 397-401 (1966).

IVERSON, L., Time compression. *Internat. J. Educ. Blind*, 5, 78-79 (1956).

STEVENS, S. S., The direct estimation of sensory magnitudes. *Amer. J. Psychol.*, 69, 1-25 (1956).

INTELLIGIBILITY OF TIME-COMPRESSED CNC MONOSYLLABLES

DANIEL S. BEASLEY

SHELLEY SCHWIMMER

WILLIAM F. RINTELMANN

The effects of time-compressed monosyllabic CNCs on the auditory discrimination performance of 96 young adults with normal hearing were studied. Five conditions of time compression, 30% through 70% in 10% steps, plus a 0% control condition were presented at four sensation levels (8, 16, 24, and 32 dB). Ear presentation and list version were counterbalanced with these factors. Results indicated that intelligibility was inversely related to time-compression ratio and directly related to sensation level. Ear and list effects were minimal.

A battery of audiological tests (including pure tone, speech audiometry, alternate binaural loudness balancing, SISI, and Bekesy audiometry) yields response patterns which are peculiarly associated with damage to a particular anatomical site within the peripheral auditory system. These tests have proven useful in the assessment of lesions in the middle ear, inner ear, and eighth cranial nerve. Lesions in the brainstem and the auditory cortex, by contrast, elude detection by existing audiometric procedures. Present evidence suggests that individuals with disorders of the higher auditory pathways often exhibit response behavior which appears essentially normal (Willeford, 1969; and Katz, 1969).

Apparently, conventional auditory tests lack the structure and sensitivity necessary for the identification of lesions in the auditory cortex. Thus, investigators have sought specially designed audiometric measures requiring the cortical integration of complex signals in order to assess the function of these higher auditory centers (Willeford, 1969; Katz, 1969; and Bergman, 1971). Such measures have often taken the form of signal distortion, as in filtered speech (Jerger, 1964; and Speaks and Jerger, 1965), periodically switched speech (Calearo and DiMitri, 1958; and Calearo, Teatini, and Pestalozza,

JOURNAL OF SPEECH AND HEARING RESEARCH, 1972, vol. 15, 340-350.

98

1962), staggered spondee word tests (Katz, 1962), and temporally distorted signals (Bordley and Haskins, 1955).

Because of the role temporal factors play in speech perception (Hirsh, 1967; Aaronson, 1967; and Beasley and Shriner, 1971), distortion in the form of time compression has significant potential as a diagnostic measure. Studies by Sticht and Gray (1969) and Luterman, Welsh, and Melrose (1966), using time-compressed CID W-22 word lists, revealed differential results for young adult listeners compared to geriatric listeners, and sensorineural hearing-impaired listeners compared to normal listeners. However, Sticht and Gray did not employ a population large enough to provide normative data for diagnostic purposes. Further, adequate response curve information necessary for diagnostic purposes was hampered by the fact that Sticht and Gray only used three levels of time compression (36%, 46%, and 59%) and Luterman et al. (1966) only used two levels (10% and 20%). In addition, neither study revealed information about the possible effects of varying sensation level upon the auditory analysis of their distorted signals. Finally, both studies used the W-22 speech discrimination test, which has been criticized on the basis that the word lists may be too easy to be effective in differential diagnosis (Carhart, 1965). Other studies which have investigated the diagnostic value of time-compressed speech (Calearo and Lazzaroni, 1957; Bocca and Calearo, 1963; and de Quiros, 1964) have not provided adequate normative data, and have not used standard time-compression procedures.

This study sought to isolate the effects of varying degrees of time compression upon the intelligibility of a clinically standardized monosyllabic auditory test, using young adults with normal hearing. In addition, these effects were investigated relative to intensity increases, right/left ear differences, and word-list differences. The findings should provide the basis for comparative studies with auditorally pathological subjects, as well as normative data for future clinical diagnostic purposes.

EXPERIMENTAL PROCEDURES

Subjects were assigned to one of six experimental conditions. Each condition was characterized by one of six levels of time compression, using four versions of a standardized word list presented at four sensation levels (SL), and according to a randomized right/left ear paradigm.

Subjects

Ninety-six normal-hearing right-handed young adults selected from a university population were randomly assigned to six groups of 16 each. The test ear for each subject was determined by random selection. Eight right ears and eight left ears were tested for each of the six groups.

Each subject was required to pass a pure-tone screening test presented bilaterally at a 20-dB hearing level (ISO, 1964) at octave intervals from 125 Hz to 8000 Hz. In addition, a live-voice presentation of the CID W-1 spondee word list was administered unilaterally to obtain the speech reception threshold for the designated test ear.

Stimulus Generation

The experimental stimuli used in this study were the four lists of Form B of the NU-6 speech discrimination test (Tillman and Carhart, 1966). Each list is composed of 50 meaningful CNC units, phonemically balanced according to the scheme advocated by Lehiste and Peterson (1959). The four-word lists were recorded at normal conversational speech and effort level by a trained white male talker who spoke General American English under controlled recording procedures used by Rintelmann and Jetty in 1968.

A copy of each of the four recorded lists was made using an Ampex Model 601 tape deck (frequency response 50-12,000 Hz ± 2 dB). These copies were then temporally processed using the Fairbanks electromechanical time compression apparatus (Fairbanks, Everitt, and Jaeger, 1954) as modified by Zemlin.[1] Each list was time compressed by 30%, 40%, 50%, 60%, and 70%. In addition, each list was passed through the time-compression apparatus under 0% time compression in order to control for the effects of possible fidelity distortion in the time-compressed tapes. This resulted in 24 experimental tape recordings, six time-compressed recordings for each of the four lists.

Copies of each experimental tape were made using an Ampex Model 601 tape recorder and an Ampex AG 500-2 tape recorder (frequency response 50-13,000 Hz, ± 2 dB), monitored by an Ampex AA 620 power amplifier. During this procedure, five seconds of silent interval response time were allotted between each stimulus item.

Presentation Procedures

The subjects were divided into six groups, corresponding to the six different percentages of time compression under study. Each subject within a single group was presented with the four lists of Form B of the NU-6 test, each list at one of four sensation levels: 8, 16, 24, and 32 dB. Within each group, the order of presentation of sensation level was rotated. In this manner, each test was presented at each sensation level a total of four times for each time-compression condition, and the sensation levels were counterbalanced to avoid possible order effects of sensation level presentation.

All subjects were tested individually in a prefabricated double-walled test chamber (IAC 1200 series) with the experimenter seated in an adjacent single-walled control room. The ambient noise in the test room was sufficiently low (45 dB on the C scale of a Bruel and Kjaer sound-level meter) so as not to interfere with testing at even the lowest sensation level.

Each subject received standard instructions. The experimental tapes were presented to the listener via a Viking Model 433 tape deck (frequency response 60-12,000 Hz, ± 2 dB) housed in a Maico MA 24 audiometric unit, through TDH 39 earphones mounted in MX 41/AR cushions.

---

[1] W. Zemlin, personal communication, University of Illinois-Urbana (1970).

RESULTS

The results support the thesis that, as the ratio of time compression increases, the intelligibility of the word lists decreases. Further, as the sensation level was increased, intelligibility increased under the several conditions of time compression. As for the interlist equivalency of the NU-6 speech discrimination test, the results showed that List I was the most difficult while List IV was the easiest. However, the effect of word lists interacted with sensation level and time compression. Finally, ear differences in this study were found to be minimal. These results are depicted in Figures 1 through 3.

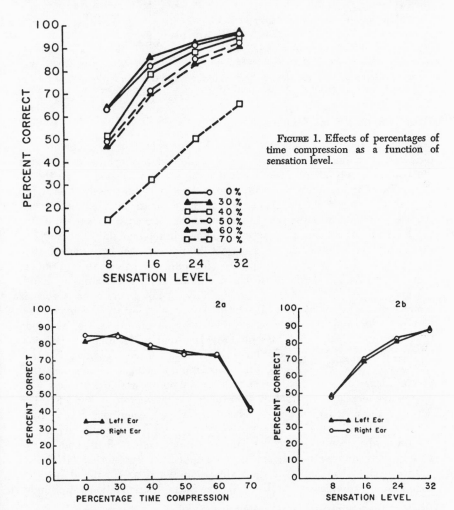

FIGURE 1. Effects of percentages of time compression as a function of sensation level.

FIGURE 2. Right/left ear differences as a function of percentage of time compression (2a) and sensation level (2b).

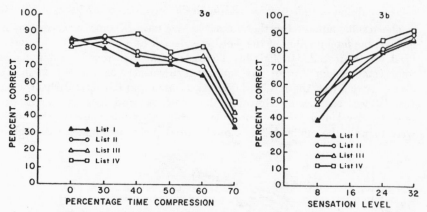

FIGURE 3. Effects of the four lists of Form B of the NU-6 test as a function of percentage of time compression (3a) and sensation level (3b).

Time Compression and Sensation Level

Figures 1 through 3 indicate that as the percentage of time compression increases, intelligibility decreases. Apparently, however, time compression did not negatively affect discrimination until 40% compression, since the 0% and 30% conditions were essentially equal at all but one sensation level (16 dB). In addition, it should be noted that the decrease in intelligibility was relatively gradual over the several conditions of time compression, until 70%, at which point there was a dramatic breakdown in intelligibility. This suggests that at high compression ratios, a normal listener may not have enough time or information to perceptually process incoming verbal stimuli (Daniloff, Shriner, and Zemlin, 1968; Beasley and Shriner, 1971; and Aaronson, 1967).

Figure 1 also shows that the intelligibility of time-compressed speech is significantly affected by sensation level. Specifically, listeners demonstrated improved discrimination at each condition of time compression as sensation level increased. This effect was most evident under 70% time compression, where the slope of the articulation curve is linear. Under the other five percentages of time compression, the articulation functions are characterized by curvilinear progressions in which discrimination scores improve less with progressive increases in intensity, approaching an asymptote at 32-dB SL. The slopes of the articulation curves generated for each condition of time compression were all found to increase between 2 and 3.5% per dB increase in intensity, when computed between the sensation levels of 8 dB and 16 dB. This is consistent with previous data compiled on undistorted NU-6 lists with respect to the slopes of the articulation functions computed between these two sensation levels.[2] At 32-dB SL, the mean discrimination scores under

---

[2]W. Rintelmann and A. Jetty, unpublished manuscript, Michigan State University (1968).

102

each condition of time compression, with the exception of 70%, were above 90% correct, which may be considered clinically normal.

Ear Effects

Figure 2 depicts the results according to right and left test ear. These data suggest that there were essentially no differences between right and left ear presentations at the several conditions of time compression and sensation level under study.

List Effects

Figure 3 illustrates the effects of the four lists of Form B of the NU-6 discrimination test at the six conditions of time compression, and the four sensation levels. Figure 3a indicates a general decrease in intelligibility for all lists, except List IV, as the time-compression ratio increases. Specifically, this effect occurs beyond 0%, whereas at 0% time compression, there is essentially no list difference (range from about 81-86%). The rather erratic configuration exhibited by List IV may be explained by simply noting that List IV will sustain a greater degree of distortion before intelligibility declines. Support for this contention is evident from Figure 3a and 3b where it can be seen that List IV is the easiest, while List I appears to be the most difficult.

Reference to Figure 3a reveals that the interlist variability is greatest for the time-compression ratios of 40%, 60%, and 70%, whereas 30% and 50% show similar range of scores with less variability. Figure 3b shows that as sensation level was increased, the interlist variability decreased. Again, List IV and List I appear to be the easiest and most difficult, respectively. Finally, there was essentially no consistent interaction between lists and test ear. However, this conclusion is tentative, due to the small and unequal number of subjects per cell for this interaction, which resulted from the fact that test ear was randomly assigned within each subject group.

DISCUSSION

Clinical Implications

The function of the auditory mechanism becomes progressively less definitive when consideration is given to the pathway central to the cochlear apparatus (Bocca and Calearo, 1963). According to Jerger (1960), the higher in the central nervous system the neurological lesion, the more subtle or complex are the stimuli required to uncover the lesion. In an analogy comparing the auditory system to a "bottleneck," he noted that once conventional auditory tests using pure tone and speech stimuli pass through the bottleneck of the peripheral auditory system up to and including the eighth nerve,

103

more difficult material is necessary to determine the existence of neurological auditory disorders. Bocca and Calearo (1963) and Bocca (1967) have suggested the value of distorted speech tests to identify the more subtle effects of lesions in the higher auditory pathways.

As one form of distorted speech signal, the potential clinical utility of time-compressed speech has been demonstrated. Calearo and Lazzaroni (1957), using time-compressed sentential material, found that among subjects with ascertained intrinsic lesions of the temporal lobe, discrimination ability was clearly worse when an accelerated message was transmitted to the ear contralateral to the lesion. Using similar stimuli, de Quiros (1964) found in various subject groups with central nervous system disorders that accelerated speech provided useful information which, when correlated with other findings, could aid in differential diagnosis of brain lesions. Further, Sticht and Gray (1969), and Luterman et al. (1966) revealed graphic differences for young and aged subjects, and normal-hearing and sensorineurally impaired subjects, respectively.

An advantage of using temporally modified speech signals over other forms of speech distortion, such as filtering, in differential diagnosis of higher auditory lesions, is that several theoretical models suggest speech perception is essentially temporally biased (Aaronson, 1967). In addition, such signals do not eliminate relevant spectral information, such as formant structure, whereas this does not hold true for filtered speech.

Although there are several methods of temporally distorting speech signals, the most efficient and controlled method to date is time compression using the electromechanical compressor. This procedure has the additional advantage of having been used in a large number of previous studies (Fairbanks, Guttman, and Miron, 1957; Fairbanks and Kodman, 1957; Daniloff, Shriner, and Zemlin, 1968; and Shriner, Beasley, and Zemlin, 1969). If this method is to be used clinically, however, it is necessary to obtain normative data using standard clinical procedures. This study has provided the necessary normative data. Before further investigations are carried out clinically, however, it is desirable to consider several pertinent points relative to the findings of the present study.

TIME COMPRESSION

This study demonstrates a gradual decrease in the intelligibility of monosyllables corresponding to progressively greater percentages of time compression over the range of 30% to 60%, with a dramatic reduction of intelligibility occurring at the 70% time-compression condition. These findings are in agreement with those of Daniloff et al. (1968), who found a significant breakdown in intelligibility to occur at 70% time compression using 11 different vowels placed in an /h-d/ context as their experimental stimuli. Fairbanks and Kodman (1957), however, found no appreciable breakdown in intelligibility of phonetically balanced monosyllables until a time-compression ratio of 80%

104

was reached. The discrepancy between the results of Fairbanks and Kodman (1957) and those of both Daniloff et al. (1968) and the present study can be accounted for in several ways.

First, Fairbanks and Kodman (1957) used a 10-msec discard interval in their method of time compression, as opposed to the 20-msec discard interval employed in the other two studies. According to Daniloff et al. (1968), this probably served to enhance the intelligibility at higher compression ratios employed in these latter two studies since smaller segments of the message, and therefore, smaller bits of information were differentially deleted. Secondly, Fairbanks and Kodman used highly trained listeners, whereas naive listeners served as subjects in the other two studies. Finally, Fairbanks and Kodman presented their stimuli at sufficiently high sensation levels (80-dB SL) to insure maximum intelligibility; whereas, in this study, the maximum intensity level employed was at a sensation level of 32 dB. At this level, maximum discrimination was not reached for 70% time-compression.

An exception to the tendency for intelligibility to decline with gradual increments in the time-compression ratio of monosyllables in this study seems to occur between the 0% and 30% time-compression conditions. Equivocal as it is, this is not the only instance in which such a finding has occured. Aaronson and Markowitz (1967) conducted a study in which the duration of the auditory test stimuli was varied for a fixed presentation rate. Spoken digits were compressed by 33% and compared to the original seven-digit sequence with respect to ease of short-term memory recall. It was found that when subjects attempted to recall a seven-digit sequence a few seconds after presentation, they did better when the sequence was time compressed by 33% than they did under conditions of 0% time compression. Aaronson considered her findings in view of short-term memory (STM) storage. That is, while a signal compressed by about 30% may be "distorted," its intelligibility is not degraded, and the short temporal load on STM may actually enhance perceptual analysis. However, future research is needed to clarify this issue.

Sensation Level

The interaction of intensity and time compression suggest a relationship between the two factors. The data indicate that for every increase in intensity, there is a corresponding increase in intelligibility of the test stimuli for all conditions of time compression employed. The effects of intensity increments lessen, as would be expected, as an optimal listening intensity is approached. This effect is readily observable from the curvilinear configuration of the articulation functions of the first five levels of compression.

The effects of intensity on the comprehension ability of normal subjects used in the studies of Calearo and Lazzaroni (1957) and of de Quiros (1964) cannot readily be compared to our findings due to the difference in speech stimuli and time-compression methods employed by each. It should be noted, however, that a tendency for intensity to neutralize the effects of speech

105

acceleration was reported by Calearo and Lazzaroni (1957) for their normal subjects. This holds true to a considerable extent in our study as well. Although the mean articulation scores for each of the first five conditions of time compression are not exactly equal even at the highest sensation level, they all fall within the "clinically normal" range. This is not the case for 70% time compression, wherein the articulation function is still linear at the highest sensation level, suggesting that sufficient intensity levels have not been reached for maximum discrimination.

Since tests of speech discrimination are usually administered in the clinical setting at sufficiently high intensity levels for the patient to perform optimally (Hirsh, 1952), it can be reasoned, on the basis of this study, that a clinical test of discrimination using time-compressed monosyllables, should not employ stimuli compressed beyond 60% at the highest sensation level examined. Further studies using pathological subjects are needed to determine the appropriate combinations of time compression and sensation levels that would be of maximum diagnostic utility. Such studies are being conducted in our laboratory.

Test Ear

In order to validly use the same test for both right and left ears, performance of normal subjects would warrant that test results between ears be essentially equal. The question of differences between ears is therefore worthy of consideration in light of the potential utility of time-distorted speech as a diagnostic tool for central auditory disorders.

Under dichotic listening conditions, right ear superiority was found for digits (Kimura, 1961; and Broadbent and Gregory, 1964), phonetically matched words (Borkowski, Spreen, and Stutz, 1965) and plosive consonants (Shankweiler and Studdert-Kennedy, 1967). Left ear performance was better for orchestrated melodies (Kimura, 1967), sonar signals (Chaney and Webster, 1966), environmental sounds (Curry, 1967), 2-click thresholds (Murphy and Venables, 1970), and rapid pitch changes (Darwin, 1969). However, studies of monotic listening tasks (Dirks, 1964; Corsi, 1967; Kimura, 1967; and Glorig, 1958) have failed to reveal clinically significant right (dominant ear effects. These monotic findings are supported by our study, suggesting that time-compressed speech can be clinically utilized in a monotic listening task without being confounded by ear laterality effects.

List Effects

All lists are essentially equal at 0% time compression, whereas higher ratios of time compression as well as low sensation levels serve to increase the interlist variability. Further, List IV overall is the easiest and List I is the hardest. It should be recognized, however, that the order of list presentation remained constant for all subjects under each condition of time compression.

Despite the fact that intensity order was counterbalanced within each of these conditions, it is possible (see Figure 3) that order effects of presentation were influential under the conditions of greater degrees of time compression, establishing Lists I, II, III, and IV as hardest to easiest, respectively. Therefore, in the formation of a clinical discrimination test using time-compressed speech stimuli, the effects of adapting to the discrimination task resulting in improved scores is worthy of further investigation.

REFERENCES

AARONSON, D., Temporal factors in perception and short term memory. *Psychol. Bull.*, 67, 130-144 (1967).

AARONSON, D., and MARKOWITZ, N., Immediate recall of normal and "compressed" auditory sequences. Paper presented to Eastern Psychol. Assn., Boston (1967).

BEASLEY, D., and SHRINER, T., Auditory analysis of time-varied sentential approximations. Presented to 82nd meeting Acoust. Soc. of Amer., Denver (1971).

BERGMAN, M., Hearing and aging: Implications of recent research findings. *J. aud. Commun.* 10, 164-171 (1971).

BOCCA, E., Distorted speech tests. In A. Graham (Ed.), *Sensorineural Hearing Processes and Disorders*. Boston: Little, Brown (1967).

BOCCA, E., and CALEARO, C., Central hearing processes. In J. Jerger (Ed.), *Modern Developments in Audiology*. New York: Academic (1963).

BORDLEY, J., and HASKINS, H., The role of the cerebrum in hearing. *Ann. Otol. Rhinol. Laryng.*, 64, 370-382 (1955).

BORKOWSKI, J., SPREEN, O., and STUTZ, J., Ear preference and abstractness in dichotic listening. *Psychonomic Sci.*, 3, 547-548 (1965).

BROADBENT, D., and GREGORY, M., Accuracy of recognition for speech presented to the right and left ears. *Quart. J. exp. Psychol.*, 14, 359-360 (1964).

CALEARO, C., and DIMITRI, T., Sulla intelligibilita della voce periodicemente alternata da un orchio all altro. Presented to Congress di Audiologica, Padova (1958).

CALEARO, C., TEATINI, G., and PESTALOZZA, G., Speech intelligibility in the presence of interrupted noise. *J. aud. Res.*, 2, 179-186 (1962).

CALEARO, C., and LAZZARONI, A., Speech intelligibility in relation to the speed of message. *Laryngoscope*, 67, 410-419 (1957).

CARHART, R., Problems in the measurement of speech discrimination. *Arch. Otolaryng.*, 82, 253-260 (1965).

CHANEY, R., and WEBSTER, J., Information in certain multidimensional sounds. *J. acoust. Soc. Amer.*, 40, 447-455 (1966).

CORSI, P., The effects of contralateral noise upon perception and immediate recall of monaurally-presented verbal materials. Master's thesis, McGill Univ. (1967).

CURRY, F., A comparison of left-handed and right-handed subjects on verbal and non-verbal dichotic listening tasks. *Cortex*, 3, 343-352 (1967).

DANILOFF, R., SHRINER, T., and ZEMLIN, W., Intelligibility of vowels altered in duration and frequency. *J. acoust. Soc. Amer.*, 44, 700-707 (1968).

DARWIN, C., Auditory perception and cerebral dominance. Doctoral dissertation, Univ. Cambridge (1969).

DE QUIROS, J., Accelerated speech audiometry, and examination of test results. (Translated by J. Tonndorf). *Transl. Beltone Inst. Hearing Res.*, No. 17, Chicago (1964).

DIRKS, D., Perception of dichotic and monaural verbal material and cerebral dominance for speech. *Acta Otolaryng.*, 58, 73-80 (1964).

THE INTELLIGIBILITY OF
TIME COMPRESSED WORDS AS A
FUNCTION OF AGE AND
HEARING LOSS

THOMAS G. STICHT

BURL B. GRAY

Speech intelligibility scores for time compressed PB words were determined for 28 young and old subjects having either normal or sensorineural hearing losses. The discrimination of time compressed words was not affected differentially by the nature of the subject's hearing ability. However, time compression attenuated the performance of the aged more than the young, and this difference increased as the amount of compression was increased.

In 1954, Fairbanks, Everitt, and Jaeger developed an electromechanical method for the time compression of speech without concomitant frequency distortion. With this method of time compression, small temporal segments of the recorded messages are deleted, and the remaining temporal segments are recorded adjacent to one another. The technique is somewhat analogous to cutting out and discarding small segments of magnetic tape, and splicing the remaining pieces together again. In either case the result is a continuous message, compressed with respect to the amount of time required to present the message, and no changes in the frequency spectrum.

Since the appearance of the work by Fairbanks and his associates, a number of studies have been performed to evaluate the intelligibility of time compressed words, and to evaluate how comprehensible such speech remains after compression resulting in very fast word rates. Much of this work has been reviewed recently (Foulke and Sticht, 1966).

With regard to the intelligibility of time compressed speech, it has been found that, for subjects with normal hearing, intelligibility may remain as high as 50% for spondaic or monosyllabic words compressed by 75-85% (Garvey, 1953; Fairbanks and Kodman, 1957). There are some indications that the intelligibility of time compressed words (or brief sentences) is severely attenuated in elderly persons having sensorineural hearing losses, in persons with

JOURNAL OF SPEECH AND HEARING RESEARCH, 1969, vol. 12, no. 2, 443-448.

temporal lobe lesions, and in persons with diffuse cerebral pathology (Bocca and Calearo, 1963; de Quiros, 1964). There are, however, some conflicting reports with respect to the relationship between age and the intelligibility of time compressed speech. Bocca and Calearo (1963) report decreased intelligibility of compressed words or short sentences with increased age. In a more recent study (Luterman, Welsh, and Melrose, 1966) a group of aged sensorineural subjects responded in a manner similar to that of young normal and young sensorineural subjects to phonetically balanced (PB) word lists subjected to 10 and 20% time compression. There were no differential effects of compression on the responses of the older subjects.

The present paper reports research in which the intelligibility of time compressed words was tested for young and old sensorineural and normal hearing subjects. None of the research reviewed has reported the effects of time compression on older subjects having normal audiograms. Such a comparison should reveal the effects of diffuse changes in the central auditory pathways, with the effects of cochlear disorders removed, or at least minimized. In addition to the inclusion of an older, normal hearing group of subjects our research differs from that of Luterman et al. in that the range of compression ratios is greater. The results of Bocca, Calearo, and their associates have shown the greatest effects of age with compression ratios over 50%. Therefore, our research has extended compression beyond 50% to maximize the possible interaction of age and compression.

METHOD

Apparatus

All the stimulus materials were delivered and controlled via Allison 22 B clinical audiometers. The latter were routinely calibrated at one month intervals. The stimulus material was presented through TDH 39 earphones. All testing was conducted in sound attenuated, double walled testing rooms.

Subjects

Fourteen normal hearing subjects (no loss greater than 15 dB ISO 1964 at 250, 500, 1 k, 2 k, and 4 kHz) and 14 subjects having sensorineural hearing loss were used. Each of the two subject groups was evenly divided into subjects under 60 years of age and those over 60 years of age.

Procedure

Subjects were drawn from the staff or the routine clinical population of the audiological testing service of the Monterey Institute for Speech and Hearing. Each prospective subject was given pure tone air conduction and bone conduction threshold tests. In addition, speech reception threshold (SRT) tests and speech discrimination tests were administered. All tests were presented to each ear unilaterally. For the purposes of the study, only one ear was selected for testing for each potential subject.

Based upon the audiological testing, 10 potential subjects were obtained for each of the four experimental categories (i.e., young and old normals and young and old sensorineurals). The experimental material was administered to this population of 40 people. This material consisted of words 1-15 and 26-40 of List 1A and words 1-15 and 26-40 of List 2A of C.I.D. Auditory Test W-22 (PB word lists). The first group of 15 words was not compressed (0% compression), while the second, third, and fourth groups of words were compressed by 36, 46, and 59% respectively. Time compression was by means of the sampling method described in Foulke and Sticht (1966), and outlined above. The four word lists were then mixed, by means of a table of random numbers, to form one list of 60 words.

TABLE 1. Mean age and scores on the discrimination and intelligibility tests used to match the groups.

Group		Age (Years)	Discrimination (% Correct)	Intelligibility (No. Wrong)
Normal	Young	27.0	96.3	0.43
	Old	64.4	97.1	0.43
Sensori-	Young	48.1	85.7	2.00
Neural	Old	69.2	85.7	2.00

The list of 60 tape recorded words was presented individually to each of the potential subjects. The list was presented at 40 dB re SRT except in cases where tolerance was a problem, in which case the words were presented at a "most comfortable" listening level. The subject was required to repeat the word upon hearing it. A record was obtained for the number of misidentifications made for the words presented at each of the four compression ratios.

Following the administration of the experimental materials to the four experimental groups, subjects from the normal hearing, young, and old groups were matched on the basis of their speech discrimination score and their score on the 0% compression experimental list. A similar procedure was then followed for the sensorineural subjects. In research by Luterman et al. (1966), old and young sensorineural subjects were matched on the basis of SRT and average three frequency loss in dB. However, their results showed that the older subjects scored lower than the younger subjects on the 0% compression (normal) condition of their study, signifying that they were, indeed, not matched for speech reception of the experimental material. Hence, in the present study, matching on the basis of the scores for the 0% compression material was accomplished. Through such matching, 7 subjects were obtained for each of the four experimental groups. Table 1 presents the average age of each group, the discrimination scores, and scores on the 0% compression experimental words. The very close matching is apparent. The difference in the mean ages between the two groups designated as young is also apparent. Some possible consequences of this difference are discussed below.

RESULTS

The average number of errors made by each of the experimental groups for the words compressed by 36, 46, and 59% was computed. These mean scores are presented along the ordinate of Figure 1, while the amount of compression is presented on the abscissa. At 0% compression, there are no differences between the age groups because they were matched on this condition prior to the analysis of results. An analysis of variance was performed on the data obtained with the 36, 46, and 59% compression ratios for each of the groups. Table 2 summarizes this analysis. As indicated, the main effects of hearing ability, age, and amount of compression are highly significant. The only significant interaction is that of age and amount of compression.

These analyses suggest that there are no differential effects of age or compression due to the two types of hearing ability. Thus, for both hearing groups, the effect of age is to increase, to a similar extent, the number of discrimination errors. However, in our study there are significant differences between the ages of the "young" normals and "young" sensorineurals. The latter are some

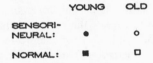

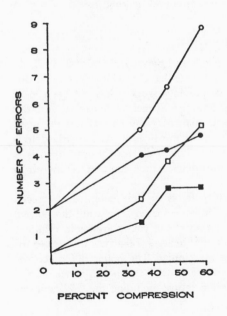

FIGURE 1. Mean number of errors on the intelligibility tests for the four experimental groups as a function of increasing amounts of time compression.

111

TABLE 2. Analysis of variance for the data obtained with the 36%, 46%, and 59% time compressed PB words.

Source	Mean Square	df	F
Between Subjects			
Normal vs.			
Sensorineural (A)	133.76	1	10.54**
Age (C)	76.19	1	6.00*
A × C	5.76	1	0.45
Within Subjects			
Compression			
(B)	34.69	2	34.15**
B × A	1.15	2	1.29
B × C	10.04	2	9.82**
A × B × C	1.15	2	1.29

*p < 0.025
**p < 0.005

20 years older than the former. Because of this difference in ages, it is best to consider this comparison with considerable reservation. With a much younger sensorineural group, the difference in error scores between the young and old sensorineurals might be greater than such differences for the normal hearing subjects. Under such circumstances, there might be found a significant age and hearing ability interaction.

Of primary interest in the study is the highly significant interaction of age and compression ratio. Inspection of Figure 1 reveals the nature of this interaction. With increased age, the ability to discriminate time compressed words diminishes as the amount of compression is increased. This is so for subjects with normal hearing and subjects with sensorineural hearing losses.

DISCUSSION

These results agree with the results of others (Bocca and Calearo, 1963; de Quiros, 1964) in indicating that elderly persons have special difficulty in discriminating rapidly produced speech. In previous work it has not been clear to what extent this difficulty might be due to presbycusis or to central auditory disorders. In the present study, the performance of the normal hearing aged subjects, who showed no audiometric signs of presbycusis, was greatly deteriorated by the process of time compression. This indicates that presbycusis is not a necessary condition of the aged in order for time compressed speech to disrupt performance.

Another suggestion that the disruptive effects of time compressed speech are of central rather than peripheral origin comes from comparing the normal and sensorineural hearing groups. The curves of the young groups in Figure 1 are similar for both sensorineural and normal hearers. Likewise, the curves for the older subjects in these two groups are similar. The major difference between the sensorineural and normal groups is that the performance of the former is attenuated across all compression ratios, including the 0% compres-

112

sion condition. Assuming that the high frequency losses in the sensorineural disorders are of a peripheral (receptor or first order neuron) nature, it would appear that such disorders serve to attenuate the baseline of performance, but are not particularly sensitive to distortions produced by the time compression of words.

A considerable amount of evidence, both of a physiological and perceptual nature, suggests that the rate of information processing over the sensory channels of the aged is reduced (Talland, 1968). Channel capacity (Miller, 1956) appears to be exceeded at lower rates of information transmission in the elderly. Stated otherwise, for a given rapid rate of information transmission, the elderly would be expected to perform more poorly than the young. Such was the observation in our study with the older subjects as compared to the younger subjects, when the rate of presentation of speech sounds was accelerated through the compression process. However, with the time compression of individual monosyllabic words, three things happen: (1) part of the speech spectrum is discarded, (2) the form of the word is changed by bringing parts of the speech spectrum together into unfamiliar patterns of temporal contiguity (determined by spectrographic analyses), and (3) the speech sounds occur at a faster rate. With individual words it is not clear which of these factors is having the greater effect on the response of the aged. Through the use of connected discourse, it is hoped that research in progress will help to elucidate this problem.

ACKNOWLEDGMENT

The audiological screening and testing of subjects was administered by Ferne Mueh and Barbara Savauge, clinical audiologists at the Monterey Institute for Speech and Hearing. We gratefully acknowledge their aid in this research.

REFERENCES

BOCCA, E., and CALEARO, C., Central hearing processes. In J. Jerger (Ed.), *Modern Developments in Audiology*. New York: Academic Press (1963).

FAIRBANKS, G., EVERITT, H., and JAEGER, R., Method for time or frequency compression-expansion of speech. *Trans. Inst. radio Engrs. Prof. Grp. Acoust.*, 7-11 (August 2, 1954).

FAIRBANKS, G., and KODMAN, F., JR., Word intelligibility as a function of time compression. *J. acoust. Soc. Amer.*, 29, 636-641 (1957).

FOULKE, E., and STICHT, T. G., A review of research on accelerated speech. In E. Foulke (Ed.), *Proc. Louisville Conf. Time Compressed Speech*. Louisville, Kentucky: Center for Rate Controlled Recordings, Univ. Louisville (1966).

GARVEY, W. D., The intelligibility of speeded speech. *J. exp. Psychol.*, 45, 102-108 (1953).

LUTERMAN, D. M., WELSH, O. L., and MELROSE, J., Responses of aged males to time-altered speech stimuli. *J. Speech Hearing Res.*, 9, 226-230 (1966).

MILLER, G. A., The magical number seven, plus or minus two: Some limits on our capacity for processing information. *Psychol. Rev.*, 63, 81-97 (1956).

TALLAND, G. A., *Human Aging and Behavior*. New York: Academic Press (1968).

QUIROS, J. B. DE, Accelerated speech audiometry, an examination of results. *Transl. No. 17, Beltone Inst. Hearing Res.* (1964).

113

A Comparative Study of Listening Rate Preferences for Oral Reading and Impromptu Speaking Tasks

NORMAN J. LASS AND C. ELAINE PRATER

Abstract

A **paired comparison** paradigm was employed to compare the listening rate preferences of 26 adult subjects for oral reading and impromptu speaking tasks. Recordings of a reading and speech were time-altered by means of a speech compressor to yield nine rates: 100, 125, 150, 175, 200, 225, 250, 275, and 300 wpm. Two master tapes were constructed, one for each of the two tasks investigated. The tapes were presented to each subject for listening rate preference judgments. Results of subjects' evaluations indicate that preferred listening rates are very similar for both oral reading and impromptu speaking tasks. The most preferred rate for both tasks was 175 wpm, and the least preferred rate for both tasks was 100 wpm. Comparison of the present findings with previous research and suggestions for future investigations are provided.

INTRODUCTION

With the development of special equipment which allows for the control of the rate of recorded speech without serious distortion in the pitch or quality of the original signal [1, 3, 5, 7] there has been an increased interest in the listener's listening rate preferences.

Three studies on listening rate preferences in normal adults appear in the literature. Hutton [10], as part of a larger psychophysical study of speech rate, investigated the listening rate preferences of a group of 50 subjects. Using 40 versions of a reading of a standard prose passage ranging in rate from 77.5 to 412.5 words per minute, and a nine-point scale ranging from "inferior" to "superior," he found that the reading rate receiving the highest ranking was 163 words per minute.

Norman J. Lass (Ph.D., Purdue University, 1968) is Assistant Professor of Speech and Hearing Sciences and Director of the Speech and Hearing Sciences Laboratory at West Virginia University.

C. Elaine Prater (B.S., West Virginia University, 1971) was formerly a student in the Speech Pathology-Audiology program and a research assistant in the Speech and Hearing Sciences Laboratory at West Virginia University. She is presently a graduate student in the Audiology and Speech Pathology program at Memphis State University.

JOURNAL OF COMMUNICATION, 1973, vol. 23, no. 1, 95-102.

Foulke and Sticht [8] studied the listening rate preferences of 100 college students for literary material of moderate difficulty. Employing a method of limits procedure in which the subject was allowed to manipulate the reading rate of the passage, they found the mean preferred listening rate for the group to be 207 words per minute.

Using a paired comparison paradigm, Cain and Lass [2] determined the listening rate preferences of a group of 100 subjects. Using nine different rates, from 100 to 300 words per minute in 25 wpm intervals, they found the most preferred rate to be 175 words per minute, and the least preferred rates were 100 and 300 words per minute.

All three studies on listening rate preferences have employed a reading passage as the material to be evaluated by their subjects. However, since there are basic differences in overall rate, pause times, and number of pauses between reading and impromptu speaking conditions [12, 15], statements on listening rate preferences for impromptu speaking tasks cannot be validly made from the existing data. The purpose of the present investigation was to compare listeners' listening rate preferences for oral reading and impromptu speaking tasks.

METHOD

Subjects

A total of 26 females served as subjects. All were students at West Virginia University and had no reported hearing difficulty. The subjects ranged in age from 18 to 36 years, and had a mean age of 20 years.

Recording Materials

The passage employed for the reading task was the first paragraph of Fairbanks' [4:127] "The Rainbow Passage." The impromptu speech employed consisted of a two-minute discussion of the historical development of a local television station. Both the reading and impromptu speech were recorded by the same individual, a professional male announcer. Recordings of the reading and speech were made in a sound-treated room using a Scully model 280 tape recorder and a Neumann model KM84i condenser microphone.

Time-Alteration Procedures

Of the six sentences in the reading passage, only the middle four sentences were employed for time-alteration purposes and used in the experiment. The first and last sentences were deleted in an attempt to avoid any possible rate variation effects associated with initiating and terminating a reading [10]. Of the two-minute impromptu speech, a middle portion was used in the study for time-alteration purposes.

The original recordings of the reading and speech were time-altered by means of a speech compressor to yield nine different rates: 100, 125, 150, 175, 200, 225, 250, 275, and 300 words per minute. The speech compressor is an electromechanical device which permits the time-compression and time-expansion of tape recorded materials without serious distortion to the pitch or quality of the recording. This is accomplished by means of a sampling technique in which brief segments of the recorded material are periodically deleted or repeated [5, 7].

Construction of Master Tapes

A paired comparison procedure [9] was employed for presentation of the different rates for preference evaluations. Two master tapes were constructed, one for the reading task and one for the impromptu speaking task. The order used in both tapes for presentation of the pairs was that experimentally established by Ross [14] for paired comparison tasks to avoid time and space errors. Each master tape contained 36 pairs, [n(n-1)/2], with each rate appearing eight times on each tape.

In the construction of the tapes, a total of 32 electronic reproductions of each of the nine rates was made. A one-second pause was employed between members of a pair, and a three-second pause was inserted between each pair. In addition to the 36 pairs, each tape included a set of pre-recorded instructions explaining the subjects' task as well as three pairs to be evaluated for practice purposes.

Listening Sessions

All 26 subjects participated in two listening sessions, with 13 subjects listening to the reading tape in the first session and the impromptu speech tape in the second session, and 13 subjects listening to the impromptu speech tape first and the reading tape

116

Table 1

Experimental proportions, summed proportions, and rank orderings of nine rates based on the evaluations of the 26 subjects listening to the reading master tape

Rates (wpm)	100	125	150	175	200	225	250	275	300
100	—	1.000	1.000	.962	.923	.962	.923	.923	.769
125	.000	—	.885	.962	.846	.692	.538	.192	.115
150	.000	.115	—	.654	.692	.385	.269	.077	.000
175	.038	.038	.346	—	.077	.192	.115	.000	.000
200	.077	.154	.308	.923	—	.462	.000	.000	.000
225	.038	.308	.615	.808	.538	—	.346	.000	.000
250	.077	.462	.731	.885	1.000	.654	—	.000	.000
275	.077	.808	.923	1.000	1.000	1.000	1.000	—	.038
300	.231	.885	1.000	1.000	1.000	1.000	1.000	.962	—
Σ p	0.538	3.770	5.808	7.194	6.076	5.347	4.191	2.154	0.922
Rank Order	9	6	3	1	2	4	5	7	8

second. The subjects' task was to determine to which of the two rates in each pair they preferred to listen. The tapes were presented binaurally to each subject by means of a Nagra model IV-D tape recorder and sets of matched Sharpe model HA-10A headphones. The listening sessions, which lasted approximately 45 minutes, were held in a sound-treated room at the West Virginia University Medical Center.

RESULTS

Results of subjects' listening rate preference judgments for the reading and impromptu speaking tasks are presented in Tables 1 and 2, respectively. The tables contain information on the mean proportions of cases in which a given rate was preferred when paired with another rate, for each of the nine different rates employed in the study. To obtain the proportions, it was necessary to construct tables for each of the 26 subjects, and to divide the frequency of judgments in a given category by the total number of judgments made. For example, in Table 1, the value .654 (column 4, row 3) is to be interpreted as follows: approximately 65 percent of the 26 subjects listening to the

117

Table 2

Experimental proportions, summed proportions, and rank orderings of the nine rates based on the evaluations of the 26 subjects listening to the impromptu speech tape

Rates (wpm)	100	125	150	175	200	225	250	275	300
100	—	1.000	1.000	.962	.962	1.000	1.000	1.000	1.000
125	.000	—	.962	1.000	.962	.923	.769	.577	.385
150	.000	.038	—	.885	.885	.423	****	.115	.038
175	.038	.000	.115	—	.346	.500	.077	.038	.000
200	.038	.038	.115	.654	—	.692	.000	.000	.000
225	.000	.077	.577	.500	.308	—	.154	.000	.000
250	.000	.231	****	.923	1.000	.846	—	.115	.000
275	.000	.423	.885	.962	1.000	1.000	.884	—	.154
300	.000	.615	.962	1.000	1.000	1.000	1.000	.846	—
Σ p	0.076	2.422	4.616	6.886	6.463	6.384	3.884	2.691	1.577
Rank Order	9	7	4	1	2	3	5	6	8

**** Due to a technical error in the preparation of the master tape, no comparison of 250 and 150 wpm was provided.

master reading tape preferred the rate of 175 wpm to the rate of 150 wpm. In Table 2, the value 1.000 (column 2, row 1) indicates that all 26 subjects preferred the speaking rate of 125 wpm when it was paired with the rate of 100 wpm.

The rank ordering of the nine rates investigated, based on all of the obtained proportions for each of the two tasks, reflects the listening rate preferences for the entire group of subjects. To obtain the rank orders for the nine rates, the proportions presented in each table were summed and the rankings were determined from the summed proportions (Σ p). The rank orderings are given at the foot of each column in the tables. They indicate that the rankings of preferred listening rates are very similar for both oral reading and impromptu speaking tasks. The most preferred listening rate for both tasks was 175 wpm, and the least preferred listening rate was 100 wpm. Some differences exist between the two tasks for rates between most and least preferred; however, the differences are frequently simple reversals in position in the rankings, and do not reflect any regular trend in the data.

The results of this investigation indicate that there are only slight differences in subjects' listening rate preferences between oral reading and impromptu speaking tasks. For both tasks, the subjects preferred 175 wpm most, 200 wpm second, and preferred least 300 and 100 wpm. Furthermore, the differences that do exist between the two tasks represent reversals in rankings. For example, the rates of 225 and 150 wpm are in positions #3 and #4, respectively, in the speaking task, while in the reading task, they are #4 and #3, respectively. However, no real trend of preferring faster rates for the speaking task is established in the data, since 200 wpm is preferred over 225, 250, 275, and 300 wpm, and 150 wpm is preferred over 250, 275, and 300 wpm, for the impromptu speaking tape. Thus, despite differences between reading and speaking tasks, listeners prefer most and least the identical rates for both tasks.

It is interesting to note that when comparing the rank orderings in the present investigation for the reading task with those obtained by Cain and Lass [2] in an earlier study, all rankings of the nine rates are found to be identical in both studies. This finding provides further support for the reliability of such listening rate preference judgments.

The finding that 175 wpm was the subjects' most preferred rate is in disagreement with Foulke and Sticht's [8] earlier results. The most preferred listening rate chosen by their subjects was 207 wpm. One possible explanation for this discrepancy is the methodological differences between the two studies. While only nine discrete rates were available to the subjects in the present investigation, Foulke and Sticht offered their subjects a range from 0 to 500 wpm. In addition, the present study employed a paired comparison technique for rate preference evaluations, while a method of limits procedure, in which the subjects were allowed to manipulate the rate of the passage, was used in the Foulke and Sticht study. Furthermore, it should be noted that the rate used in the present study which came closest to Foulke and Sticht's figure of 207 wpm was 200 wpm, which was the second most preferred rate.

In comparing the most preferred rate of the subjects in the current study with the most preferred rate reported by blind listeners, the difference is large. Foulke [6], in conducting a survey of the acceptability of time-compressed speech by blind students, found that when presented with a variety of samples of accelerated speech, they preferred a rate of 275 wpm most often. This difference between the listening rate preference of the blind and the sighted is not unexpected. Since blind students receive most of their information by listening, while sighted students receive it through visual reading, it is only natural that the blind could tolerate and prefer a faster listening rate than the sighted.

The influence of experience in listening to time-compressed speech material on the individual's preferred listening rates has been implied by the findings of Iverson [11] and Foulke [6]. It is suggested that future research explore this issue in detail to determine if subjects' listening rate preferences can be altered through appropriate experiences with time-compressed speech.

It is also suggested that future research explore the listening rate preferences of children in an attempt to determine if differences exist in such preferences between children and adult listeners.

A final suggestion for future inquiry is the investigation of listening rate preferences of groups of individuals with various speech defects and the comparing of such preferences with those of "normal" individuals. This comparison would be especially interesting in the case of stutterers, where a disturbance in the rate-rhythm patterns of the stutterer may have some influence on his preferred listening rates.

REFERENCES

1. Breuel, J. W., and L. M. Levens. "The A.F.B. Harmonic Compressor." In *Proceedings of the Second Louisville Conference on Rate and/or Frequency Controlled Speech* (edited by E. Foulke). Louisville, Kentucky: University of Louisville, 1970, 185–192.
2. Cain, C. J., and N. J. Lass. "Listening Rate Preferences of Adults." In *Time-Compressed Speech* (edited by S. Duker). Metuchen, New Jersey: Scarecrow Press, (in press).
3. Campanella, S. J. "Signal Analysis of Speech Time-Compression Techniques." In *Proceedings of the Louisville Conference on Time-Compressed Speech* (edited by E. Foulke). Louisville, Kentucky: University of Louisville, 1967, 108–114.
4. Fairbanks, G. *Voice and Articulation Drillbook.* New York: Harper and Row, 1960.

5. Fairbanks, G., W. L. Everitt, and R. P. Jaeger. "Method for Time or Frequency Compression-Expansion of Speech." *Transactions of the Institute of Radio Engineers Professional Group on Audio*, AU 2, 1954, 7–12.

6. Foulke, E. "A Survey of the Acceptability of Rapid Speech." *New Outlook for the Blind*. 60:261–265, 1965.

7. Foulke, E. "Methods of Controlling the Word Rate of Recorded Speech." *Journal of Communication*, 20:305–314, 1970.

8. Foulke, E., and T. G. Sticht. "Listening Rate Preferences of College Students for Literary Material of Moderate Difficulty." *Journal of Auditory Research*, 6:397–401, 1966.

9. Guilford, J. P. *Psychometric Methods*. New York: McGraw-Hill Book Co., 1954, 154–177.

10. Hutton, C. L. "A Psychophysical Study of Speech Rate." Doctoral dissertation, University of Illinois, 1954.

11. Iverson, L. "Time Compression." *International Journal of Education of the Blind*, 5:78–79, 1956.

12. Lass, N. J., and J. D. Noll. "A Comparative Study of Rate Characteristics of Cleft Palate and Noncleft Palate Speakers." *Cleft Palate Journal*, 7:275–283, 1970.

13. Mattingly, I. G. "Speech Synthesis by Rule as a Research Technique." *Journal of the Acoustical Society of America*, 41:1588, 1967.

14. Ross, R. T. "Optimal Orders for the Presentation of Pairs in the Method of Paired Comparisons." *Journal of Educational Psychology*, 25:375–382, 1934.

15. Snidecor, J. C. "A Comparative Study of the Pitch and Duration Characteristics of Impromptu Speaking and Oral Reading." *Speech Monographs*, 10:50–56, 1943.

VERBAL TRANSFORMATION EFFECT

VERBAL TRANSFORMATION EFFECT AND AUDITORY PERCEPTUAL MECHANISMS [1]

RICHARD M. WARREN

Continued listening to recorded repetitions of a single word or phrase induces illusory changes. These "verbal transformations" (VT's) may range from a word that rhymes with the actual stimulus to extreme phonetic distortions. The VT effect has revealed semanitc and phonetic aspects of verbal organizational processes. It is suggested that the strategies employed for the perception of connected discourse change in a regular manner throughout the normal life span. Some aspects of VT's appear related to other perceptual phenomena including aphasia and both auditory and visual illusions induced by unchanging patterns of sensory input.

It has been known for some time that repeating a word to oneself results in a lapse of meaning: "Repeat aloud some word—the first that occurs to you; *house,* for instance—over and over again; presently the sound of the word becomes meaningless and blank; you are puzzled and a morsel frightened as you hear it [Titchener, 1915, pp. 26–27]." This lapse of meaning upon repetition is now generally called semantic or verbal satiation and is the subject of much current interest (see Amster, 1964, for a review of this literature). If, rather than repeating a word to oneself, one listens to a recording of a word repeated over and over, a different effect occurs. Abrupt illusory changes are experienced, frequently involving considerable phonetic distortion. It is usually difficult to believe that the stimulus is not changing, even when the listener knows that all repetitions are identical. This "verbal transformation effect" has revealed some rather unexpected characteristics of speech perception and has suggested mechanisms underlying the perception of connected discourse.

Verbal transformations were discovered while looking for an auditory analogue of visual reversible figures. The classical reversible stimuli are ambiguous stimuli (e.g., the Necker cube, Rubin's figure-ground illusions), and perceptual organization fluctuates from

one interpretation to the other. It seemed that it should be possible to create ambiguous auditory configurations through repetition of certain words. For example, if the word "say" were repeated over and over without pause, it would be equivalent to repetitions of the word "ace." Would perceptual alternation occur between these two plausible interpretations of the stimulus? If these changes took place, would verbal satiation eventually cause both forms to disintegrate into a meaningless jumble of sounds, or would these changes inhibit such disintegration? In order to answer these questions, it was necessary to provide identical repetitions, equivalent in duration, emphasis, and pronounciation. As a preliminary experiment, Warren and Gregory (1958) prepared short endless loops of recorded tapes. When the experimenters played these tapes to themselves and to others at the Cambridge University Psychology Laboratory, they found that changes of the sort anticipated did occur, and that the loss of semantic organization associated with verbal satiation was avoided. But surprisingly, compelling illusory changes in phonetic structure were observed as well, even though the words were played clearly. The experimenters' bias was such that the note describing their observations was entitled "An Auditory Analogue of the Visual Reversible Figure" (Warren & Gregory, 1958).

However, after some further preliminary work, the present author became convinced that this verbal transformation (VT) effect was not analogous to classical visual reversals. The differences are great:

[1] Preparation of this paper was partially supported by a grant from the Graduate School, University of Wisconsin, Milwaukee, and by National Institutes of Health Grant NB 05998. The author expresses his gratitude to R. P. Warren for her helpful criticisms and suggestions.

1. The visual illusions occur with only a few special configurations, while VT's occur with all words.

2. The visual illusions most often involve reinterpretation without appreciable distortion of the stimulus configuration, while VT's usually involve considerable distortion of clearly pronounced stimuli.

3. Each of the visual illusions generally involves the same perceptual forms for different people, while the auditory forms vary greatly with individuals.

4. The visual illusions generally involve transitions between two (occasionally three or four) forms, while VT's usually involve more than four (sometimes more than a dozen) forms during a period of 2 or 3 minutes.

NATURE OF VERBAL TRANSFORMATIONS

The first systematic study of the VT effect employed British sailors as subjects (Warren, 1961a). Stimuli were prepared by recording single vocal statements which were then spliced to form a loop of tape. Each loop was played back and rerecorded on a conventional reel to give a stimulus which could be played for 3 minutes. The verbal stimuli (words, phrases, and short sentences) were chosen to allow a broad coverage of phonetic, semantic, and temporal factors. Some of the findings are given below, following a short description of testing and scoring procedures.

The subject listened to the repeating stimulus through headphones, tapping on the table and calling out what he heard as soon as he could (the experimenter recorded the time and transcribed the response). The subject continued listening for 3 minutes, tapping and calling out each time the voice seemed to change what it was saying. The subject's record was scored both for numbers of forms (different words or other perceptual organizations) and numbers of transitions (changes from one form to another). The characteristics of the stimuli and the response scores are given in Table 1.

Stimulus complexity. The greatest distortion tended to occur with the simpler stimuli; responses with the two phoneme stimulus SEE included such severely distorted forms as "this," and even "next please." An example of one subject's responses to a more complex stimulus containing four phonemes, TRESS, played loudly and clearly for 3 minutes is as follows (all responses listed in the order reported): "stress, dress, stress, dress, Jewish, Joyce, dress, Jewess, Jewish, dress, floris, florist, Joyce, dress, stress, dress, purse" (16 transitions, 8 forms). This sequence illustrates the variety of phonetic and semantic linkages encountered frequently for VT's with single word stimuli. With still greater phonetic complexity, distortions tended to become less. VT's of repeated short sentences usually preserved the syllabic structure and most of the phonemes. While the grammatic structure and meaning of individual words in the sentence were transformed (occasionally by homonymic change), there was a pronounced tendency to maintain a meaning related to the general topic of the actual sentence (e.g., the stimulus OUR SIDE IS RIGHT undergoing VT to "I'll side his right").

Time course for transitions and for new forms. Transitions occurred at almost the same rate throughout the 3-minute test, but the appearance of new forms tended to decrease rapidly from an initially high rate. For the single words repeated without pause, an asymptote was reached by the middle of the test. It seemed as if once a repertoire of perhaps 5 or 6 words was acquired, additional forms were added at a steady slow rate.

Indistinct speech. The effect of repetition upon perception of indistinct speech is rather interesting. Of course, if just one statement of an indistinct utterance is heard, people generally recognize their inability to identify what is being said. Skinner (1936) employed a device which he called "the verbal summator" to repeat a collection of unintelligible speech sounds over and over. He found that subjects organized the stimuli into words and phrases with considerable confidence concerning the accuracy of their reports, despite the fact that these bore little resemblance to the actual stimulus. Skinner shut off the recording as soon as the subject responded. Had he continued to play the record, VT's no doubt would have been observed by him. VT's, curiously, occur at a lower rate for an indistinct stimulus than for the same stimulus played clearly (see Table 1). If we were to consider that semantic satiation is involved in VT's,

TABLE 1

CHARACTERISTICS OF REPEATING STIMULI AND MEANS OF RESPONSES OF 18 SUBJECTS
DURING 3-MINUTE TEST PERIOD

Repeated stimulus word(s)	Listening conditions	Number of repetitions in 3 minutes	Transitions reported (M)	Different forms (M)
1. TRESS	Faint speech, masking noise	429	15.3	4.8
2. LAME-DUCK	Loud and clear	279	19.7	5.0
3. TRESS	Loud and clear	429	33.6	7.2
4. SEE	Loud and clear	387	13.9	5.0
5. TRESS	Faint but distinct	429	28.9	7.2
6. SEESHEE	Loud and clear	228	13.5	5.8
7. TREK (0.2 sec. pause)	Loud and clear	492	23.7	6.1
8. SEESHAW	Loud and clear	225	9.9	3.8
9. TREK (0.9 sec. pause)	Loud and clear	168	8.4	3.0
10. LAME-DUCK	Loud and clear	279	14.6	3.7
11. TRESS	Faint speech, masking noise	429	14.1	4.6
12. OUR SIDE IS RIGHT	Loud and clear	126	12.7	1.9
13. TRICE	Loud and clear	444	19.6	5.8
14. FILL-UP	Loud and clear	339	16.1	3.6
15. TRUCE	Loud and clear	417	16.5	4.8
16. OUR SHIP HAS SAILED	Loud and clear	120	15.4	2.3
17. TREK (4 sec. pause)	Loud and clear	42	9.5	2.0
18. RIPE	Loud and clear	390	21.6	4.0
19. TRUCE	Loud and clear	417	22.2	5.0
20. RAPE	Loud and clear	435	22.0	5.3

Note.—From Warren, 1961a.

we might reason that following perceptual organization, repetition progressively satiates this organization, decreasing its cohesiveness and clarity until eventually it disintegrates and is replaced. With masking noise, since the stimulus is less clear to start with, it would be anticipated that the time required for "satiation" should be less, and hence VT's would occur at a more rapid rate. The increase in perceptual stability with noise suggests that either the concept of semantic satiation needs to be refined further, or that it is not applicable to this illusion. Other inadequacies of this concept as related to VT's will be discussed subsequently.

Cochlear and afferent neural changes. Changing the intensity of stimulation does not seem to affect either the rate or variety of VT's once a level adequate for intelligibility is reached (compare Stimuli 3 and 5 in Table 1). This suggests that peripheral factors such as cochlear or afferent neural fatigue are relatively unimportant when compared with central processes in governing this illusion. If central perceptual mechanisms are indeed of major importance, we would also expect that monotic and diotic stimulation would produce equivalent VT's, which, in fact, later work did reveal (Warren, 1961b).

Repetition rate. Do repeated words seem to change because of a mechanism related to a generalization of the seventeenth century philosopher John Locke that, *"The mind cannot fix long on one invariable idea* [Locke, 1894, p. 244, italics his]"? He concluded that if an individual attempted to restrict his mind to one idea, he would fail, and new ideas or modifications of the old "will constantly succeed one another in his thoughts, let him be as wary as he can [p. 245]." If this were so, and if the length of time which could be devoted to a particular perceptual organization were the limiting factor, then we would expect that the rate at which a word was repeated would have a relatively minor effect upon the rate of VT's. On the other hand, it is conceivable that the amount of redundant information is the rate determining factor; that reprocessing of identical auditory input in an identical manner can be performed only so many times. If this latter statement were valid, we would expect that the rate of VT's should be a function of the number of repetitions rather than the stimulation time. In order to change the repetition rate, three recordings of the same word (TREK) were prepared (see Table 1). Each recording was made from the same u'terance, and differed only in the duration of the silent interval between repetitions. It was found that when the presentation rate was changed from about three per second to one per second, responses were a function solely of the number of repetitions and not stimulation time. In other words, in terms of transitions and different forms, 1 minute at the faster rate was quantitatively equivalent to 3 minutes at the slower rate. When the repetition rate was decreased further to one statement every 4 seconds, the number of different forms reported still seemed to depend upon the number of stimulus repetitions, but the number of transitions was the same as that obtained for an equal time interval at a repetition rate of one per second. These quantitative results seem of interest, and should be replicated and extended with stimuli of graded complexity and different repetition rates.

There is a related point that should be noted. The more complex stimuli required fewer repetitions to produce illusory changes. For those stimuli repeated clearly without pauses, the most repetitions were required for the simplest stimulus SEE (28 repetitions per VT); intermediate numbers of repetitions for more complex single words (13 to 25 repetitions per VT); and the least numbers of repetitions for the two sentences (7.8 and 9.9 repetitions per VT).

Age differences in verbal transformations. In preliminary testing it was observed that elderly people did not experience VT's in the same fashion that the young adults did. This was unexpected, since there was little evidence for major differences between the young and the aged for illusions involving visual reorganization. For example, Miles (1934) tested over 1000 subjects varying in age from 25 years to 90 years with a dynamic visual reversible stimulus (the shadow of a rotating two-bladed fan) and found no significant age differences in reports of illusory changes.

Experiments (Warren, 1961b; Warren, 1962; Warren & Warren, 1966) have demonstrated major age differences both in the frequency and in the nature of VT's. By preparing a series of five stimulus tapes of single repeated words which were used throughout this cross-sectional investigation, it was insured that the differences observed resulted from factors associated with age and not with the stimuli. The words used were: TRESS, SEE, FLIME, POLICE, and TRICE, presented in the order listed. In the first study it was found that aged adults (mostly retired professional men and their wives, ages 62–86) were much less susceptible to VT's than young adults (junior college students, ages 18–25). Next, a study with nursery school children (age 5) showed that they resembled the aged in generally not experiencing VT's. This was followed by a study of primary school children (3 groups—age 6, 8, and 10 years, respectively) which showed that individuals become susceptible to VT's at the age of 6 or 7. By age 8 all children experienced VT's, and did so at the same rate as 10-year-old children and young adults. Studies by other investigators have generally employed young adults of college age. However, Taylor and Henning (1963) employed subjects averaging 35 years of age, and they reported that scores for both transitions and forms fell between those of the younger and older adults reported by Warren (1961b).

The cross-sectional studies revealed age differences not only in the numbers, but in the types of forms. Children reported not only English words, but English-Not-Words (nonsense words with speech sounds grouped according to the rules of English), and English-Non-Syllables (English speech sounds clustered in a manner not found in English, such as an initial "sr" as in "srime"). Young adults occasionally reported English-Not-Words, but never English-Non-Syllables. The aged restricted their responses almost entirely to English words. Even when presented with an English-Not-Word stimulus (FLIME), the aged typically did not report this stimulus, but rather distorted it into an English word (e.g., "flying"), and then continued to hear this word throughout the 3-minute test. (An interesting exception is the English-Not-Word, the incorrect past participle "flyed," reported frequently by the aged.)

Thus, the VT effect suggests that as people age, their units for organization of speech become progressively larger. These perceptual units appear to be individual phonemes for children, English phoneme clusters for young adults, and English words for the aged.

While the aged do very poorly in identifying an English-Not-Word, they actually have a more veridical perception of the repeated English words than do the younger subjects. The aged typically identified these words properly, and then kept on perceiving the actual stimulus throughout the entire 3-minute test. When the old people did experience an illusory change, it often involved a gradual change requiring many stimulus repetitions for completion .(e.g., the initial phoneme T in TRICE might seem to get fainter and fainter until it disappeared and the subject perceived only "rice"). Young adults and children heard abrupt changes without transitional states. When the extent of phonemic differences between successive forms reported by individual subjects was examined, a consistent change with age was noted. For all groups (ranging from 6 through 86 years of age) the number of phonemic changes decreased with increasing age. In other words, perceptual reorganizations involved ever finer distinctions with advancing years. However, the slight phonemic changes associated with VT's in well-preserved aged are not in evidence when symptoms of senility are present. A study just completed in the author's laboratory by Obusek (1968) found that the extent of phonemic changes from one form to the next for a senile group was comparable to the level reported for 10-year-old children. On the other hand, the numbers of transitions and different forms reported by the deteriorated aged were below those obtained for well-preserved subjects of the same age—as if in this respect the senile had aged more.

The studies of age differences have suggested that the VT effect reflects skilled reorganizational mechanisms normally aiding comprehension of connected discourse for all but young children and the aged. More will be said about this in the following discussion.

FAILURE OF SATIATION THEORY

It was pointed out earlier in this article that the concept of cortical satiation does not seem consistant with the observation that VT's decrease if a repeated word is made indistinct with masking noise. Studies from other laboratories have in general also indicated that the concept of satiation leads to predictions contrary to the facts.. Thus, Paul (1964) reasoned that if satiation be considered a type of cortical inhibition, then a central nervous system (CNS) depressant (phenobarbital) should increase the rate of VT's, and a CNS stimulant (dexedrine) should decrease the rate. Paul found an effect just opposite to that predicted from satiation theory; that is, phenobarbital decreased, and dexedrine increased the rate of VT's relative to a control group receiving a placebo pill.

Axelrod and Thompson (1962), using a single group of subjects, determined scores not only for VT's, but also for two visual illusions (perspective reversals of a Necker cube, and changes in apparent motion of an ambiguous rotating pattern). The correlation between numbers of illusory changes experienced by individuals, though positive, was so low that Axelrod and Thompson concluded that it did not appear that these illusions all reflected a single process such as satiation.

INSTRUCTIONAL BIAS

There is a subtle bias involved in conducting any experiment on the VT effect. The very fact that the subject is required to continue to listen to the stimulus suggests that there is a reason for listening (i.e., that the stimulus might change). However, the existence of illusory changes does not seem to rest upon this suggestion. People who have prepared the tapes and worked as experimenters still experience VT's. Warren (1961a) and Natsoulas (1965) found that subjects who were told beforehand that each stimulus consisted solely of the same word repeated over and over nevertheless reported illusory changes. The effect of such knowledge upon the rate of VT's was investigated by Natsoulas and Levy who instructed one group that repetitions were identical and that any changes heard by subjects occurred within their own perceptual systems, while a second group was led to believe that changes were occurring on the tape (unpublished experiment described by Natsoulas, 1967). The group aware of the true nature of the stimulus reported fewer changes, and Natsoulas concluded that this was not surprising since, " 'Hearing things' is not an admired ability among people in our culture [p. 270]."

Taylor and Henning (1963) designed a study to investigate the effect of instructional bias concerning non-English forms upon VT's. All subjects were instructed that they would be listening to real changes; one group was told that only English words would be spoken, a second "unrestricted" group was told that both English and nonsense words would be spoken. In order to enhance this instructional bias, subjects were exposed to "practice" tapes, in which real changes occurred in what the voice was saying in keeping with the particular instructions given to the subjects. They found that both instructional groups reported the same number of English words, but that the group told that they would hear only English did not report nonsense forms as did the unrestricted group. It was concluded that the absence of nonsense words in the restricted group represented "perceptual suppression" (i.e., subjects never perceived non-English forms) rather than "response suppression" (i.e., subjects perceived but did not report non-English forms). The reasoning used to determine the nature of suppression depended upon the validity of a general rule proposed for VT's: that is, the number of transitions experienced, T, is proportional to the number of possible transitions among reported forms, F, so that

$$T = kF(F - 1)$$

where k is an empirical constant. However, testing this rule using raw data from our published experiments revealed that this relation did not apply, and hence Taylor and Henning's (1963) suggested reasons for attributing their observed instructional bias to perceptual suppression rather than response suppression seem weakened.

MEANINGFULNESS OF STIMULI

Natsoulas (1965) determined the effect of the meaningfulness of repeated words upon VT's. He employed four pairs of stimuli: one member of each pair was a common English word (e.g., PARROT), while for the other member the speaker interchanged the initial and final consonant of this word producing a stimulus (e.g., TARROP) containing the same phonemes but lacking meaning as an English word. Subjects were informed that the stimuli would be repeated without change, and told that they might or might not hear changes which really did not exist, with assurances that there was nothing preferable about hearing or not hearing them.

Natsoulas was especially interested in the time required for the first transition to occur. He found that this time was greater for the meaningful member for three of the four pairs he employed, with two of these three differences being statistically significant. Natsoulas indicated that the increase in time required for meaningful words to change was due to two effects: (a) the "auto-inhibition" produced by repetition must overcome a tendency to hear a word veridically, which is greater for more familiar words; (b) the English word has been heard under many conditions and with different pronunciations, and hence should be recognized despite some degree of distortion. Once the first change had occurred, then the rate of transitions was the same for each member of the pair, so that meaningfulness was no longer a rate-determining factor for transformations. It was also found that the meaningful members of each of the four pairs gave rise to fewer forms than the non-English member, the difference being statistically significant in two cases. This observation was in keeping with studies (Warren, 1961b, Warren & Warren, 1966), in which it was found that with each age group, FLIME gave rise to more different forms than did the other four stimuli (all of which were meaningful words).

Semantic Binding of Responses

The meaning of a stimulus word favors perceptual reorganization to words having a related meaning. However, difficulties arise when one tries to measure the semantic linkage between words. Also, some words may have linkages for the subject due to associations not known to the experimenter. But, by choosing a stimulus word having strong emotional content, it is possible to exert considerable control over the semantic nature of the subject's responses. In the study with British sailors (Warren, 1961a), RAPE was used as a stimulus word, and responses were obtained suggesting a violent sexuality, with successive forms frequently showing a close association in meaning accompanied by considerable change in phonetic structure. An example of one subject's responses over 3 minutes (presented fully in the order reported) is: "rape, wait, rake, break, rape, break, rape, break, rape, go ahead, break, rape, break, go ahead, rape, break, rape, break, rape, go ahead, rape, break, leg-break, rape, go ahead, break, go ahead, rape, go out, sprout, go out, sprout, go ahead, rape, go out, go ahead, break, rape, go ahead, leg-break, go ahead, go out, sprout, spread out, leg-break." It was observed that the subjects do not believe that they are revealing anything about themselves by their responses, but that they are simply reporting the sometimes foolish things the voice is saying quite clearly.

Skinner (1936) considered his verbal summator (which repeated a series of indistinct speech sounds until the subject reported a word or phrase) to be "a sort of verbal inkblot." Later investigators have used this device in the manner he proposed as an apperceptive test (Grings, 1942; Shakow & Rosenzweig, 1940; Trussel, 1939). The VT effect with clearly pronounced words would seem to lend itself to a somewhat different projective test, a *bound association* test consisting of multiple responses directed and held to a theme corresponding to the stimulus word.

Phonetics of Verbal Transformations

The most detailed phonetic analysis of the VT effect was that of Barnett (1964). She employed stimuli chosen for their differences in phonetic grouping, phonetic complexity, and frequency of occurrence in English (including, as the lower limit, English-Not-Words). Her 12 repeated stimulus words, in the order presented, were: CHANGE, LUDDY, ICE, JOY, FLIME, REVERE, HISTORY, ZOOMARTHI, AMPLY, IMPORTANT, WASHABLE, and KIRK.

Barnett transcribed subjects' responses phonetically as they were called out. While her detailed analysis of the data was limited to speech sounds, she found an intrusion of semantics which complicated the study. One word, PUSS, was in her preliminary list of stimuli, but had to be eliminated because of "interesting perceptions" and "emotional connotations." Another word which served as an experimental stimulus and caused semantic difficulties was HISTORY. It was reported frequently as [pɪst] by some, and, according to Barnett, gave some evidence of being heard but not reported by others.

After a phonetic analysis of VT's, she concluded that the articulatory position of both vowels and consonants were relatively labile and subject to frequent illusory changes. Relative stability was noted for the voiced/voiceless property of consonants, and for the type of movement characteristic of each particular consonant and vowel. Intervowel glides were stable both in position and type of movement with the exception of [ɔɪ].

Illusion, Pathology, and Normal Function

Illusions, especially visual ones, are well known to the public. They are interesting and entertaining, harmless deceptions much like a magic show. The VT effect is also readily appreciated by an unsophisticated audience, and indeed stimulus tapes demonstrating this illusion were prepared by British Broadcasting Company engineers and broadcast in Great Britain over the Third Programme in 1962.

However, it is the hope of most investigators working with illusions that they are not studying isolated idiosyncratic phenomena, but that their research will help the understanding of normal function. It is the author's opinion that VT's provide information relevant to normal perception of connected discourse, reflecting skilled reorganizational mechanisms employed by all, except the very young and

130

the aged, as a means to enhance the comprehension of speech.

Recently, Howes (1964) stated:

aphasia is practically unique in providing us with an objective means of determining the natural lines along which language decomposes. . . . In other approaches we impose our own logical methods of analysis upon language; only in aphasia does nature herself clearly show her hand [p. 51].

The VT effect appears to be a technique for attaining the goals Howes reserves for studies of aphasia, except that normal people may be used and language skills may be disrupted by the experimenter in a highly selective fashion. We may consider that exposure to repeated speech sounds produces, in effect, a functional lesion which is temporary and reversible.

While the study of the VT effect is still in its infancy, nevertheless it does give rise to suggestions concerning the mechanisms for perception of connected discourse.

Mechanisms for verbal transformations. What processes underly VT's? The evidence seems to indicate that at least two successive steps are involved: first perceptual organization, and then perceptual decay. Each of these opposing forces can be observed separately by changing conditions somewhat from those producing VT's. As mentioned earlier, by actively repeating a word to oneself, we can observe a lapse of meaning, a progressive disorganization until we are left with a meaningless jumble of speech sounds. It seems that the neuromuscular activity of producing speech sounds prevents VT's by inhibiting illusory phonetic changes. On the other hand, if we start with a recording of what is actually a meaningless jumble of speech sounds, playing this over and over results in organization into words or phrases (Skinner's verbal summator). When we allow both organization and decay to occur (continued stimulation by externally generated repeated stimuli—either words or indistinct speech sounds), then VT's are found. This description of sequential processes is not offered as an explanation of VT's. It simply indicates that mechanisms involved in this illusion may be manifest in other illusions as well. It is comforting that the VT effect is not completely isolated, but we are still left with important basic questions.

Comparison with visual effects. When one continues to stare at a printed word, changes analogous to VT's do not occur. Rather, a type of verbal satiation occurs; the meaning of the word evaporates and the symbols seem unfamiliar (Don & Weld, 1924; Severance & Washburn, 1907). Of course, while staring at a word, involuntary eye movements are constantly occurring, so that the brain receives neurologically different but perceptually equivalent input. It is possible to cancel out the effect of eye movements with appropriate optical systems (Ditchburn & Fender, 1955; Riggs, Ratliff, Cornsweet, & Cornsweet, 1953). When an unchanging pattern of visual stimulation is maintained in this manner, portions of the stopped visual image fade and reappear, with a tendency for meaningful perceptual organizations to dominate (Pritchard, Heron, & Hebb, 1960), producing changes similar in some respects to those observed for VT's. In an example given by Pritchard (1961), the printed word BEER viewed as a stopped retinal image went through a series of changes involving whole letters or parts of letters, with a tendency for the portion remaining to form a word; so that reports might include PEER, PEEP, BEE, and BE. VT's also involve changes which tend to preserve or create meaning, but in the auditory domain, perceptual blotting out of portions of the stimulus is rare, and generally illusory forms have a complexity equivalent to that of the stimulus.

Skilled verbal reorganization. There are, it seems, good reasons for believing that VT's reflect skilled reorganizational mechanisms for auditory perception of language. The studies of Bryan and Harter (1897, 1899) are relevant to this contention. They claimed that a "telegraphic language" existed for skilled telegraphers which was similar in many respects to other languages. It was pointed out that mastery required several years of continual application, perhaps 10 years for the degree of speed and accuracy required for a press dispatcher. When this degree of expertness was attained, the receiver could work effortlessly and automatically, often transcribing complex messages while thinking about something entirely different. It was found that the expert telegrapher usually delayed 6–12 words before transcribing. In other words, he stored the information, and so could correct and reorganize the information if subsequent portions of the message indicated an error. A process similar to this storage must occur for perception of speech as well. As Brain has pointed out (1962), "the meaning of a word which appears earlier in a sentence may depend upon the words which follow it. In such a case, the n.eaning of the earlier word is held in suspense, as it were, until the later words have made their appearance [p. 209]." Lashley (1951, p. 120) has given an excellent example of this process in an address. He first spoke of the process of "rapid writing," and then after creating this set for the meaning of "writing," several sentences later stated, "Rapid righting with his uninjured hand saved from loss the contents of the capsized canoe." He pointed out that the context necessary for the proper meaning of the sounds corresponding to "righting" are not activated for 3–5 seconds after hearing the word.

It is not only meaning that waits upon future context. Identification of particular speech sounds also requires storage and comparison with subsequent auditory stimulation. Chistovich (1962) has noted that subjects, who repeated speech heard through headphones as quickly as possible, make many errors in phonemes. He suggested that these erorrs reflect the temporal course of speech identification. Of course, an appreciable delay before response can eliminate these errors. Miller (1962) and Lieberman (1963) have emphasized that skilled speech perception cannot be a simple Markovian chain process with perception occurring first on phonemic and then on higher levels. Such a process does not take advantage of the redundancy of the message, and does not allow for a correction of errors. Thus, an error once committed would provide incorrect context and hence cause other errors until perception was completely disrupted.

The need for reorganizational mechanisms is not always the consequence of errors committed by listener or speaker. Clear messages may be encountered in laboratory studies, but under usual listening conditions we have to cope with a noisy environment (e.g., a cough, the movement of a chair, footsteps in the cor-

ridor, other voices) which is capable of effectively masking the distinctive features of an utterance.

It is the author's opinion that individuals invoke verbal reorganization of connected discourse whenever the preliminary organization of speech sounds into words and phrases is not confirmed by subsequent context. Of course, when presented with a repeating word, there can be no confirmation by context, no fitting into a stabilizing grammatical and semantic environment provided by the surrounding words. Hence the repeated word is subject to successive reorganizations, none of which can possibly receive contextual confirmation. It should be kept in mind that the suggested mechanism is not accessible to introspection, and it can be studied only through its effects.

The age differences which have been observed for the VT effect are consistent with the explanation just offered. If we consider that VT's reflect skilled reorganizational processes, they could not appear in children until language skills had attained a certain level. The requisite level seems to be attained normally by the age of 6 or 7 (Warren & Warren, 1966). Why is it then that the aged (those over 60) do not report VT's, in spite of their mastery of language? The answer may be that they lack the requisite capacity for short-term storage of verbal information. It is well established that especial difficulty is encountered by the aged for complex storage tasks involving intervening activity (Welford, 1958). In view of their limitations, their optimal strategy as listeners may be to organize speech directly into English words, with very little short-term storage suitable for reorganization, and hence very few VT's.

Despite a superficial similarity in language proficiency over the greater part of our life span, it seems that considerable changes occur with age in the mechanisms employed for speech perception. A percepual homeostasis may be achieved through the appearance of skills appropriate to changes in functional capacity.

REFERENCES

AMSTER, H. Semantic satiation and generation: Learning? Adaptation? *Psychological Bulletin,* 1964, 62, 273–286.

AXELROD, S., & THOMPSON, L. On visual changes of reversible figures and auditory changes in meaning. *American Journal of Psychology*, 1962, 75, 673–674.

BARNETT, M. R. *Perceived phonetic changes in the verbal transformation effect.* (Doctoral dissertation, Ohio University) Ann Arbor, Mich.: University Microfilms, 1964. No. 64–7328.

BRAIN, W. R. Recent work on the physiological basis of speech. *Advancement of Science*, 1962, 19, 207–212.

BRYAN, W. L., & HARTER, N. Studies in the physiology and psychology of the telegraphic language. *Psychological Review*, 1897, 4, 27–53.

BRYAN, W. L., & HARTER, N. Studies on the telegraphic language. The acquisition of a hierarchy of habits. *Psychological Review*, 1899, 6, 345–375.

CHISTOVICH, L. A. Temporal course of speech sound perception. In, *Proceedings of the 4th International Commission on Acoustics.* (Article H 18) Copenhagen, 1962.

DICHTBURN, R. W., & FENDER, D. H. The stabilized retinal image. *Optica Acta*, 1955, 2, 128–133.

DON, V. J., & WELD, H. P. Minor studies from the psychological laboratory of Cornell University. LXX. Lapse of meaning with visual fixation. *American Journal of Psychology*, 1924, 35, 446–450.

GRINGS, W. W. The verbal summator technique and abnormal mental states. *Journal of Abnormal and Social Psychology*, 1942, 37, 529–545.

HOWES, D. H. Application of the word-frequency concept to aphasia. In A. V. S. de Rueck & M. O'Conner (Eds.), *Ciba foundation symposium on disorders of language.* Boston: Little, Brown, 1964.

LASHLEY, K. S. The problem of serial order in behavior. In L. A. Jeffress (Ed.), *Cerebral mechanisms in behavior: The Hixon symposium.* New York: Wiley, 1951.

LIEBERMAN, P. Some effects of semantic and grammatical context on the production and perception of speech. *Language and Speech*, 1963, 6, 172–187.

LOCKE, J. *Concerning human understanding.* London: Holt, 1690. Book 2, Chapt. 14, Section 13. (Reprinted: Oxford: Clarendon Press, 1894. Vol. 1.)

MILES, W. R. Age and the kinephantom. *Journal of General Psychology*, 1934, 10, 204–207.

MILLER, G. A. Decision units in the perception of speech. *IRE Transactions on Information Theory*, 1962, IT-8, 81–83.

NATSOULAS, T. A study of the verbal-transformation effect. *American Journal of Psychology*, 1965, 78, 257–263.

NATSOULAS, T. What are perceptual reports about? *Psychological Bulletin*, 1967, 67, 249–272.

OBUSEK, C. J. A study of speech perception in the aged by means of the verbal transformation effect. Unpublished master's thesis, University of Wisconsin, Milwaukee, 1968.

PAUL, S. K. Level of cortical inhibition and illusory changes of distinct speech upon repetition. *Psychological Studies*, 1964, 9, 58–65.

PRITCHARD, R. M. Stabilized images on the retina. *Scientific American*, 1961, 204, 72–78.

PRITCHARD, R. M., HERON, W., & HEBB, D. O. Visual perception approached by the method of stabilized images. *Canadian Journal of Psychology*, 1960, 14, 67–77.

RIGGS, L. A., RATLIFF, F., CORNSWEET, J. C., & CORNSWEET, T. N. The disappearance of steadily fixated visual test objects. *Journal of the Optical Society of America*, 1953, 43, 495–501.

SEVERANCE, E., & WASHBURN, M. F. Minor studies from the psychological laboratory of Vassar College. IV. The loss of associative power in words after long fixation. *American Journal of Psychology*, 1907, 18, 182–186.

SHAKOW, D., & ROSENZWEIG, S. The use of the tautophone ("verbal summator") as an auditory apperceptive test for the study of personality. *Character and Personality*, 1940, 8, 216–226.

SKINNER, B. F. The verbal summator and a method for the study of latent speech. *Journal of Psychology*, 1936, 2, 71–107.

TAYLOR, M. M., & HENNING, G. B. Verbal transformations and an effect of instructional bias on perception. *Canadian Journal of Psychology*, 1963, 17, 210–223.

TITCHENER, E. B. *A beginner's psychology.* New York: Macmillan, 1915.

TRUSSEL, M. A. The diagnostic value of the verbal summator. *Journal of Abnormal and Social Psychology*, 1939, 34, 533–538.

WARREN, R. M. Illusory changes of distinct speech upon repetition—The verbal transformation effect. *British Journal of Psychology*, 1961, 52, 249–258. (a)

WARREN, R. M. Illusory changes in repeated words: Differences between young adults and the aged. *American Journal of Psychology*, 1961, 74, 506–516. (b)

WARREN, R. M. An example of more accurate auditory perception in the aged. In C. Tibbitts & W. Donahue (Eds.), *Social and psychological aspects of aging.* New York: Columbia University Press, 1962.

WARREN, R. M., & GREGORY, R. L. An auditory analogue of the visual reversible figure. *American Journal of Psychology*, 1958, 71, 612–613.

WARREN, R. M., & WARREN, R. P. A comparison of speech perception in childhood, maturity, and old age by means of the verbal transformation effect. *Journal of Verbal Learning and Verbal Behavior*, 1966, 5, 142–146.

WELFORD, A. T. *Ageing and human skill.* London: Oxford University Press, 1958.

133

THE USE OF ISOLATED VOWELS AS AUDITORY STIMULI IN ELICITING THE VERBAL TRANSFORMATION EFFECT

NORMAN J. LASS AND SHEILA S. GOLDEN

ABSTRACT

The purpose of this investigation was to determine the effectiveness of single isolated vowels as auditory stimuli in eliciting perceptual illusory changes in subjects, a phenomenon referred to by Warren (1961a) as the "verbal transformation effect." Three vowels, /i/, /æ/, and /u/, were individually presented to a group of 24 normal adult listeners in a single experimental session. Each vowel was repeatedly presented by means of headphones for a period of five minutes. Results indicate that single isolated vowels are capable of eliciting verbal transformations in normal listeners. However, the transformations reported often differed from those obtained in previous studies which used more phonetically complex auditory stimuli. The nature of the verbal transformations, average number of alternate forms perceived and transitions employed, and average number of repetitions of the stimuli prior to the onset of the subjects' first verbal transformations were discussed. Comparisons with findings of previous investigations and suggestions for future research were provided.

CONTINUED LISTENING TO recorded repetitions of a stimulus has been found to produce perceptual illusory changes in normal listeners (Barnett, 1964; Naeser & Lilly, 1970; Natsoulas, 1965; Obusek, 1968; Taylor & Henning, 1963; Warren, 1961a, 1961b; Warren, 1968; Warren & Gregory, 1958; Warren & Warren, 1966). This phenomenon was labelled by Warren (1961a) as the "verbal transformation effect."

The verbal transformation effect has been found to occur for a variety of speech stimuli, from a word with two sounds to complete sentences. However, single isolated vowels have never been employed to specifically elicit verbal transformations in listeners. The purpose of the present investigation was to determine the effectiveness of single isolated vowels as auditory stimuli in eliciting the verbal transformation effect in normal adult subjects.

METHOD

Subjects

Twenty-four individuals, three males and 21 females, served as subjects. All were students in the Speech Pathology-Audiology program at West Virginia University. They ranged in age from 19 to 24 years, with a mean age of 20 years. All subjects reported no hearing difficulty and had normal neurological history and status as determined by a questionnaire.

CANADIAN JOURNAL OF PSYCHOLOGY, 1971, vol. 25, 349-359.

Recording procedure

Three sustained isolated vowels, /i/, /æ/, and /u/, were recorded by a male speaker using a Nagra IV tape recorder and an Altec model 681A condenser microphone. The recording was made in a sound-treated room at the West Virginia University Medical Center. An attempt was made to control for the consistency of the frequency and sound pressure levels of the speaker's productions of the vowels. To maintain a constant frequency, the output of a Beltone model 15cx pure-tone oscillator set at 125 Hz was monitored by the speaker through a single headphone. Simultaneously, the speaker monitored the sound pressure level of his voice on a General Radio model 1551-c sound level meter in an attempt to maintain a constant reading of 65 db on the meter.

Construction of stimulus tapes

To facilitate construction of electronic reproductions of the stimuli, from each of the three sustained vowels, a 200-msec segment of the original recording was cut and spliced into an otherwise blank tape loop. The tape loop was repeatedly played on an Ampex model 602 tape recorder and electronically reproduced on a Wollensak model T-1500 tape recorder. The taped segments were cut and spliced into a second tape loop. This tape loop contained 200 msec vowel segments plus 500 msec pauses between the vowel segments. Because of the relatively short duration of the vowels and pauses, it was found necessary to employ a total of six vowel and pause segments to construct the tape loop. In the above manner, three master tape loops were constructed, one for each of the three vowels under investigation. Each of the three tape loops was played repeatedly for a five-minute period on an Ampex model 602 tape recorder and electronically reproduced on a Wollensak model T-1500 tape recorder to produce the three master stimulus tapes. On each tape, the vowel was repeated at a rate of 86 times per minute, for a total of 430 repetitions in the allotted five-minute period.

Experimental procedure

The following set of instructions was orally presented to each subject:

You will hear a voice through a set of earphones. Listen carefully to the voice and tell me what it seems to be saying as soon as you can. After you call out what you hear, keep on listening carefully. If you think you hear a change to a different stimulus, call out what you hear as soon as the change occurs. If there is a change back to the original stimulus or to another different stimulus, call it out as soon as the change occurs. Any change to a new stimulus or to a stimulus previously heard should be called out immediately upon hearing it. Even if the change is momentary, that is, involving just one repetition, be certain to call it out. Do not wait to confirm the change by listening further. Do not worry about whether what you hear is meaningful or familiar. Do not worry about being right or wrong. What I want to know is what the stimulus seems like to you under these special conditions. Don't forget to call out immediately every time you hear a change, whether to something new or whether the change is back to a stimulus which you called out before. However, if you hear no change in the stimulus, you will remain silent. Are there any questions?

In an attempt to familiarize the subject with the experimental task, a two-minute practice stimulus tape was played for him. This tape was constructed in the same manner as the experimental stimulus tapes. The vowel employed in the practice tape was /ɔ/. Upon completion of the practice tape, the three experimental stimulus tapes were played. The subject was told to tap on the base of the microphone upon hearing the first stimulus on each tape. Each of the three tapes was presented to the subject binaurally by means of a Nagra IV tape recorder and a set of matched Beyer DT-48-S headphones. The subject's responses were recorded on an Ampex model 602 tape recorder using an Altec model 681A condenser microphone. The examiner listened to the subject's responses by means of a set of Beyer DT-48-S headphones and recorded each response on a sheet of paper. All phonetic forms were recorded using the International Phonetic Alphabet. Upon completion of each stimulus tape, the examiner's list of responses was presented to the subject to verify the correctness of the listed responses. Any necessary changes were made at that time.

All three stimulus tapes were presented to each subject individually in a single experimental session. The order of presentation of the three stimulus tapes was counterbalanced so that six orders were used, with four subjects in each of the six order groups. Therefore, all possible orders for presentation of the three auditory stimuli were employed. A three-minute rest period was provided between each stimulus tape. The session, which lasted approximately 30 minutes, was held in a sound-treated room at the West Virginia University Medical Center.

Data analysis

To determine the exact transformations as well as the number of new forms and transitions employed by each subject, one of the investigators listened to the subject's response tape via headphones and verified what was written down during the listening sessions. The number of repetitions of the stimulus prior to the onset of each subject's first transformation was determined in the following manner: (1) the subject's response tape was played through a General Radio model 1521-B graphic level recorder having a paper speed of 31.75 mm per second and a writing speed of 100 mm per second; (2) the examiner placed a mark at the beginning of the stimulus tape (which was indicated by the sound of a tapping on the base of the microphone made by the subject) and at the occurrence of the first verbal transformation reported; (3) a line was drawn perpendicular to the baseline of the graphic level tracing at these two points; (4) the distance between the two points was measured in millimeters; (5) the stimulus tapes were played through the graphic level recorder; (6) the mm distance obtained from each subject's response tape was marked on the tracings of the stimulus tapes and the number of repetitions of the stimulus was counted up to that point on the tracing. In the above manner, the number of repetitions prior to the onset of the first verbal transformation of each of the 24 subjects was determined for each of the three vowels employed in the study.

RESULTS

Forms, transitions, and repetitions prior to first verbal transformations. Table I contains the average number of different forms (different perceptual phenomena) and transitions (changes from one form to another) as well as the average number of repetitions of each stimulus prior to the onset of the subjects' first verbal transformations. The table indicates that there are some differences among the three vowels investigated. It appears that the vowel /u/ yielded the largest average number of different forms in the five-minute listening period, and required the fewest average number of repetitions prior to eliciting the subjects' first verbal transformations.

136

TABLE I

MEAN NUMBER OF DIFFERENT FORMS AND TRANSITIONS AND
MEAN NUMBER OF REPETITIONS OF STIMULI PRIOR TO THE
ONSET OF THE SUBJECTS' FIRST VERBAL TRANSFORMATIONS
FOR EACH OF THE THREE VOWELS

Stimulus	Different Forms	Transitions	Number of repetitions prior to 1st VT
/i/	5.1	11.3	62.9
/æ/	6.2	12.6	59.7
/u/	6.8	10.5	57.1

TABLE II

MEAN NUMBER OF NEW FORMS AND TRANSITIONS FOR EACH OF FIVE ONE-MINUTE
PORTIONS OF THE LISTENING PERIOD

Stimulus	New Forms					Transitions				
	1	2	3	4	5	1	2	3	4	5
/i/	1.5	1.3	1.3	0.5	0.5	2.5	3.0	3.6	1.3	0.9
/æ/	1.6	1.8	1.3	1.0	0.5	2.2	3.5	3.2	2.8	0.9
/u/	1.5	1.5	1.4	1.3	1.1	1.7	2.0	2.0	2.5	2.3

However, /u/ also produced the fewest average number of transitions of all three vowels. The vowel /æ/ elicited the largest average number of transitions.

Table II contains the average number of different forms and transitions employed by the 24 subjects for each of five one-minute portions of the listening period of each vowel. It shows that for all three vowels investigated, the average number of new forms was greatest for the first or second minute and progressively decreased for the next three minutes. However, the trend for new transitions was less consistent. For the stimulus /i/, the average number of new transitions increased for the first three minutes of the listening period, with a sharp decrease during the last two minutes of the period. /æ/ showed the largest average number of transitions in the second one-minute segment, a gradual decrease over the next two minutes, and a sharp decrease in the last minute of the period. The vowel /u/ manifested an increase in average number of transitions over the first four minutes, with a slight reduction in the last one-minute portion.

Inferential statistical analysis, consisting of two two-factor analyses of variance (Vowels × One-Minute Time Segments) (Winer, 1962), one for number of new forms and one for number of transitions, were employed to determine if the observed differences among the three auditory stimuli were statistically significant or chance occurrences. Results of these analyses indicate the following:

137

(1) there are no significant differences among the three vowels in number of forms ($F = 1.07$, $df = 2$ and 46) and number of transitions ($F = 1.09$, $df = 2$ and 46) elicited;

(2) there is a significant time effect operating for all three vowels in number of forms ($F = 9.38$, $df = 4$ and 276) and transitions ($F = 11.16$, $df = 4$ and 276) at the .001 level of significance;

(3) there is no significant vowel × time interaction in forms ($F = 1.02$, $df = 8$ and 276) and transitions ($F = 1.12$, $df = 8$ and 276).

Nature of verbal transformations. Apparently due to the nature of the stimuli employed, some of the transformations reported in this study appear to be rather unique and have not been frequently reported by subjects in previous investigations concerned with the verbal transformation effect. Table III contains the total number of forms as well as the exact forms which were reported by more than one subject for each of the three stimuli. The table shows that the vowel /æ/ elicited the largest number of forms, /u/ the next largest, and /i/ the fewest number of forms.

Table IV contains a classification of the type of transformations elicited by the three auditory stimuli. The classification employed was based on the different forms reported by all subjects. The table indicates that a large number of transformations for all three vowels investigated were phonetic in nature. That is, the subjects' transformations often involved a perceptual change in the phonetic structure of the repeating stimuli. These phonetic transformations included the following types: (1) the substitution of one speech sound for the stimulus sound (e.g., /I/ for /i/; /ʌ/ for /æ/;

TABLE III

FORMS REPORTED FOR EACH OF THE THREE AUDITORY STIMULI BY MORE THAN ONE SUBJECT. (THE NUMBER OF SUBJECTS REPORTING A PARTICULAR FORM IS GIVEN IN THE PARENTHESES PRECEDING THE FORM. PHONETIC SYMBOLS ARE USED FOR ALL FORMS IN BRACKETS.)

/i/
44 forms: (6) /I/; (5) /ip/; (4) /bip/; (6) /bi/; (2) /bI/; (2) /it/; (4) /mi/; (3) /ni/; (9) "faster"; (4) "slower"; (11) "louder"; (2) "softer"; (5) "lower in pitch"; (4) "higher in pitch"; (4) "longer in duration"; (3) "staccato"; (2) "change in stress pattern"; (3) "nasal quality"; (2) "hoarse quality"; (3) "distorted".

/æ/
58 forms: (5) /ʌ/; (2) /ʌp/; (3) /æp/; (2) /ɔ/; (3) /æt/; (2) /bæp/; (2) /bʌp/; (2) /bæ/; (3) /bip/; (9) "louder"; (13) "faster"; (5) "slower"; (6) "lower in pitch"; (7) "higher in pitch"; (3) "staccato"; (6) "change in stress pattern"; (4) "shorter in duration"; (3) "longer in duration"; (2) "sounds like a frog"; (2) "sounds like a buzzer"; (2) "fuzzy"

/u/
53 forms: (8) /ʌ/; (3) /ən/; (6) /ʌm/; (2) /ip/; (2) /bIp/; (4) /I/; (2) /Im/; (4) /bip/; (2) /i/; (12) "slower"; (5) "faster"; (5) "louder"; (7) "softer"; (6) "higher in pitch"; (15) "lower in pitch"; (8) "longer in duration"; (3) "shorter in duration"; (5) "change in stress pattern"; (2) "sounds like a busy signal"; (3) "nasal quality"; (2) "hazy".

TABLE IV

NUMBER AND PERCENTAGE OF TYPES OF VERBAL TRANSFORMATIONS REPORTED BY THE 24 SUBJECTS FOR EACH OF THE THREE VOWELS INVESTIGATED

Types of Transformations

Stimulus		Phonetic	Pitch	Rate	Duration	Loudness	Rhythm	Clarity	Quality	Familiar Sounds	Other
/i/	N	51	9	13	7	13	5	5	5	1	1
	per cent	46.4	8.2	11.8	6.4	11.8	4.5	4.5	4.5	0.9	0.9
/æ/	N	48	13	18	7	10	10	4	0	11	2
	per cent	39.0	10.6	14.6	5.7	8.1	8.1	3.3	0.0	8.9	1.6
/u/	N	57	21	17	11	12	7	4	5	3	4
	per cent	40.4	14.9	12.1	7.8	8.5	5.0	2.8	3.5	2.1	2.8

/ʌ/ for /u/); (2) the addition of one phoneme to the original stimulus sound (e.g., /ip/ for /i/; /æt/ for /æ/; /u-I/ for /u/); and (3) the substitution of more than one non-existent sounds for the stimulus sound (e.g., /nʌ/ for /i/; /ʌ p/ for /æ/; /ip / for /u/).

It was found that the majority of the phonetic types of transformations reported by subjects for all three vowels (86, 92, and 91 per cent for /i/, /æ/, and /u/, respectively) involved single-syllable forms which were semantically as meaningless as the original repeating stimuli. However, relatively few transformations (12, 21, and 30 per cent for /i/, /æ/, and /u/, respectively) involved the perception of single isolated vowels. That is, the majority of the subjects' phonetic transformations were phonetically more complex than the original stimuli.

In addition to phonetic transformations, other transformations, such as those involving perceptual changes in the rate, duration, loudness, pitch, quality, clarity, and rhythm of the repeating stimuli, were frequently reported by the subjects. In fact, these transformations, as a group, accounted for the majority of all transformations reported (52, 50, and 58 per cent of all transformations for /i/, /æ/, and /u/, respectively).

A differentiation was made by subjects in their reports of transformations between the "Rate" of the stimulus presentation (i.e., inter-stimulus pause time appeared to them to be altered) and "Duration" of each stimulus heard (i.e., stimulus time appeared to have changed). Transformations of "Quality" usually involved reports of changes in the nasal quality of the signal. "Rhythm" transformations were often expressed as changes in the stress pattern of the repeating stimuli. The "Clarity" category involved perceptual changes to either a "clearer", "sharper" signal or to a less clear, more "fuzzy" or "hazy" signal. The category of "Familiar Sounds" included transformations such as "doorbell", "duck", "buzzer", "frog", and "busy signal." The stimulus /æ/ elicited the largest number of transformations of this kind. The category "Other" in Table IV contains transformations which could not be placed into any of the existing categories. For example, on several occasions some of the subjects could not verbally express the change which they perceived, but were certain that some change had occurred in their perception of the repeating stimuli. Such transformations were placed in this category.

DISCUSSION

Nature of verbal transformations. Results of this study indicate that single isolated vowels are effective in eliciting verbal transformations in normal adult listeners. However, it was found that the transformations reported often differed from those obtained with more phonetically complex audi-

140

tory stimuli. Although a large number of transformations reported in this study for all three vowels involved perceptual changes in the phonetic structure of the repeating stimuli (as was found most often in previous studies employing more phonetically complex stimuli), the majority of transformations involved changes concerned with the various parameters of the auditory stimuli. These transformations included perceptual changes in the pitch, loudness, duration, rate, rhythm, quality, and clarity of the repeating stimuli. In addition, some transformations involved the perception of various familiar sounds, and some were not capable of description by the listeners. Few transformations of these types have been reported in previous studies concerned with the verbal transformation effect. Furthermore, many of the perceived phonetic changes reported in the present study were more distorted (i.e., the reported changes were phonetically more complex than the original repeating stimuli) than those obtained in previous investigations. These findings are considered by the present writers to be the result primarily of the phonetic simplicity of the repeating stimuli, and are in agreement with the findings of previous studies (Warren, 1961a, 1961b; Warren & Warren, 1966) in which it was observed that "... the greatest distortion tended to occur with the phonetically simpler stimuli ..." (Warren, 1968, p. 262.)

However, another factor must also be considered in attempting to explain the nature of the reported transformations in the present study. This factor pertains to the group of listeners employed. The subjects in this study were all familiar with the International Phonetic Alphabet and used this alphabet in their training as speech pathologists. In addition, through their coursework and clinical experiences, they were taught to listen carefully and to thoroughly analyze what they heard. Perhaps this background and training can at least partially account for the unique types of transformations reported as well as for the phonetic variations reported in the study.

Nature of auditory stimuli. The stimuli in the present study can be classified as "nonsense" stimuli in view of the fact that they have no semantic meaning in the English language. As meaningless stimuli, the three vowels elicited transformations from the subjects which are similar in one respect to those obtained in previous investigations employing nonsense stimuli. Warren (1961a, p. 255) found that "Many subjects never reported the speech sounds correctly when presented with a repeating unfamiliar or nonsense stimulus." In the present study, 83 per cent of the subjects identified /i/ correctly on their initial response, 38 per cent identified /æ/ correctly, and only 17 per cent properly identified /u/. In fact, two of the 24 subjects never reported /i/, six never reported /æ/, and 19 never reported /u/ correctly throughout the entire listening sessions.

This finding may be related to the use of segments excised from steady state vowels as the auditory stimuli in the present study. Warren and Warren (1970) have shown that for short utterances of vowels (150 to 200 msec), onset and decay characteristics are important perceptual cues. Since the 200 msec segments from the steady state vowels employed in the present study lack these onset and decay characteristics, it would be logical to expect the result to be artificial sounding vowels. Perhaps this artificiality contributed in some cases to the incorrect identification of the vowels.

Morton and Carpenter (1962) also observed difficulty by some of their subject groups in identifying segments from steady state vowels. However, in comparing the identification of the vowel /u/ by their experienced group (comparable to the phonetically-trained subjects in the present study), which is the only vowel used in both studies, they found that 100 per cent correct identification was achieved, while only 20 per cent of our subjects correctly reported /u/.

The transformations reported by the subjects in the present investigation were frequently nonsense, meaningless utterances (85, 76, and 84 per cent for /i/, /æ/, and /u/, respectively). This finding is not in agreement with Warren's (1961a, p. 255) results; he found that a meaningless stimulus "... seemed to undergo readily a distortion to a frequently encountered word or meaningful phrase." Perhaps this difference in findings is also related to differences in the listeners employed in the two studies. Warren used subjects with no phonetic training, while the listeners in the present study all had been trained to use the International Phonetic Alphabet and thus were probably more capable of, and experienced in, thoroughly analyzing what they heard.

Number of forms and transitions. Despite differences in the phonetic complexity of the stimuli employed in the two studies, the number of forms elicited by the vowels in the present study is similar to the number of forms reported by Warren (1961a) for comparable repetitions of his stimuli. For example, Warren reports the average number of forms for 444 repetitions of the stimulus "trice" to be 5.8; 435 repetitions of "rape" elicited an average of 5.3 forms; an average of 7.2 forms was obtained for 429 repetitions of "tress." These numbers are similar to the 5.1, 6.2, and 6.8 average number of forms reported for /i/, /æ/, and /u/, respectively.

However, the numbers reported for transitions for the three vowels in the present investigation are much smaller than the numbers reported by Warren. An average of 19.6 transitions was reported for "trice"; 22.0 was the average number of transitions reported for "rape"; "tress" produced an average of 33.6 transitions. The present study produced an average of 11.3, 12.6, and 10.5 transitions for /i/, /æ/, and /u/, respectively, far fewer than those reported by Warren.

The relationship proposed by Taylor and Henning (1963) to exist between number of forms and number of transitions, $T = kF (F - 1)$, where "k" is an empirical constant, "T" is the number of experienced transitions, and "F" is the number of reported forms, was not supported by the data from the present study. This finding is in agreement with Warren's (1968), whose data could also not support the proposed quadratic relationship.

Suggestions for future research. (1) The durations employed for stimulus and inter-stimulus pauses were arbitrarily determined by the experimenters. It is suggested that future research investigate systematically the effects of variations in stimulus and pause times on the verbal transformations of listeners.

(2) Since the current study dealt exclusively with adult listeners, and since it has been shown that there are some basic differences in the verbal transformations reported between different age groups (Warren, 1961b; Warren & Warren, 1966), it is suggested that this experiment be repeated using a group of children and a group of aged adults as listeners. Such a study would determine if individuals who differ in age from those in the present study would respond differently to the repetitive playing of isolated vowels.

REFERENCES

BARNETT, M. R. Perceived phonetic changes in the verbal transformation effect. Unpublished PH.D dissertation, Ohio University, 1964.

MORTON, J., & CARPENTER, A. Judgement of the vowel colour of natural and artificial sounds. *Language and Speech*, 1962, 5, 190–204.

NAESER, M. A. & LILLY, J. C. Preliminary evidence for a universal feature detector system: perception of the repeating word. Paper presented at the 79th Meeting of the Acoustical Society of America, April 21–24, 1970, Atlantic City, New Jersey.

NATSOULAS, T. A study of the verbal-transformation effect. *Amer. J. Psychol.*, 1965, 78, 257–263.

OBUSEK, C. J. A study of speech perception in the aged by means of the verbal transformation effect. Unpublished MS thesis, University of Wisconsin-Milwaukee, 1968.

TAYLOR, M. M. & HENNING, G. B. Verbal transformations and an effect of instructional bias on perception. *Canad. J. Psychol.*, 1963, 17, 210–223.

WARREN, R. M. Illusory changes of distinct speech upon repetition – the verbal transformation effect. *Brit. J. Psychol.* 1961a, 52, 249–258.

WARREN, R. M. Illusory changes in repeated words: differences between young adults and the aged. *Amer. J. Psychol.* 1961b, 74, 506–516.

WARREN, R. M. Verbal transformation effect and auditory perceptual mechanisms. *Psychol. Bull.*, 1968, 70, 261–270.

WARREN, R. M. & GREGORY, R. L. An auditory analogue of the visual reversible figure. *Amer. J. Psychol.*, 1958, 71, 612–613.

WARREN, R. M., and WARREN, R. P. A comparison of speech perception in childhood, maturity, and old age by means of the verbal transformation effect. *J. verb. Learn. verb. Behav.*, 1966, 5, 142–146.

WARREN, R. M. & WARREN, R. P. Auditory illusions and confusions. *Scientific American*, 1970, 223, 30–36.

WINER, B. J. *Statistical Principles in Experimental Design*. New York: McGraw-Hill Book Co., 1962.

THE VERBAL TRANSFORMATION EFFECT: CONSISTENCY OF SUBJECTS' REPORTED VERBAL TRANSFORMATIONS

MARY E. TEKIELI AND NORMAN J. LASS

A. INTRODUCTION

The phenomenon in which continued listening to recorded repetitions of a stimulus produces perceptual illusory changes in listeners is called the "verbal transformation effect" (10). This perceptual phenomenon, including the phonetic nature of the reported verbal transformations (1, 4), and the effects of such variables as stimulus complexity (3, 10), repetition rate of stimulus (10), meaningfulness of stimulus (5), loudness and clarity of stimulus (10), instructional bias (8), and age differences of listeners (6, 11, 12), have been studied by a number of investigators.

However, except for a single statement by Warren (10), the consistency of subjects' reported verbal transformations has never been systematically investigated. Warren (10, p. 257) claims that when a few of his subjects were presented with the same repeating stimulus that was heard by them three weeks earlier, ". . . the forms reported were almost identical with those heard previously, frequently appearing in almost the same order."

The purpose of this investigation was to extend Warren's observations and to study systematically the consistency of subjects' reported verbal transformations in terms of the number of forms and transitions elicited, number of repetitions of the stimulus prior to the onset of the subjects' first verbal transformations, types of transformations reported, exact forms employed, and order of reported verbal transformations.

B. METHOD

1. Subjects

Twenty-four adult females served as subjects. All were students in the Speech Pathology-Audiology program at West Virginia University. They

JOURNAL OF GENERAL PSYCHOLOGY, 1972, vol. 86, 231-245.

ranged in age from 19 to 24 years, with a mean age of 20 years. All subjects had normal articulation, hearing, and neurological status, and reported no physical or emotional problems.

2. Auditory Stimuli

A total of six experimental stimuli were employed in the study: (a) a nonsense syllable—/ko/; (b) a one-syllable meaningful word—"see"; (c) a two-syllable nonsense word—/ikfrɛ/; (d) a two-syllable meaningful word—"police"; (e) a four-syllable nonsense phrase—/trɛ os ri fæ/; (f) a four-syllable, four-word meaningful sentence—"our ship has sailed."

The six stimuli were chosen in order to explore consistency in stimuli varying in both meaningfulness and phonetic complexity.

3. Recording Procedure

The stimuli were recorded by a professional male announcer using an Ampex model 602 tape recorder and an Altec model 681A condensor microphone. The recordings were made in a sound-treated room at the West Virginia University Medical Center. Preceding the production of each stimulus the speaker used the carrier phrase "Say the word _____" which he monitored at zero on the volume unit meter of the tape recorder.

4. Construction of Stimulus Tape

Electronic reproductions of the original recordings of the stimuli were made with a Nagra IV tape recorder and an Ampex model 602 tape recorder. The reproductions of each stimulus were cut and spliced into a tape loop having interstimulus pause times of 500 msec. Because of the relatively short duration of the stimuli employed in the study, it was necessary to use more than one reproduction of the stimulus in order to construct the tape loops. In addition, since the stimuli differed in duration, the exact number of reproductions of the stimuli used was not identical in all tape loops. In the above manner, six master tape loops were constructed, one for each of the six stimuli under investigation. Each of the tape loops was played repeatedly for a 1.5 minute period on a Nagra IV tape recorder and electronically reproduced on an Ampex model 602 tape recorder to produce a master stimulus tape containing 1.5 minute samples of the six stimuli. A one second, 500 Hz tone generated by a General Radio model 1310 pure-tone oscillator was recorded on an Ampex model 602 tape recorder and cut and spliced into the master tape before each of the six stimuli in order to prepare the listener for the stimulus that followed.

145

5. Procedure

Each subject participated in four sessions: one screening and three experimental sessions. The screening session involved procedures for the selection of subjects. The three experimental sessions were used to obtain information on subject consistency in reporting verbal transformations. The time interval between experimental sessions was carefully controlled: a minimum of two days and a maximum of five days were allowed between sessions.

6. Screening Session

The following tasks were included in the screening session: (*a*) a pure tone and speech audiometric screening evaluation on a Beltone model 15CX clinical audiometer and a Grason-Stadler model 162 speech audiometer; (*b*) administration of a sentence screening articulation test (9); and (*c*) completion of questionnaires on neurological history and status, and general health status. Individuals who exhibited any speech, hearing, neurological, or health problems were excluded as subjects from the study.

At the conclusion of the screening session, the examiner orally presented to the subject a list of requirements for participating in each experimental session. The purpose of this list of requirements was to identify and eliminate factors that could possibly interfere with the subject's ability to attend to the listening task. These factors included the following: (*a*) insufficient sleep, (*b*) acute emotional or physical problems, (*c*) the influence of medication, and (*d*) the immediate influence of alcoholic beverages.

7. Experimental Sessions

The following set of instructions was orally presented to each subject:

> I am going to play a tape recording through these headphones (present headphones). When the tape starts, click your fingers near the microphone as soon as you hear the voice (demonstrate). I want you to listen carefully to the voice and tell me what it seems to be saying as soon as you can. After you call out what you hear, keep on listening carefully. If you think you hear a change to a different stimulus, call out what you hear as soon as the change occurs. If there is a change back to the original stimulus or to another different stimulus, call it out as soon as the change occurs. Any change to a new stimulus or to a stimulus previously heard should be called out immediately upon hearing it. Even if the change is momentary—that is, involving just one repetition—be certain to call it out. Do not wait to confirm the change by listening further. Do not worry about whether what you hear is meaningful or

146

familiar. Do not worry about being correct or incorrect. What I want to know is what the stimulus seems like to you under these special conditions. Don't forget to call out immediately every time you hear a change, whether to something new or whether the change is back to a stimulus which you called out before. However, if you hear no change in the stimulus, please remain silent. You will hear a tone immediately prior to the onset of the stimulus. Attempt to maintain your maximum concentration during the entire experimental task. Are there any questions?

In an attempt to familiarize the subject with the experimental task, a 1.5 minute practice stimulus ("the word") was played for her. The tape of this stimulus was constructed in the same manner as the experimental stimuli used in the study. Upon completion of the practice stimulus tape and the answering of the subjects' questions, all six experimental stimuli were played to the subject binaurally by means of a Nagra IV tape recorder and a Grason-Stadler model 162 speech audiometer at an intensity of 82 dB (re: .0002 dyne/cm²). The subject listened to the stimuli through a pair of matched TDH-39 headphones with MX41AR cushions. Her responses were recorded on a Wollensak model T-1500 tape recorder and microphone system. The examiner listened to the subject's responses through headphones and recorded each response on a sheet of paper. All phonetic forms were recorded with the use of the International Phonetic Alphabet (IPA). Upon completion of each stimulus, the examiner's list of subject responses was presented to the subject to verify the correctness of the listed responses. Any necessary changes were made at that time. A five-minute rest period was allowed between the presentation of each stimulus (2).

The above instructions and procedures were used for all three experimental sessions. The order of presentation of the stimuli was based on a modified system of counterbalancing so that six orders were used, with four subjects in each of the six order groups. However, each subject received the same order of presentation for all three experimental sessions. Each session, which lasted approximately 45 minutes, was held in a two-room sound-treated suite (IAC model 402A) at the West Virginia University Speech and Hearing Clinic.

8. Data Analysis

To determine the exact transformations, as well as the number of forms and transitions employed by each subject, one of the investigators listened to each subject's response tape via headphones and verified what had been written down during the experimental sessions. The number of repetitions of each stimulus prior to the onset of the subject's first verbal transformation was determined in the following manner: (*a*) the examiner listened to the response tape of each subject and by means of a stopwatch determined the duration from the beginning of the stimulus tape (which was indicated by the sound of a click of the fingers made by the subject) to the subject's first reported verbal transformation; (*b*) the stimulus tape was played through a General Radio model 1521-B graphic level recorder having a paper speed of 31.75 mm per second and a writing speed of 100 mm per second; (*c*) the time (in seconds) between the beginning of the stimulus tape and the subject's first reported verbal transformation (obtained from the subject's response tape) was converted to a distance measurement (in millimeters), and the millimeter distance equivalent was marked on the graphic level recorder tracing obtained from the stimulus tape; and (*d*) the number of repetitions of the stimulus was counted up to the marked point on the tracing of the stimulus tape. In the above manner, the number of repetitions of the stimulus prior to the onset of the first verbal transformation of each of the 24 subjects was determined for each of the six auditory stimuli in each of the three experimental sessions.

C. RESULTS

1. *Number of Forms, Transitions, and Repetitions Prior to Subjects' First Verbal Transformations*

Table 1 contains the average number of different forms (different perceptual phenomena), transitions (changes from one form to another), and repetitions of each stimulus prior to the onset of the subjects' first verbal transformations, for each of the three experimental sessions. The table indicates the following: (*a*) for all six stimuli investigated, the subjects as a group exhibited the greatest consistency for average number of forms reported and the poorest consistency for average number of repetitions of a stimulus prior to eliciting the first verbal transformations; (*b*) in each of the three sessions, the subjects consistently exhibited a larger average number of transitions than forms for all six stimuli; (*c*) the largest average number of forms and transitions was consistently reported for one of the two phonetically simplest stimuli employed (/ko/) and the smallest average number of forms and transitions was consistently elicited by one of the two phonetically most complex stimuli ("our ship has sailed"); (*d*) a larger average number of forms, transitions, and repetitions of a stimulus prior to the subjects' first verbal transformations was elicited by the three meaningless nonsense stimuli employed in the study (1.7 forms, 3.2 transitions, and 16.7 repetitions) than by the three meaningful stimuli (1.4 forms, 2.3 transitions, and 14.7 repeti-

TABLE 1
MEAN NUMBER AND MEAN DISCREPANCY SCORES FOR NUMBER OF FORMS, TRANSITIONS, AND REPETITIONS OF THE STIMULUS PRIOR TO SS' FIRST VERBAL TRANSFORMATIONS FOR EACH OF THE SIX STIMULI

Stimulus	Session #	Forms	Transitions	Repetitions
		Mean number in each of the three sessions		
/ko/	1	1.9	3.2	19.7
	2	1.8	4.5	13.7
	3	2.0	4.4	15.4
"see"	1	1.7	2.8	21.1
	2	1.5	2.4	21.6
	3	1.5	3.0	15.3
/ikfrɛ/	1	2.0	3.2	19.5
	2	1.8	3.5	15.1
	3	1.8	3.4	17.9
"police"	1	1.5	2.2	14.1
	2	1.8	2.8	14.6
	3	1.8	2.4	11.6
/trɛ os ri fæ/	1	1.2	1.6	18.4
	2	1.3	1.8	17.2
	3	1.6	2.8	13.0
"our ship has sailed"	1	.8	1.2	14.0
	2	1.0	2.2	11.4
	3	1.0	2.0	9.0
		Mean discrepancy scores		
/ko/		1.4	2.8	11.4
"see"		1.4	3.0	17.8
/ikfrɛ/		1.0	2.5	13.0
"police"		.8	2.0	9.1
/trɛ os ri fæ/		1.0	2.1	13.8
"our ship has sailed"		.8	1.8	8.5

tions); (*e*) for all three experimental sessions, the average number of repetitions of a stimulus prior to the first verbal transformations was consistently least for one of the two phonetically most complex stimuli ("our ship has sailed") and greatest for one of the two phonetically simplest stimuli ("see"); and (*f*) for all six stimuli investigated, a smaller average number of repetitions of the stimulus was consistently required to elicit the subjects' first verbal transformations in the last experimental session than was needed in the first session.

Mean discrepancy scores were employed to estimate intrasubject consistency in the study. Such scores were used because of their clarity in describing variability in subjects' performances. In addition to these discrepancy scores, estimations of the variance components (7, 13) were also computed to verify the results obtained with the discrepancy scores. In all cases, the variance estimates and mean discrepancy scores agreed with each other in regard to the trends observed in the data. However, since the discrepancy scores are more meaningful in a descriptive analysis of the data, only they will be reported here.

A separate discrepancy score was computed for each of the 24 subjects' responses to each of the six stimuli. This discrepancy score is a measure of the amount of variability exhibited by each subject for a given measure (forms, transitions, etc.) across the three experimental sessions. It was computed as follows: (a) the difference between the lowest and highest of the three values of a measure (one value for each of the three sessions) reported by the subject was determined; this figure represents each subject's discrepancy score; and (b) the discrepancy scores of all 24 subjects were summed and divided by 24 to yield a group mean discrepancy score.

Table 1 contains the mean discrepancy scores for number of forms, transitions, and repetitions of the stimulus prior to the subjects' first verbal transformations, for each of the six stimuli under investigation. The table indicates the following: (a) for all six stimuli, within-subject variability was consistently greatest for number of repetitions of the stimulus prior to the subjects' first verbal transformations, and least for number of forms reported; that is, the subjects were more consistent in the number of forms that they reported for a given stimulus from session to session than they were for the number of repetitions of a stimulus that were needed to elicit their first verbal transformations; (b) a comparison of the subjects' responses to the phonetically simplest stimuli (/ko/ and "see") and their responses to the phonetically most complex stimuli (/trɛ os ri fæ/ and "our ship has sailed") indicates that the subjects consistently exhibited a smaller amount of variability in number of forms, transitions, and repetitions of the stimulus for the phonetically most complex stimuli; and (c) the subjects consistently manifested slightly larger mean discrepancy scores for the three meaningless stimuli as a group (1.1 forms, 2.5 transitions, and 12.7 repetitions) than for the three meaningful stimuli (1.0 forms, 2.3 transitions, and 11.8 repetitions).

2. Types of Verbal Transformations

Table 2 contains a classification of the types of verbal transformations elicited by the six stimuli for each of the three experimental sessions. The classification employed here was based on the different forms reported by all subjects. The table indicates that (a) for the three meaningless stimuli employed in the study, the type of transformation consistently reported most frequently for all three sessions was a change in the phonetic structure of the

150

repeating stimulus; (b) for two of the three meaningful stimuli ("see" and "police"), the type of change reported most frequently for all three sessions pertained to the duration of the stimulus; "our ship has sailed" yielded the largest number of transformations in the phonetic category; (c) the smallest number of subjects' verbal transformations for all six stimuli was consistently of the "Clarity," "Familiar Sounds," and "Other" categories; and (d) for all six stimuli, the largest total number of transformations was of the phonetic type, 206; while "Familiar Sounds" category contained the smallest number of transformations (one).

The "Phonetic" category in this table pertains to transformations involving a perceptual change in the phonetic structure of the repeating stimulus. It is interesting to note that not only did the meaningless stimuli elicit more phonetic types of transformations than the meaningful stimuli, but they also yielded more distorted perceptual changes. That is, the reported transformations were more frequently phonetically more complex than the original repeating stimulus for the meaningless stimuli. The category "Other" in the table contains transformations that could not be placed into any of the existing categories. On several occasions some of the subjects could not verbally express the change that they perceived, but were certain that some change had occurred in their perception of the repeating stimulus. Such transformations were placed in this category.

Table 2 contains the mean discrepancy scores for the different types of verbal transformations reported by the 24 subjects for each of the six stimuli. The table indicates that (a) phonetic types of transformations consistently exhibited the largest mean discrepancy scores for the phonetically most complex stimuli (/trɛ os ri fæ/ and "our ship has sailed"), while for the phonetically simplest stimuli (/ko/ and "see"), the largest mean discrepancy scores were manifested in the transformations involving a change in the duration of the repeating stimulus; (b) for all six stimuli, the subjects consistently exhibited the smallest amount of variability across the three sessions in their use of transformations involving changes in the perceived pitch of the repeating stimulus; and (c) overall, intrasubject discrepancy appears to be very small for types of verbal transformations reported, with no category yielding a mean discrepancy score of more than .8; that is, the subjects appear to be highly consistent in terms of the types of verbal transformations that they report for a given stimulus from session to session.

3. Identical Forms

Table 3 contains all identical forms that were reported by more than one subject in each of the three experimental sessions. The table shows that (a)

151

TABLE 2

Number and Mean Discrepancy Scores for Types of Verbal Transformations for Each of the Six Stimuli

Stimulus	Session #	Phonetic	Pitch	Rate	Duration	Loudness	Stress	Clarity	Quality	Familiar Sounds	Other
		Number reported by the 24 subjects in each of the three sessions									
/ko/	1	14	2	14	7	13	3	0	3	0	0
	2	16	0	8	14	8	4	0	4	1	0
	3	13	0	12	9	11	5	0	8	0	1
"see"	1	2	2	12	13	11	5	0	2	0	0
	2	2	0	9	16	5	6	0	3	0	0
	3	3	0	9	13	8	3	2	4	0	0
/ikfɾɛ/	1	33	2	6	7	3	2	0	0	0	0
	2	35	0	6	3	1	0	0	0	0	1
	3	27	0	7	8	5	1	0	0	0	1
"police"	1	2	1	3	21	1	5	0	8	0	1
	2	3	2	7	12	2	11	0	9	0	3
	3	2	2	2	14	4	6	0	10	0	1
/tɾɛ os ri fæ/	1	8	3	8	9	0	4	0	0	0	0
	2	13	2	9	6	0	5	0	0	0	1
	3	15	1	10	10	2	6	0	0	0	1
"our ship has sailed"	1	5	4	5	3	3	1	1	0	0	1
	2	6	4	4	3	2	2	2	2	0	1
	3	7	4	7	1	7	1	1	0	0	0
		Mean discrepancy scores									
/ko/		.4	.1	.5	.7	.6	.3	a	.4	.1	.1
"see"		.1	.1	.5	.8	.7	.3	.1	.2	a	a
/ikfɾɛ/		.8	.1	.4	.4	.3	.1	a	a	a	.1
"police"		.2	.1	.4	.8	.2	.4	a	.3	a	.2
/tɾɛ os ri fæ/		.7	.1	.3	.3	.1	.3	a	a	a	.1
"our ship has sailed"		.3	.0	.3	.2	.3	.1	.1	.1	a	.1

a None reported.

152

there is a progressive decrease in number of identical forms (and number of subjects reporting the forms) in all three sessions from the phonetically simplest to the phonetically most complex stimuli; /ko/ yielded the largest number of identical forms and "our ship has sailed" the smallest; and (b) the meaningless stimuli as a group elicited a larger number of identical forms in all three sessions than did the meaningful stimuli.

TABLE 3

IDENTICAL FORMS REPORTED IN EACH OF THE THREE EXPERIMENTAL SESSIONS BY MORE THAN ONE SUBJECT (The number of subjects reporting a particular form is given in parentheses preceding the form. Phonetic symbols are used for all forms in brackets.)

Stimulus	Sessions		
	#1	#2	#3
/ko/	(5) /kol/	(5) /kol/	(5) /kol/
	(3) /ko-ə/	(3) /ko-ə/	(3) /ko-ə/
	(2) /kow/	(4) /kow/	(2) /kow/
	(7) "louder"	(3) "louder"	(5) "louder"
	(5) "faster"	(4) "faster"	(4) "faster"
	(4) "slower"	(3) "slower"	(5) "slower"
	(2) "longer"	(2) "longer"	(2) "longer"
"see"	(2) "prolonged /i/"	(4) "prolonged /i/"	(3) "prolonged /i/"
	(4) "prolonged /s/"	(5) "prolonged /s/"	(6) "prolonged /s/"
	(5) "faster"	(4) "faster"	(6) "faster"
	(5) "louder"	(5) "louder"	(3) "louder"
/ikfrɛ/	(5) /ikfrɛr/	(4) /ikfrɛr/	(3) /ikfrɛr/
	(2) /ikəfrɛ/	(2) /ikəfrɛ/	(2) /ikəfrɛ/
	(5) /ikfrejə/	(4) /ikfrejə/	(4) /ikfrejə/
	(3) /ikfrʌ/	(3) /ikfrʌ/	(2) /ikfrʌ/
"police"	(10) "prolonged /s/"	(5) "prolonged /s/"	(7) "prolonged /s/"
	(3) "distorted /s/"	(2) "distorted /s/"	(2) "distorted /s/"
/trɛ os ri fæ/	(5) "faster"	(5) "faster"	(6) "faster"
	(2) "slower"	(2) "slower"	(3) "slower"
"our ship has sailed"	(2) "slower"	(4) "slower"	(3) "slower"

Table 4 contains the number and percentage of identical forms reported in all three sessions, in two of the three sessions, and in only one of the three sessions. The table shows the following: (a) one of the two phonetically simplest stimuli (/ko/) yielded the largest number of identical forms reported in all three sessions, while subjects reported the fewest number of identical forms in all three sessions for one of the two phonetically most complex stimuli investigated ("our ship has sailed"); (b) the three meaningless stimuli as a group produced more identical forms in all three sessions, 49, than did the three meaningful stimuli, 29; and (c) for each of the six stimuli investigated, the majority of forms were reported in only one of the three sessions; an average of 57.3 percent of all forms were reported in only one of the three sessions, while an average of 24.5 percent of the forms were reported in two of the three sessions, and an average of 18.2 percent were used in all three sessions.

TABLE 4

NUMBER AND PERCENTAGE OF IDENTICAL FORMS, IDENTICAL ORDERS FOR TYPES OF VERBAL TRANSFORMATIONS, AND IDENTICAL ORDERS FOR IDENTICAL FORMS REPORTED BY THE 24 Ss IN ALL THREE SESSIONS, IN TWO OF THE THREE SESSIONS, AND IN ONLY ONE OF THE THREE SESSIONS

Stimulus	Sessions		
	1 of 3	2 of 3	3 of 3
	Identical forms		
/ko/	41(53%)	16(21%)	20(26%)
"see"	41(58%)	19(27%)	11(15%)
/ikfrɛ/	42(52%)	19(24%)	19(24%)
"police"	49(65%)	16(21%)	11(14%)
/trɛ os ri fæ/	43(63%)	16(23%)	10(14%)
"our ship has sailed"	24(53%)	14(31%)	7(16%)
	Identical orders for types of VTs		
/ko/	8(40%)	10(50%)	2(10%)
"see"	12(63%)	6(32%)	1(5%)
/ikfrɛ/	6(30%)	7(35%)	7(35%)
"police"	9(47%)	7(37%)	3(16%)
/trɛ os ri fæ/	4(20%)	14(70%)	2(10%)
"our ship has sailed"	4(27%)	9(60%)	2(13%)
	Identical orders for identical forms		
/ko/	13(65%)	7(35%)	0(0%)
"see"	14(74%)	5(26%)	0(0%)
/ikfrɛ/	14(70%)	5(25%)	1(5%)
"police"	9(47%)	10(53%)	0(0%)
/trɛ os ri fæ/	10(50%)	9(45%)	1(5%)
"our ship has sailed"	7(47%)	7(47%)	1(6%)

4. Identical Orders of Reported Verbal Transformations

The consistency of the order of subjects' reported verbal transformations for types and identical forms was also investigated. Table 4 contains the number and percentage of identical orders for types of verbal transformations used in all three sessions, in two of the three sessions, and in only one of the three sessions. The table indicates that (*a*) the stimuli /ikfrɛ/ and "police" yielded the largest number and percentage of identical orders for all three sessions; (*b*) the three meaningless stimuli as a group elicited more identical orders, 11, than did the three meaningful stimuli, 6; and (*c*) for all six

154

stimuli investigated, an average of 47.4 percent of all orders were used in two of the three sessions, 37.8 percent were reported in one of the three sessions, and 14.8 percent were employed in all three sessions.

Table 4 also reports on the number and percentage of identical orders used for exact forms. It indicates that (*a*) none of the six stimuli elicited more than one identical order for all three sessions; and (*b*) for all six stimuli, an average of 58.8 percent of all orders were used in only one of the three sessions, 38.4 percent in two of the three sessions, and 2.8 percent in all three sessions.

D. DISCUSSION

1. *Overall Consistency*

The findings of this study indicated that overall consistency of subjects' reported verbal transformations was not equal for all measures investigated. Intrasubject consistency was found to be high for number of forms and transitions employed, as well as for types of verbal transformations reported by the subjects. The group mean discrepancy score for all six stimuli investigated was only 1.1 for number of forms, 2.4 for number of transitions, and .3 for types of reported verbal transformations, an indication of a small amount of variability for these measures.

However, the subjects appear to vary considerably from session to session in terms of the number of repetitions of the stimulus that they require before reporting their initial verbal transformations (a group mean discrepancy of 12.3). In addition, there is little consistency exhibited by the subjects for a given stimulus in terms of the exact forms and orders employed from session to session. This finding is in disagreement with Warren's (10, p. 257) earlier observation on a few of his subjects that, when they were presented with the same repeating stimulus that they had heard three weeks earlier, ". . . the forms reported were almost identical with those heard previously, frequently appearing in almost the same order." In the present study, for all six stimuli investigated, an average of only 18.2 percent of all forms used were reported in all three sessions, while 57 percent were used in only one of the three experimental sessions. For orders of types of reported transformations, while 37.8 percent of all orders were used in one of the three sessions, only 14.8 percent were reported in all three sessions. For orders of exact forms, only 2.8 percent of all subjects' employed orders were reported in all three sessions, and 58.8 percent were found in one of the three sessions.

The finding that subjects vary considerably from session to session with re-

155

gard to these three measures leads the current writers to conclude that caution must be exercised in making generalizations from the data pertaining to order employed, exact forms reported, and number of repetitions of the stimulus required prior to the subjects' first verbal transformations, in studies concerned with the verbal transformation effect phenomenon. The implication here is that a subject may report a particular form, order, etc. on one occasion, but not necessarily use that same form, order, etc. when presented with the same repeating stimulus on a second occasion, or on a third occasion, etc. Generalizations on these measures are, therefore, very difficult to make with any assurance. However, since the types of forms, as well as the number of forms and transitions used, appear to be more consistent than the exact forms and orders reported, generalizations regarding these measures can be made with more confidence.

2. Nature of Auditory Stimuli

As was true for overall consistency in this study, no single statement can be made regarding consistency of subjects' reported verbal transformations as a function of the meaningfulness or phonetic complexity of the repeating stimulus. For number of forms, transitions, and repetitions prior to the subjects' first verbal transformations, the meaningless stimuli as a group yielded slightly poorer consistency than the meaningful stimuli investigated (combined mean discrepancy scores of 1.1 forms, 2.5 transitions, and 12.7 repetitions for the meaningless stimuli as compared to 1.0 forms, 2.3 transitions, and 11.8 repetitions for the meaningful stimuli). For some types of verbal transformations, consistency was higher for the meaningless stimuli (duration, loudness, and stress), while for other types it was higher for the meaningful stimuli (phonetic and pitch). For the measures of exact forms, order of types of transformations, and order of exact forms, the subjects exhibited greater consistency for the meaningless than for the meaningful stimuli. A total of 64 percent of all forms elicited by the meaningless stimuli were reported in all three experimental sessions, while 45 percent of all forms obtained from the meaningful stimuli were used in all three sessions. The same trend is evident for orders of types of reported verbal transformations. A total of 55 percent of all orders elicited by the meaningless stimuli were used in all three sessions, while 34 percent of the orders obtained from the meaningful stimuli were found in all three sessions. For order of exact forms, 10 percent of all orders obtained from the meaningless stimuli were present in all three sessions, while only 6.6 percent of the orders obtained from the meaningful stimuli were employed in all three sessions.

In terms of phonetic complexity of the stimuli employed, the phonetically most complex stimuli (/trɛ os ri fæ/ and "our ship has sailed") yielded a higher degree of consistency than the phonetically simplest stimuli (/ko/ and "see") employed in the study for number of forms, transitions, and repetitions prior to the subjects' first verbal transformations. The phonetically most complex stimuli yielded combined mean discrepancy scores of 1.8 forms, 3.9 transitions, and 22.3 repetitions, while the combined mean discrepancy scores for the simplest stimuli were 2.8 forms, 5.8 transitions, and 29.2 repetitions. For all but one type of transformation (phonetic), the phonetically most complex stimuli exhibited the greater consistency. For exact forms employed, greater intrasubject consistency was manifested for the simplest stimuli. A combined total of 41 percent of all forms used for the simplest stimuli were found in all three experimental sessions, while 30 percent of the forms reported by the most complex stimuli were used in all three sessions. However, for order of types of transformations reported by the subjects, the most complex stimuli showed the greater consistency. A total of 23 percent of all orders used for the complex stimuli were employed in all three sessions, and 15 percent of all orders for the simple stimuli were reported in all sessions. The same trend existed for order of exact forms employed. A total of 7.1 percent of the orders for the most complex stimuli were reported in all three sessions, while none of the orders elicited by the simplest stimuli was found in all three sessions. From these findings it must be concluded that no single statement can be made concerning the consistency of subjects' reported verbal transformations as a function of either the meaningfulness or phonetic complexity of the repeating stimulus.

3. Nature of Reported Verbal Transformations

The majority of transformations (72 percent) reported in this study involved perceptual changes in the various parameters of the repeating auditory stimuli, including the pitch, rate, duration, loudness, stress, clarity, and the quality of the signal. Except for one other study (3), few transformations of these types have been reported in previous investigations concerned with the verbal transformation effect phenomenon. The other study in which such similar types of reported transformations were found was concerned with isolated vowels as the repeating auditory stimuli. The authors attributed their subjects' unique types of transformations to two factors: (a) the phonetic simplicity of the repeating stimuli, and (b) the phonetic training and experiences of the subjects in their study. The listeners were all majoring in speech pathology and, in addition to their use of the International Phonetic

157

Alphabet, they were experienced in listening to and analyzing what they heard. The stimuli in the present study were phonetically more complex than the vowels used by Lass and Golden. However, since the subjects in both studies had the same phonetic training and experiences (although no individual served as a subject in both studies), and since similar types of unique verbal transformations were reported in both studies, the factor of listener training and experience appears to deserve further exploration.

REFERENCES

1. BARNETT, M. R. Perceived phonetic changes in the verbal transformation effect. Unpublished Ph.D. dissertation, Ohio University, Athens, 1964.
2. BEVAN, W., AVANT, L. L., & LANKFORD, H. G. The influence of interpolated periods of activity and inactivity upon the vigilance decrement. *J. Appl. Psychol.*, 1967, 51, 352-356.
3. LASS, N. J., & GOLDEN, S. S. The use of isolated vowels as auditory stimuli in eliciting the verbal transformation effect. *Can. J. Psychol.*, 1971, 25, 349-359.
4. NAESER, M. A., & LILLY, J. C. Preliminary evidence for a universal feature detector system: Perception of the repeating word. Paper presented at the 79th Meeting of the Acoustical Society of America, Atlantic City, New Jersey, April 21-24, 1970.
5. NATSOULAS, T. A study of the verbal-transformation effect. *Amer. J. Psychol.*, 1965, 78, 257-263.
6. OBUSEK, C. J. A study of speech perception in the aged by means of the verbal transformation effect. Unpublished Master's thesis, University of Wisconsin, Milwaukee, 1968.
7. SNEDECOR, G. W. Statistical Methods. Ames, Iowa: Iowa State Coll. Press, 1956. Pp. 259-262.
8. TAYLOR, M. M., & HENNING, G. B. Verbal transformations and an effect of instructional bias on perception. *Can. J. Psychol.*, 1963, 17, 210-223.
9. TEMPLIN, M. C., & DARLEY, F. L. The Templin-Darley Tests of Articulation. Iowa City: Bur. Educ. Res. & Serv., Exten. Div., Univ. Iowa, 1960.
10. WARREN, R. M. Illusory changes of distinct speech upon repetition—The verbal transformation effect. *Brit. J. Psychol.*, 1961, 52, 249-258.
11. ———. Illusory changes in repeated words: Differences between young adults and the aged. *Amer. J. Psychol.*, 1961, 74, 506-516.
12. WARREN, R. M., & WARREN, R. P. A comparison of speech perception in childhood, maturity, and old age by means of the verbal transformation effect. *J. Verb. Learn. & Verb. Behav.*, 1966, 5, 142-146.
13. WINER, B. J. Statistical Principles in Experimental Design. New York: McGraw-Hill, 1962. Pp. 46-70.

THE VERBAL TRANSFORMATION EFFECT: A COMPARATIVE STUDY OF THE VERBAL TRANSFORMATIONS OF PHONETICALLY TRAINED AND NON-PHONETICALLY TRAINED SUBJECTS

By NORMAN J. LASS AND RICHARD M. GASPERINI

The purpose of this investigation was to determine if there are differences between phonetically trained and non-phonetically trained subjects in terms of their reported verbal transformations. A total of seven auditory stimuli, representing variations in meaningfulness and phonetic complexity, were presented to 28 phonetically trained and 28 non-phonetically trained listeners. Results indicate that there are both similarities and differences between the two groups. The differences that exist are quantitative, and not qualitative, in nature. The phonetically trained group reported more forms and transitions, and required fewer repetitions of the stimulus prior to their first verbal transformations, than the non-phonetically trained subjects. However, both groups reported the same types of transformations and, in many instances, identical forms as well.

The observation that continued listening to recorded repetitions of a stimulus produces perceptual illusory changes in normal listeners was first made by Warren & Gregory (1958) and later labelled by Warren (1961a) as the 'verbal transformation effect'.

The majority of studies concerned with this phenomenon have employed subjects with no phonetic training or extensive listening experience (Warren & Gregory, 1958; Warren, 1961a, b; Taylor & Henning, 1963; Natsoulas, 1965; Warren & Warren, 1966; Obusek, 1968; Warren, 1968). However, in a preliminary study concerned with providing evidence for a universal feature detector system, Naeser & Lilly (1970) used a group of phonetically trained linguists and a group of non-phonetically trained non-linguists as listeners in a task involving continued listening to the word 'cogitate'. One of their findings was that of the five types of verbal transformations analysed, over 60 per cent reported by the group of linguists were non-dictionary types and approximately 30 per cent were of the dictionary variety. However, for the group of non-linguists, only 30 per cent of the reported transformations were of the non-dictionary type, while almost 50 per cent were dictionary types. Naeser & Lilly considered the factor of phonetic training as a possible explanation for their findings. They commented that 'perhaps the fact that the linguists were using IPA [International Phonetic Alphabet] and the non-linguists only traditional English orthography made the difference' (p. 6).

Further support for this hypothesis of the importance of phonetic training on the listener's verbal transformations came from a study by Lass & Golden (1971) concerned with the effectiveness of single isolated vowels as auditory stimuli in eliciting the verbal transformation effect. Their subjects had phonetic training and used the International Phonetic Alphabet regularly in their training as speech pathologists. They found that the verbal transformations of their subjects often differed from those

BRITISH JOURNAL OF PSYCHOLOGY, 1973, vol. 64, no. 2, 183-192.

reported in previous investigations. In addition to the transformations involving perceptual changes in the phonetic structure of the repeating stimulus (the type reported most often in previous studies), the majority of their subjects' transformations involved changes in the various parameters of the auditory stimulus, such as the loudness, duration, quality and clarity of the signal. The authors attributed some of these differences between their findings and those obtained in previous studies to the phonetic training and listening experience of their subjects. They state that: 'Perhaps this background and training can at least partially account for the unique types of transformations reported...' (p. 356).

Additional support for the importance of the phonetic training factor was provided by a study of the consistency of subjects' reported verbal transformations by Tekieli & Lass (1972). Employing subjects with the same phonetic training and experience as those in the Lass & Golden (1971) study, and using stimuli varying in meaningfulness and phonetic complexity, they also found that: 'The majority of transformations (72 per cent) reported in this study involved perceptual changes in the various parameters of the repeating auditory stimuli, including the pitch, rate, duration, loudness, stress, clarity, and the quality of the signal' (p. 244). They concluded that 'since the subjects in both studies [their study and Lass & Golden's study] had the same phonetic training and experiences...and since similar types of unique verbal transformations were reported in both studies, the factor of listener training and experience appears to deserve further exploration' (p. 245).

The purpose of the present investigation was to pursue further the issue of phonetic training in listeners by comparing the verbal transformations of a group of phonetically trained subjects with those of a group of non-phonetically trained subjects, and thus to determine if this subject variable is an important one in the study of the verbal transformation effect phenomenon.

METHOD

Subjects

A total of 56 individuals, 28 in each of two groups, served as subjects. All were students at West Virginia University. The non-phonetically trained group consisted of students from various programmes throughout the university. None of the subjects in this group had had phonetic training or listening experience of any kind. This group comprised 19 males and nine females, ranging in age from 19 to 23 years, with a mean age of 20 years.

The phonetically trained group consisted of students in the Speech Pathology-Audiology programme at West Virginia University. All subjects in this group were thoroughly familiar with the International Phonetic Alphabet and used it routinely in their training as speech pathologists. In addition, through their course work and clinical experiences, they had experience in listening to, and thoroughly analysing, what they heard. There were three males and 25 females in this group. The age range was 19–22 years, and the mean age was 20 years.

No subject in either listener group reported hearing difficulty and all had normal neurological history and status as determined by a questionnaire. It is obvious that there is a disproportionate number of males and females in the two subject groups in the study. However, the sex of the subject was not thought to be an important factor in the present investigation or in a number of previous studies on the verbal transformation effect phenomenon (Warren & Warren, 1966; Lass & Golden, 1971; Perl, 1970; Lass et al., 1973).

Recording procedure

A total of seven auditory stimuli was employed in the study: (1) an isolated vowel, /i/; (2) a nonsense syllable, /ko/; (3) a one-syllable meaningful word, 'see'; (4) a two-syllable nonsense word, /ikfrɛ/; (5) a two-syllable meaningful word, 'police'; (6) a four-syllable nonsense phrase, /trɛ os ri fæ/; (7) a four-syllable, four-word meaningful sentence, 'our ship has sailed'.

The stimuli used were chosen in order to compare the two groups' verbal transformations for stimuli varying in both meaningfulness and phonetic complexity.

Recording procedure

Recordings of all stimuli were made by a professional male announcer with an Ampex model 602 tape-recorder and an Altec model 681A condenser microphone. The recordings were made in a sound-treated room at the West Virginia University Medical Center. Preceding the production of each stimulus the speaker used the carrier phrase 'Say the word —', which he monitored at zero on the VU meter of the tape-recorder.

In the production of the isolated vowel, /i/, an attempt was made to control for the consistency of the frequency and sound-pressure level of the speaker's phonation. To maintain a constant frequency, the output of a Beltone model 15CX pure-tone oscillator set at 125 Hz was monitored by the speaker through a single headphone. Simultaneously, the speaker monitored the sound-pressure level of his voice on a General Radio model 1551-C sound-level meter in an attempt to maintain a constant reading of 65 db on the meter.

Construction of stimulus tapes

Each of the seven recorded stimuli was cut and spliced into a separate tape loop. The loops were played repeatedly on a Nagra model IV-D tape-recorder and electronically reproduced on an Ampex model 602 tape-recorder. Each of the stimuli was then cut and spliced into a second tape loop containing 500 msec. pauses between stimuli. In the case of the isolated vowel, /i/, a 200 msec. segment was excised from the original sustained phonation of the vowel. Because of the relatively short duration of the utterances, it was necessary to use more than one reproduction of the stimulus in order to construct the tape loop. In the above manner, seven master tape loops were constructed, one for each of the seven stimuli under investigation in the study. Each tape loop was played repeatedly for a 3 min. period on a Nagra model IV-D tape-recorder and electronically reproduced on an Ampex model 602 tape-recorder to produce seven master stimulus tapes.

Experimental procedure

The following set of instructions was orally presented to each subject: 'I am going to play a tape-recording through these headphones [present headphones]. When the tape starts, click your fingers near the microphone as soon as you hear the voice [demonstrate]. I want you to listen carefully to the voice and tell me what it seems to be saying as soon as you can. After you call out what you hear, keep on listening carefully. If you think you hear a change to a different stimulus, call out what you hear as soon as the change occurs. If there is a change back to the original stimulus or to another different stimulus, call it out as soon as the change occurs. Any change to a new stimulus or to a stimulus previously heard should be called out immediately upon hearing it. Even if the change is momentary, that is, involving just one repetition, be certain to call it out. Do not wait to confirm the change by listening further. Do not worry about being correct or incorrect. Do not worry about whether what you hear is meaningful or familiar. What I want to know is what the stimulus seems like to you under these special conditions. Don't forget to call out immediately every time you hear a change, whether to something new or whether the change is back to a stimulus which you called out before. However, if you hear no change in the stimulus, please remain silent. You will hear a tone immediately prior to the onset of the stimulus. Attempt to maintain your maximum concentration during the entire listening task. Are there any questions?'

In an attempt to familiarize the subject with the experimental task, a 1·5 min. practice stimulus tape was played for him. This tape was constructed in the same manner as the experimental stimulus tapes. The stimulus employed in the practice tape was 'the word'. Upon completion of the practice tape, the seven experimental stimulus tapes were played to the subject binaurally by means of a Nagra model IV-D tape-recorder and a set of matched Sharpe model HA-10A headphones. The subject's responses were recorded on an Ampex model 602 tape-recorder using an Altec model 681A condenser microphone. The examiner listened to the sub-

Table 1. *Mean number of forms, transitions and repetitions of the stimuli prior to the onset of the first verbal transformations for the phonetically trained and non-phonetically trained listener groups*

	Phonetically trained group			Non-phonetically trained group		
Stimulus	Forms	Transitions	Repetitions	Forms	Transitions	Repetitions
/i/	2·8	6·7	44·5	1·5	3·2	56·1
/ko/	3·1	7·2	30·0	2·6	3·8	31·5
'see'	2·6	7·1	24·4	2·2	4·0	21·7
/ikfrɛ/	3·2	6·8	25·8	2·2	3·6	27·6
'police'	2·9	4·8	19·3	1·8	2·5	32·8
/trɛ os ri fæ/	2·0	3·9	25·2	1·9	2·6	25·3
'our ship has sailed'	2·4	4·8	16·7	2·1	2·9	17·6

ject's responses by means of a set of headphones and recorded each response on a sheet of paper. All phonetic forms were recorded using the International Phonetic Alphabet. Upon completion of each stimulus tape, the examiner's list of subject responses was presented to the subject to verify the correctness of the listed responses.

All seven stimulus tapes were presented to each subject individually in a single experimental session. The order of presentation of the seven stimulus tapes was counterbalanced so that seven orders were used, with four subjects from each of the two listener groups in each of the seven order conditions. A rest period of approximately 3 min. was provided between each stimulus tape. The session, which lasted approximately 40 min., was held in a sound-treated room at the West Virginia University Medical Center.

Data analysis

To determine the exact transformations as well as the number of forms and transitions reported by each subject, one of the investigators listened to the subject's response tape via headphones and verified what had been recorded during the listening sessions. The number of repetitions of the stimulus prior to the onset of each subject's first verbal transformation was determined in the following manner: (1) the subject's response tape was played through a General Radio model 1521-B graphic level recorder having a paper speed of 31·75 mm per sec. and a writing speed of 100 mm per sec.; (2) the examiner placed a mark at the beginning of the stimulus tape (which was indicated by the sound of the clicking of the subject's fingers near the microphone) and at the occurrence of the first verbal transformation reported; (3) a line was drawn perpendicular to the baseline of the graphic level recorder tracing at these two points; (4) the distance between the two points was measured in millimetres; (5) the stimulus tapes were played through the graphic level recorder; and (6) the millimetre distance obtained from each subject's response tape was marked on the tracings of the stimulus tapes and the number of repetitions of the stimulus, which was visible from the tracings, was counted up to that point on the tracing. In the above manner, the number of repetitions prior to the onset of the first verbal transformations of each of the 56 subjects was determined for each of the seven stimuli employed in the study.

RESULTS

Forms, transitions and repetitions prior to first verbal transformations

Table 1 contains the average number of forms (different perceptual phenomena), transitions (changes from one form to another), and repetitions of each stimulus prior to the onset of the subjects' first verbal transformations, for the phonetically trained and non-phonetically trained groups in the study. The table indicates the following: (1) for each of the seven auditory stimuli investigated, the phonetically trained group of subjects reported more forms and transitions, and required fewer repetitions of the stimulus prior to their first verbal transformations (except for 'see') than the non-phonetically trained group; (2) the largest differences between the two groups for numbers of forms and transitions reported occurred for the phonetically simplest stimulus employed in the study (/i/), while the smallest differences between the two groups was for one of the phonetically most complex stimuli (/trɛ os ri fæ/); (3) both subject groups manifested a larger average number of transitions than forms for all stimuli employed in the study; and (4) for both groups, one of the two phonetically most complex stimuli ('our ship has sailed') required the fewest average number of repetitions to elicit the subjects' first verbal transformations, and the phonetically simplest stimulus (/i/) required the largest number of repetitions.

Inferential statistical analysis, consisting of Mann–Whitney U tests (Siegel, 1956), was employed to determine if the observed differences between the two subject groups were statistically significant or simply chance occurrences. Results of the analyses indicate the following: (1) for all seven stimuli as a group, there are no significant differences between the phonetically trained and non-phonetically trained listeners in number of forms reported ($z = 1.75$) and significant differences in number of transitions ($z = 1.98$; $P < 0.05$) and repetitions of the stimulus prior to eliciting their first verbal transformations ($z = 2.07$; $P < 0.05$); (2) for the meaningful stimuli in the study ('see', 'police' and 'our ship has sailed'), the two groups do not differ significantly in number of elicited forms ($z = 1.58$) and transitions ($z = 1.32$), but show significant differences for number of stimulus repetitions ($z = 2.27$; $P < 0.05$); (3) for the meaningless stimuli as a group (/i/, /ko/, /ikfrɛ/, and /trɛ os ri fæ/), there are significant differences between the phonetically trained and non-phonetically trained subjects in forms ($z = 2.01$; $P < 0.05$) and no significant differences in transitions ($z = 1.70$) and repetitions ($z = 1.67$); (4) the phonetically trained and non-phonetically trained groups show no significant differences for phonetically simple stimuli in the study (/i/, /ko/, and 'see') in number of forms ($z = 1.95$) and repetitions ($z = 1.93$) which they exhibit, and significant differences in number of reported transitions ($z = 2.11$; $P < 0.05$); (5) for stimuli of intermediate phonetic complexity (/ikfrɛ/ and 'police'), the differences between the two groups are significant in forms ($z = 2.43$; $P < 0.05$) and repetitions ($z = 2.59$; $P < 0.01$) and not significant in reported transitions ($z = 1.70$); and (6) the two groups show no significant differences in number of forms ($z = 0.39$), transitions ($z = 1.37$), and repetitions ($z = 0.01$) for the phonetically complex stimuli (/trɛ os ri fæ/ and 'our ship has sailed') employed in the study.

Types of verbal transformations

Table 2 contains a classification of the types of verbal transformations elicited by the seven auditory stimuli from the two listener groups. The classification employed was based on the different forms reported by all subjects in both groups.

The *phonetic* category in this table pertains to transformations involving a perceptual change in the phonetic structure of the repeating stimulus. A differentiation was made by subjects in both groups in their reports of transformations between the *rate* of the stimulus presentation (i.e. inter-stimulus pause time appeared to them to be altered) and *duration* of each stimulus heard (i.e. stimulus time appeared to have changed). Transformations of *quality* usually involved reports of changes to a 'hoarse', 'raspy' or 'throaty' quality of the signal. *Rhythm* changes were often expressed as

Table 2. *Percentage of types of verbal transformations reported by the phonetically trained and non-phonetically trained listener groups for each of the seven stimuli employed in the study*

Stimulus	Phonetic	Pitch	Rate	Duration	Loudness	Stress	Clarity	Quality	Other
			Phonetically trained group						
/i/	33·3	7·7	33·3	5·1	6·4	6·4	3·8	3·8	0·0
/ko/	21·1	3·2	11·8	16·8	22·1	9·5	3·2	11·6	1·1
'see'	19·4	4·2	15·3	8·3	29·2	11·1	4·2	8·3	0·0
/ikfrɛ/	16·9	5·6	7·9	11·2	25·8	18·0	4·5	9·0	1·1
'police'	6·8	2·7	18·9	35·1	10·8	23·0	2·7	0·0	0·0
/trɛ os ri fæ/	11·3	5·7	18·9	11·3	17·0	26·4	5·7	3·8	0·0
'our ship has sailed'	16·7	13·6	9·1	15·2	16·7	22·7	4·5	1·5	0·0
			Non-phonetically trained group						
/i/	12·2	9·8	22·0	4·9	24·4	12·2	7·3	2·4	4·9
/ko/	18·1	0·0	9·7	20·8	18·1	11·1	4·2	16·7	1·4
'see'	7·9	0·0	15·9	17·5	36·5	7·9	4·8	4·8	4·8
/ikfrɛ/	10·5	5·3	12·3	12·3	33·3	14·0	3·5	3·5	5·3
'police'	2·1	2·1	18·8	37·5	20·8	10·4	6·3	2·1	0·0
/trɛ os ri fæ/	20·4	0·0	6·1	12·2	26·5	24·5	6·1	2·0	2·0
'our ship has sailed'	10·9	1·8	3·6	10·9	27·3	27·3	10·9	7·3	0·0

changes in the stress pattern of the repeating stimulus. The *clarity* category involved perceptual changes to either a 'clearer' signal or to one which was 'blurry' or 'distorted'. The category *other* in Table 2 includes transformations which could not be placed into any of the existing categories. It included those transformations which were perceived by the subjects but which they could not verbally express. That is, they were certain that some change had occurred in their perception of the repeating stimulus, but could not describe the change.

Table 2 shows the following: (1) across all stimuli investigated, the subjects in the phonetically trained group reported a greater percentage of phonetic, pitch, rate and stress types of transformations than did those in the non-phonetically trained group, while the non-phonetically trained subjects reported a greater percentage of duration, loudness, clarity, quality and other types of transformations than did those in the phonetically trained group; (2) across all seven stimuli, the largest differences in percentages between the two listener groups were those involving changes in the loudness and phonetic structure of the repeating stimulus (8·4 and 6·2 per cent differences, respectively), while the smallest differences occurred for quality types of transformation (0·1 per cent difference); (3) the average difference between the phonetically trained and non-phonetically trained subjects across all stimuli as well as across all categories of transformations was 3·3 per cent; (4) the majority of transformations reported by both groups of subjects were those involving perceptual changes in the various parameters of the auditory signal (i.e. changes in the pitch, rate, duration, loudness, etc., of the repeating stimulus) rather than in its phonetic structure; (5) for five of the seven stimuli in the non-phonetically trained group (/i/, 'see', /ikfrɛ/, /trɛ os ri fæ/ and 'our ship has sailed'), and for three of the seven stimuli in the phonetically trained subjects (/ko/, 'see' and /ikfrɛ/), the largest percentage of verbal transformations involved perceptual changes in the loudness of the repeating stimulus; and (6) the non-phonetically trained subjects in the study were

more often unable to verbally express the changes that had occurred in their perception of the repeating stimulus than were those in the phonetically trained group.

Exact forms

Table 3 includes the exact forms which were reported by more than one subject in
each of the two listener groups for the seven stimuli employed in the study. The
table indicates that: (1) while the phonetically trained subjects reported phonetic
types of transformations for all but one of the seven stimuli ('police'), the non-
phonetically trained group reported such transformations for three of the meaningless stimuli (/ko/, /ikfrɛ/ and /trɛ os ri fæ/) and none for the meaningful stimuli in
the study; (2) the phonetic transformations included the substitution of a single
phoneme for one of the stimulus sounds (e.g. /I/ for the stimulus /i/; /ikfrʌ/ and
/ikfrə/ for the stimulus /ikfrɛ/; /krɛ os ri fæ/, /prɛ os ri fæ/, /trʌ os ri fæ/, and /træ os
ri fæ/ for the stimulus /trɛ os ri fæ/) as well as the addition of one or more phonemes
to the original stimulus (e.g./ip/ for the stimulus /i/; /kowʌ/ and /kol/ for the stimulus
/ko/; /sijʌ/ and /si-I/ for the stimulus 'see'; /ikfrʌm/ and /ikfrɛm/ for the stimulus
/ikfrɛ/); (3) the phonetic transformations reported by the non-phonetically trained
group were identical forms to those reported by the phonetically trained subjects;
and (4) the non-phonetic verbal transformations, those involving perceptual changes
in the various parameters of the auditory signals, were very similar, and in many
cases identical, for both subject groups.

DISCUSSION

The results of this study indicate that there are both similarities and differences
between phonetically trained and non-phonetically trained subjects in terms of their
reported verbal transformations. Furthermore, the differences that exist between
these two groups are more quantitative than qualitative in nature. The subjects in
the phonetically trained group reported more forms and transitions than those who
were not phonetically trained, and required fewer repetitions of the stimulus before
reporting their first verbal transformations for all but one of the seven stimuli
employed in the study. They also reported more phonetic types of transformations,
those involving changes in the phonetic structure of the repeating stimulus, for all
stimuli than the non-phonetically trained subjects. On the other hand, the subjects
in the non-phonetically trained group reported more often that they could not verbally express the changes that they had perceived in the repeating stimuli.

The findings that the phonetically trained subjects reported more forms and
transitions, required fewer repetitions of the stimulus prior to their first verbal
transformations, and reported more phonetic types of transformations, are not
surprising in view of their training and background. All the subjects in this group
were very familiar with the International Phonetic Alphabet and used it regularly
in their training as speech pathologists. Furthermore, through their course work and
clinical experience, they were taught to use this knowledge of phonetics to listen to,
and analyse, what they heard. The non-phonetically trained subjects lacked this
phonetic training and experience and thus did not report as many forms and transitions, required more repetitions of the stimulus before reporting transformations,

165

(The number of subjects reporting a particular form is given in the parentheses preceding the form. Phonetic symbols are used for all forms in brackets.)

Stimulus	Phonetically trained group	Non-phonetically trained group
/i/	(16) /bip/	(4) 'slower'
	(2) /I/	(6) 'faster'
	(6) /ip/	(4) 'cannot describe change'
	(3) /Ip/	(2) 'higher in pitch'
	(8) 'slower'	(2) 'lower in pitch'
	(16) 'faster'	(7) 'louder'
	(3) 'rhythm change'	(3) 'softer'
	(3) 'lower in pitch'	(3) 'rhythmic beat'
	(2) 'higher in pitch'	(3) 'blurry'
	(3) 'softer'	
	(3) 'louder'	
	(2) 'shorter in duration'	
	(2) 'less distinct'	
/ko/	(7) /kol/	(5) /kol/
	(4) /kowʌ/	(6) 'increase in stress'
	(10) 'longer /o/'	(13) 'longer in duration'
	(2) 'shorter /o/'	(3) 'shorter in duration'
	(15) 'louder'	(2) 'faster'
	(3) 'softer'	(4) 'slower'
	(2) 'longer in duration'	(10) 'louder'
	(8) 'faster'	(5) 'lower in pitch'
	(2) 'slower'	(2) 'raspy quality'
	(4) 'glottal /o/'	(3) 'clearer'
	(5) 'increased stress on /k/'	(5) 'cannot describe change'
	(3) 'increased stress on /o/'	
'see'	(6) /sijʌ/	(4) 'longer /i/'
	(3) /si-I/	(6) 'longer /s/'
	(2) 'longer /i/'	(2) 'change in rhythm'
	(2) 'shorter /i/'	(8) 'softer'
	(4) 'increased stress'	(15) 'louder'
	(5) 'faster'	(10) 'cannot describe change'
	(3) 'slower'	(4) 'shorter in duration'
	(5) 'shorter in duration'	(2) 'longer in duration'
	(3) 'longer /s/'	(2) 'slower'
	(15) 'louder'	(5) 'faster'
	(2) 'softer'	
	(2) 'change in quality'	
	(2) 'lower in pitch'	
/ikfrɛ/	(7) /ikfrɛm/	(2) /ikfrɛm/
	(2) /ikfrʌm/	(4) 'cannot describe change'
	(9) /ikfrʌ/	(2) 'change in quality'
	(5) /ikfrə/	(12) 'louder'
	(11) 'increased stress on /frɛ/'	(9) 'softer'
	(2) 'increased duration of /f/'	(3) 'slower'
	(2) 'shorter duration on /ik/'	(4) 'faster'
	(5) 'faster'	(2) 'lower in pitch'
	(13) 'louder'	(2) 'higher in pitch'
	(3) 'softer'	(2) 'shorter in duration'
	(5) 'longer in duration'	(2) 'longer in duration'
	(3) 'higher in pitch'	
	(4) 'lower in pitch'	
	(2) 'softer /k/'	
'police'	(6) 'shorter /s/'	(9) 'prolonged /s/'
	(16) 'longer /s/'	(5) 'prolonged /o/'
	(8) 'increased stress on "lice"'	(3) 'distorted /s/'

Table 3 (*cont.*)

Stimulus	Phonetically trained group	Non-phonetically trained group
	(5) 'increased stress on "po"'	(2) 'longer in duration'
	(3) increased duration of /s/	(2) 'shorter in duration'
	(2) 'shorter in duration'	(3) 'slower'
	(5) 'longer in duration'	(2) 'faster'
	(7) 'faster'	(6) 'louder'
	(4) 'slower'	
	(5) 'louder'	
/trɛ os ri fæ/	(2) /krɛ os ri fæ/	(2) /krɛ os ri fæ/
	(2) /prɛ os ri fæ/	(3) 'longer in duration'
	(2) /trʌ os ri fæ/	(3) 'shorter in duration'
	(2) /træ os ri fæ/	(3) 'increased stress on /os/'
	(2) 'increased stress on /fæ/'	(3) 'clearer /os/'
	(6) 'increased stress on /os/'	(2) 'change in stress'
	(2) 'increased stress on /trɛ/'	(9) 'louder'
	(7) 'louder'	
	(2) 'softer'	
	(4) 'faster'	
	(2) 'slower'	
	(5) 'shorter in duration'	
	(3) 'longer pause between /os/ and /ri/'	
	(5) 'lower in pitch'	
	(2) 'higher in pitch'	
'our ship has sailed'	(5) 'ore ship has sailed'	(3) 'ore ship has sailed'
	(3) 'slower'	(11) 'louder'
	(3) 'faster'	(4) 'softer'
	(5) 'louder on "has sailed"'	(5) 'increased duration of /d/'
	(4) 'increased duration of /d/'	(2) 'increased duration of pause between "ship" and "has"'
	(2) 'shorter in duration'	(3) 'increased stress on "ship"'
	(2) 'longer in duration'	(2) 'clearer'
	(9) 'louder'	(2) 'distorted "ship"'
	(2) 'increased stress on "has"'	(2) 'decreased duration of pause between "has" and "sailed"'
	(3) 'increased stress on "ship"'	(3) 'lower in pitch'
	(2) 'lower in pitch'	(2) 'faster'
	(3) 'higher in pitch'	(2) 'shorter in duration'
	(2) 'more distinct on "has sailed"'	(2) 'change in stress pattern'

and reported fewer phonetic types of transformations. In addition, the fact that the non-phonetically trained group reported more often that they were unable to verbally express the change which they perceived, but were certain that some change had occurred in their perception of the repeating stimulus, is also not surprising in view of their lack of the 'tools' (namely the phonetic training and experiences) for expressing what they heard.

However, both groups of subjects reported the same *types* of transformations. In addition to phonetic types of verbal transformations, both groups reported changes in the various parameters of the auditory signal, including changes in the pitch, rate, duration, loudness, stress, clarity and quality of the repeating stimuli. In fact, the majority of all transformations for both subject groups were not phonetic in nature but rather involved such changes in the signals' parameters. Furthermore, the phonetic types of transformations which were reported by the non-phonetically trained subjects were identical to those reported in the phonetically trained group.

Therefore the findings of the present investigation do not corroborate earlier hypotheses by Naeser & Lilly (1970), Lass & Golden (1971) and Tekieli & Lass (1972) that the phonetic training of the subject may have a significant effect on the types of verbal transformations that he reports. All types of transformations reported by the phonetically trained group were also reported by the non-phonetically trained group of subjects as well. Furthermore, the phonetic types of transformations, and many of the non-phonetic types were identical for both listener groups. Thus, the effect of phonetic training appears to influence the quantity, but not the quality, of such reported transformations.

REFERENCES

LASS, N. J. & GOLDEN, S. S. (1971). The use of isolated vowels as auditory stimuli in eliciting the verbal transformation effect. *Can. J. Psychol.* **25**, 349–359.

LASS, N. J., WEST, L. K. & TAFT, D. D. (1973). A non-verbal analogue to the verbal transformation effect. *Can. J. Psychol.* (in press).

NAESER, M. A. & LILLY, J. C. (1970). Preliminary evidence for a universal feature detector system: perception of the repeating word. (Paper read to the Acoustical Society of America, Atlantic City, N.J.)

NATSOULAS, T. (1965). A study of the verbal-transformation effect. *Am. J. Psychol.* **78**, 257–263.

OBUSEK, C. J. (1968). A study of speech perception in the aged by means of the verbal transformation effect. (Unpublished Master's thesis, University of Wisconsin–Milwaukee.)

PERL, N. T. (1970). The application of the verbal transformation effect to the study of cerebral dominance. *Neuropsychologia* **8**, 259–261.

SIEGEL, S. (1956). *Nonparametric Statistics for the Behavioural Sciences.* New York: McGraw-Hill.

TAYLOR, M. M. & HENNING, G. B. (1963). Verbal transformations and an effect of instructional bias on perception. *Can. J. Psychol.* **17**, 210–223.

TEKIELI, M. E. & LASS, N. J. (1972). The verbal transformation effect: consistency of subject's reported verbal transformations. *J. gen. Psychol.* **86**, 231–245.

WARREN, R. M. (1961a). Illusory changes of distinct speech upon repetition: the verbal transformation effect. *Br. J. Psychol.* **52**, 249–258.

WARREN, R. M. (1961b). Illusory changes in repeated words: differences between young adults and the aged. *Am. J. Psychol.* **74**, 506–516.

WARREN, R. M. (1968). Verbal transformation effect and auditory perceptual mechanisms. *Psychol. Bull.* **70**, 261–270.

WARREN, R. M. & GREGORY, R. L. (1958). An auditory analogue of the visual reversible figure. *Am. J. Psychol.* **71**, 612–613.

WARREN, R. M. & WARREN, R. P. (1966). A comparison of speech perception in childhood, maturity, and old age by means of the verbal transformation effect. *J. verb. Learn. verb. Behav.* **5**, 142–146.

A NON-VERBAL ANALOGUE TO THE VERBAL
TRANSFORMATION EFFECT

NORMAN J. LASS, LINDA K. WEST, AND DIANE D. TAFT

ABSTRACT

The purpose of this investigation was to determine the effectiveness of non-speech sounds as auditory stimuli in eliciting a non-verbal analogue to the verbal transformation effect phenomenon. A total of five stimuli, three pure tones (250, 1000, and 4000 Hz), white noise, and a five-note musical motif, were presented to 25 adult listeners. Results indicate that the transformations elicited by the non-speech stimuli are similar in number of forms elicited, specific forms, and types of transformations to those produced by speech stimuli. Implications of these findings to the proposed mechanisms underlying the perception of speech are discussed.

THE VERBAL TRANSFORMATION EFFECT (Warren, 1961), the phenomenon in which continued listening to recorded repetitions of a stimulus produces perceptual illusory changes in normal listeners, has been found to occur for a variety of speech stimuli, including isolated vowels, consonant-vowel nonsense syllables, words, phrases, and sentences.

In addition, several studies have explored the effectiveness of non-speech stimuli in eliciting this type of perceptual phenomenon. Elliott (1963) employed repeating noise bursts at a rate of 20–160 per second and found that her subjects frequently reported increases in the rate and loudness of the bursts. Taylor and Henning (1963) used a beep pattern consisting of a 650 Hz tone switched on four times per second and reported the number of forms and transitions reported by their subjects. Fenelon and Blayden (1968) used a 1000 Hz pure tone as the repeating stimulus but only scored changes in the pitch of the tone as transformations. In applying the verbal transformation effect phenomenon to the study of cerebral dominance, Perl (1970) employed a 1000 Hz pure tone as the repeating stimulus, but reported only number of transformations. Obusek (1971) used a musical phrase and found that the majority of transformations reported involved changes in the *rhythm* or *tempo* of the stimulus.

In the studies cited above, only one type of non-speech stimulus was used in any single study. Furthermore, the studies differ in analysis procedures; some counted only certain types of reported changes as transformations, some reported only number of transformations, while others provided some description of the types of reported changes. Thus, comparison of findings from these investigations is frequently difficult and sometimes impossible to make.

CANADIAN JOURNAL OF PSYCHOLOGY, 1973, vol. 27, no. 3, 40-47.

The purpose of the present investigation was to explore further the effectiveness of non-speech auditory stimuli, including pure tones, white noise, and a musical motif, in eliciting transformations analogous to those reported for speech stimuli, in an attempt to determine if there exists a non-verbal analogue to the verbal transformation effect phenomenon.

METHOD

Subjects

A total of 25 individuals, 15 females and 10 males, served as subjects. All were students at West Virginia University. They ranged in age from 18 to 29 years, and had a mean age of 21 years. All subjects reported no hearing difficulty.

Auditory Stimuli

A total of five non-speech stimuli were employed in this investigation: (1) a 250 Hz pure tone; (2) a 1000 Hz pure tone; (3) a 4000 Hz pure tone; (4) white noise; and (5) a musical motif.

The pure tones were generated by a Hewlett-Packard model 200ABR pure-tone oscillator and passed through a Grason-Stadler model 162 speech audiometer. The white-noise signal was generated from the Grason-Stadler speech audiometer. The musical motif was generated by a Putney model VCS3 synthesizer and passed through the Grason-Stadler speech audiometer. All stimuli were recorded at 60 dB (re: 0.0002 microbar) using a Nagra model IV-D tape recorder.

Construction of Stimulus Tape

Electronic reproductions of the original recordings of the five stimuli were made using a Nagra model IV-D tape recorder and an Ampex model 602 tape recorder. From the electronic reproductions of the pure tones and white noise, 300 msec segments of each stimulus were cut and spliced into a tape loop with 500 msec pauses between stimuli on the loop. For the musical motif, each complete five-note motif, which was 1200 msec in duration, was cut and spliced into a tape loop with 500 msec pauses between motifs on the loop. In the above manner, a total of five tape loops were constructed, one for each of the five stimuli under investigation. Each tape loop was played repeatedly for a five-minute period on a Nagra model IV-D tape recorder and electronically reproduced on an Ampex model 602 tape recorder to produce the master stimulus tape.

Experimental Procedure

After orally presenting a set of instructions to the subject, the examiner played a practice tape of saw-tooth noise to familiarize the subject with the experimental task. Upon completion of the practice tape, the five experimental stimuli were played to the subject binaurally by means of a Nagra model IV-D tape recorder and a set of matched Sharpe model HA-10A headphones. All responses of the subject were recorded.

All five stimuli were presented to each subject individually in a single experimental session. The order of presentation of the stimuli was counterbalanced so that five orders were used, with five subjects in each of the five order groups. All sessions lasted approximately 45 minutes and were held in a sound-treated room at the West Virginia University Medical Center.

TABLE I

MEAN NUMBER OF FORMS, TRANSITIONS, AND REPETITIONS OF
EACH STIMULUS PRIOR TO THE SUBJECTS' FIRST
TRANSFORMATIONS

Stimulus	Forms	Transitions	Repetitions
250 Hz pure tone*	4.0	7.0	94.7
1000 Hz pure tone*	4.2	9.4	83.8
4000 Hz pure tone*	3.7	5.4	91.5
White noise*	5.3	11.9	67.8
Musical motif**	4.1	7.8	34.6

*375 repetitions in five minutes.
**250 repetitions in five minutes.

RESULTS

Number of Forms, Transitions, and Repetitions prior to First Transformations

Table I contains the average number of different forms (different perceptual phenomena), transitions (changes from one form to another), and repetitions of each stimulus prior to the subjects' first transformations. The table indicates the following: (1) there are only slight differences among the five stimuli in average number of forms elicited (a ratio of 1.43:1), while the differences for the average number of transitions are considerably larger (2.20:1), and those for the average number of repetitions are very large (2.74:1); (2) white noise elicited the largest average number of forms and transitions, while the fewest were produced by the 4000 Hz stimulus; (3) a larger average number of transitions than forms was elicited by all five stimuli; (4) an identical progression, from smallest to largest values, exists for forms and transitions for all stimuli, i.e., the stimulus yielding the fewest average number of forms (4000 Hz tone) elicited the fewest average number of transitions as well, etc.; and (5) the musical motif required the fewest average number of repetitions before eliciting the subjects' first transformations, while the largest average number of repetitions occurred for the 250 Hz pure tone stimulus.

Inferential statistical analysis, consisting of the use of sign tests (Siegel, 1956), was performed on the data. Results of this analysis indicate the following: (1) there are no significant differences among the five stimuli in number of forms which they elicited; (2) only one significant difference exists among stimuli for number of transitions reported: the white noise stimulus yielded a significantly larger number of transitions ($p <$ 0.05) than the 4000 Hz pure tone; and (3) all three pure tones and the white noise required a significantly larger number of repetitions ($p <$

0.01) before eliciting the subjects' first transformations than the musical motif stimulus.

Nature of Transformations

Table II contains a classification of the types of transformations elicited by the five stimuli. The classification employed was based on the different forms reported by all subjects in the study. The table indicates that the type of transformation reported most frequently for all stimuli involved a perceptual change in the pitch of the repeating signal, while changes in its phonetic structure were reported least frequently. The musical motif elicited no phonetic transformations by any of the subjects. Phonetic transformations that were reported often involved single-syllable forms, such as /b ʌ p/, /ik/, and /ip/, which were semantically as meaningless as the original repeating stimuli.

The category *Other* in Table II contains transformations which could not be placed into any of the existing categories. For example, sometimes the subjects could not express verbally the changes which they had perceived, but were certain that some change had occurred in their perception of the repeating stimuli. The musical motif stimulus produced the largest number of such transformations.

Discussion

The results of this study indicate that non-speech stimuli are effective in eliciting transformations from normal adult listeners. Furthermore, despite the apparent differences between the speech stimuli employed in previous studies and the non-speech material of the present investigation, there are many similarities in the elicited transformations.

The number of forms produced by the non-speech stimuli is similar to those obtained with speech material for a comparable number of repetitions. For example, Warren (1961) reports an average of 5.0 forms for 387 repetitions of *see*; an average of 4.0 forms was reported for 390 repetitions of the stimulus *ripe*; and the average based on all stimuli in Warren's study was 4.6 forms. This figure is very similar to the 4.3 average number of forms elicited by the five non-speech stimuli.

However, the numbers reported for transitions for the non-speech stimuli are much smaller than those reported by Warren (1961). An average of 13.9 transitions was reported for *see*, and *ripe* elicited an average of 21.6 transitions. The average number of transitions for all of Warren's stimuli was 17.6, much larger than the average of 8.3 transitions for the non-speech stimuli in the present investigation.

TABLE II

NUMBER AND PERCENTAGE OF TYPES OF TRANSFORMATIONS REPORTED BY THE 25 SUBJECTS FOR EACH OF THE FIVE NON-SPEECH STIMULI

Stimulus		Phonetic	Pitch	Rate	Duration	Loudness	Rhythm	Clarity	Quality	Familiar sounds	Other
250 Hz pure tone	N	6	73	33	19	33	9	6	4	5	2
	%	3.2	38.4	17.4	10.0	17.4	4.7	3.2	2.1	2.6	1.0
1000 Hz pure tone	N	5	119	31	30	19	7	16	8	6	6
	%	2.0	48.2	12.6	12.2	7.7	2.8	6.5	3.2	2.4	2.4
4000 Hz pure tone	N	2	60	15	32	18	4	4	13	9	6
	%	1.2	36.8	9.2	19.6	11.0	2.5	2.5	8.0	5.5	3.7
White noise	N	1	135	27	28	74	7	5	21	12	5
	%	0.0	42.9	8.6	8.9	23.5	2.2	1.7	6.7	3.8	1.7
Musical motif	N	0	76	13	21	45	16	2	8	9	9
	%	0.0	38.2	6.5	10.6	22.6	8.0	1.1	4.0	4.5	4.5

The majority of the non-speech stimuli required a larger average number of repetitions before eliciting the subjects' first transformations than did the speech stimuli in previous studies. In the Lass and Golden (1971) study, the average number of repetitions for the three isolated vowels employed as stimuli was 59.9. This figure is well below those reported for all three pure tones in the present study, similar to the number necessary for eliciting transformations from white noise, and considerably larger than the number needed for the musical motif stimulus.

In comparing the types of transformations reported in the present study with those reported in previous investigations employing speech stimuli, it is apparent that there are more similarities than differences between them. The categories which were originally established for speech stimuli (Lass & Golden, 1971; Lass & Gasperini, 1973; Tekieli & Lass, 1972) were identical with those used in the present study. Furthermore, reports of very similar, and in many cases identical, forms were obtained with both speech and non-speech stimuli. This finding indicates that listeners appear to be using the same criteria for signalling a change in this experiment with non-speech stimuli as they use when listening to speech stimuli; no apparent criteria shift occurs.

There are some differences between speech and non-speech repeating stimuli in the frequency of occurrence of some types of transformations, notably phonetic and pitch changes. In the Lass and Golden (1971) study, an average of 41.9% of all transformations reported for the three vowels were of the phonetic type and 11.2% involved pitch changes. In the present experiment, only 1.3% of all transformations were phonetic in nature, while 40.9% involved changes in the pitch of the repeating stimuli. However, there are also many similarities in the frequency of occurrence of the types of transformations for speech and non-speech stimuli: 3.0% of the non-speech transformations and 3.5% of the speech transformations involved the clarity of the repeating signal; 3.8% and 4.0% of all transformations involved changes to familiar sounds for the non-speech and speech stimuli, respectively; and 2.7% of the non-speech transformations and 1.8% of the vowel transformations reported by Lass and Golden could not be verbally expressed by the listeners and thus were placed in the *Other* category.

Obusek and Warren (1972, p. 10) indicate that "... there is as yet no convincing evidence that perceptual transformations analogous to VT's (verbal transformations) exist for repeated sequences of non-speech sounds." The findings of the present investigation indicate the existence of a non-verbal analogue to the verbal transformation effect phenomenon. Transformations are indeed elicited by non-speech stimuli and the number of forms, specific forms, and types of transformations which are reported are very similar to those elicited by speech stimuli.

Previous research on the verbal transformation effect phenomenon has suggested the existence of skilled reorganizational mechanisms which aid in the perception of speech (Warren, 1968). Verbal information appears to be stored and then confirmed on the basis of contextual cues. However, if the preliminary organization of speech sounds into words and phrases disagrees with subsequent contextual information, a reorganization of these sounds occurs. The absence of context causes a repeating word to continue to induce these skilled reorganizations which have been called *verbal transformations* (Warren, 1961). The findings in the present investigation, which indicate that such reorganizations also occur for non-speech stimuli, warrant further consideration of these proposed mechanisms underlying perception to include non-speech as well as speech sounds.

REFERENCES

ELLIOTT, L.L. Apparent change of repetitive noise bursts. *J. Acoust. Soc. Amer.*, 1963, 35, 1917–1923.

FENELON, B., & BLAYDEN, J.A. Stability of auditory perception of words and pure tones under repetitive stimulation in neutral and suggestibility conditions. *Psychon. Sci.*, 1968, 13, 285–286.

LASS, N.J., & GASPERINI, R.M. The verbal transformation effect: a comparative study of the verbal transformations of phonetically trained and non-phonetically trained subjects. *Brit. J. Psychol.*, 1973, 64, 183–192.

LASS, N.J., & GOLDEN, S.S. The use of isolated vowels as auditory stimuli in eliciting the verbal transformation effect. *Canad. J. Psychol.*, 1971, 25, 349–359.

OBUSEK, C.J. An experimental investigation of some hypotheses concerning the verbal transformation effect. Unpublished Ph.D. dissertation, University of Wisconsin-Milwaukee, 1971.

OBUSEK, C.J., & WARREN, R.M. Relation of the verbal transformation and the phonemic restoration effects. Unpublished manuscript, University of Wisconsin-Milwaukee, 1972.

PERL, N.T. The application of the verbal transformation effect to the study of cerebral dominance. *Neuropsychologica*, 1970, 8, 259–261.

SIEGEL, S. *Nonparametric Statistics for the Behavioral Sciences.* New York: McGraw-Hill, 1956.

TAYLOR, M.M., & HENNING, G.B. Transformations of perception with prolonged observation. *Canad. J. Psychol.*, 1963, 17, 349–360.

TEKIELI, M.E., & LASS, N.J. The verbal transformation effect: consistency of subjects' reported verbal transformations. *J. gen. Psychol.*, 1972, 86, 231–245.

WARREN, R.M. Illusory changes of distinct speech upon repetition – the verbal transformation effect. *Brit. J. Psychol.*, 1961, 52, 249–258.

WARREN, R.M. Verbal transformation effect and auditory perceptual mechanisms. *Psychol. Bull.*, 1968, 70, 261–270.

ORAL SENSATION AND PERCEPTION

A Theory Of The Speech Mechanism

As A Servosystem

Grant Fairbanks

EXPERIMENTAL phonetics is the study of the biological action known as *speaking* which produces the acoustical time-series known as *speech*. Numerous biological systems are involved in this action, but it is possible to consider them collectively as a single, larger, bio-acoustical system which is a proper object of study as such. It is this system, the *speaking system*, as a system, that I propose to discuss. While it is impractical to cite all my sources here, I want to mention my reliance upon the writings of MacCóll (*3*), Wiener (*9, 10*) and Trimmer (*8*) in the fields of control theory and cybernetics, and to make special acknowledgement of the personal influences of Seashore, Tiffin and Travis, who originally aroused my interest in the speaking system almost 20 years ago.

By way of review I will first show without discussion five diagrams of communication systems. Figure 1 is from Scripture (*5*), Figure 2 from Shannon (*6*), Figure 3 from Davis (*2*), and Figure 4 from Peterson (*4*).

Figure 5 shows Bott's (*1*) unpublished *speaker-listener causal series*, which has been passed on by word of mouth. As nearly as I can determine, it must have been formulated about 1930, antedating the four others. The diagram, which shows only structural elements, does not attempt to do justice to the complete statement.

Figure 6 shows an extension of the Bott scheme to a two-way speaker-listener system. Note that the brain of Speaker 1, B_1 at the left, is the source of Message 1, M_1, and also the destination of M_2, with B_2 serving analogous functions. Note also that each speaker is equipped with a transmitter and a receiver. Reflect that a given receiver, such as E_1, is operative at all times, even when its related transmitter, S_1, is producing signal intended for the independent receiver, E_2. M_1, in the form that it issues from S_1 under orders from B_1, is simultaneously relayed back to B_1 through E_1. In short, Speaker 1 hears himself as he talks. In Figure 7 we divide the diagram down the middle, make certain adaptations, and arrive at a more

JOURNAL OF SPEECH AND HEARING DISORDERS, 1954, vol. 19, 133-139.

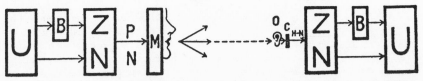

Figure 1. Diagram of the speech system. U, das Unbewusste; B, Bewusstsein; ZN, Zentralnervensystem; PN, peripheres Nervensystem; O, Ohr; C, Endorgan im Ohr; HN, Hörnerv. From Scripture (5).

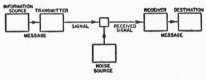

Figure 2. Schematic diagram of a general communication system. From Shannon (6).

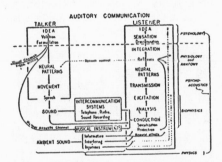

Figure 3. Diagram of the process of auditory communication. From Davis (2).

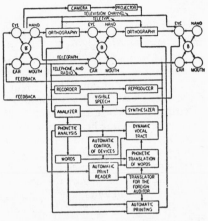

Figure 4. Fundamental systems in communication technology. From Peterson (4).

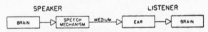

Figure 5. Structures of the speaker-listener causal series. After Bott (1).

complete diagram of the situation at the time S_1 is transmitting.

The return of M_1 to B_1 has often been referred to in such words as *auditory monitoring*, and interpreted as a sort of 'checking up' on what the speaking apparatus *has* produced. There is nothing wrong with this view of matters as far as it goes, but it seems to me that it misemphasizes the significance of self-hearing during speaking. It stresses the past. The essence of a speaking system, however, is control of the output, or prediction of the output's future. In this kind of system the significance of data about the past is that they are used for prediction of the future.

The 'monitoring' interpretation also suggests that the ear is a receiver in a listening system rather than a component of a speaking system. Theorists emphasize two different kinds of purposes for which measurements are made by the same instruments. Trimmer (7) illustrates this by comparing the use of the same scales, first to determine the unknown weight of a watermelon and then to weigh out exactly five pounds of sugar. In the

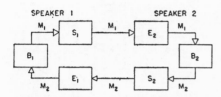

SPEAKER 1   SPEAKER 2

FIGURE 6. Two-way speaker-listener system. B, brain; S, speaking mechanism; M, message; E, ear.

case of the watermelon, the purpose was *estimation* of weight; in the case of the sugar it was *control* of weight. In Figure 7, E_1 and B_1 are measuring M_1 for purposes of control. In Figure 6 they are measuring M_2 for purposes of estimation. When I say a word and you repeat it, your hearing apparatus measures my word for purposes of estimation and then your word (the same word) for purposes of control. When we are referring to the control functions of the auditory signal, I suggest *auditory feedback* as the term of choice.

The speaking system does not seem to be what is called an *open cycle* control system. In open cycle control the device that produces the output is controlled by some quantity that is independent of the output. Devices such as alarm clocks, in which an event is controlled by time, are familiar examples. The speech synthesizers that I have seen employ this form of control. A deaf child, while being taught to speak by a deaf therapist who pursues the method of phonetic placement with a tongue blade, is almost entirely under open cycle control.

A *closed cycle* system, or *servosystem*, on the other hand, employs feedback of the output to the place of control, comparison of the output to the input, and such manipulation of the output-producing device as will cause the output to have the same

functional form as the input. The system performs its task when, by these means, it produces an output that is equal to the input times a constant. Examples of such systems are the heating plants of our homes and the homeostatic mechanisms of our bodies. It seems evident that the speaking system has at least the rudiments of a servosystem. In Figure 8 we explore this further with the model shown in block diagram.

If we start with the *effector unit*, shown at the top, we observe a *motor*, a *generator* and a *modulator* connected as shown. These are the respiratory, vibratory and resonation-articulatory structures, respectively. (The model deliberately simplifies. If it were more elaborate, the generator, for instance, would be shown as a multi-unit device capable of producing various types of inputs for the modulator, and in part located physically within the latter.) The *output* is shown by the heavy arrow at the right. The heavy lines and arrows at the top symbolize the effector's motor innervation.

The *sensor unit* at the bottom is so-labelled to emphasize its control function. (If its function were estimation, it would be called a *receiver*.) *Sensor 1* is the primary component for output take-off, the ear. The output is conducted to sensor 1 over two

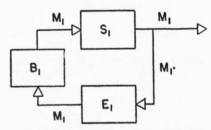

FIGURE 7. Elements of the control system for speaking. B, brain; S, speaking mechanism; M, message; E, ear.

180

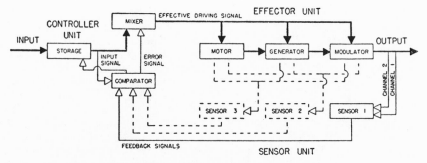

FIGURE 8. Model of a closed cycle control system for speaking.

separate channels, representing the acoustic pathways to the ear through the air and through the body tissues. *Sensor 2* and *sensor 3* symbolize the tactile and proprioceptive end-organs. These supply data about the mechanical operation of the effector, but not directly about its output. Although correlated with the output data taken off through sensor 1, these data are comparatively fragmentary. The sensor unit relays its data to the *controller unit* in the form of *feedback signals*.

The controller is an automatic device that issues specific orders to the effector. It does not originate the message, but receives its instructions from a separate unit not shown. We are concerned here with a speaking system and assume an input, although plausible extensions along these same lines may be made to a model of a language system which also originates messages.

The anatomical analogy is less definite here than for the effector and sensor, and my tendency is to keep it so for the time being. This indefiniteness does not, however, restrain us from fruitful discussion of an automatic controller in terms of functional units, and, of course, we should remind ourselves all along that this is a model, not a replica.

While a closed cycle heating system, for example, may be required only to maintain a constant pre-set temperature, the speaking system must vary its output as a function of time, according to instructions laid down at the input. The output consists of qualitatively different units that must be displayed in a time sequence that is unique. The selection and ordering of units are carried on in advance, usually for a number of units, and represent a set of input instructions. As speaking continues, each set is replaced by another. As the first component of the controller, therefore, we provide a *storage* device, which receives and stores the input and gives off an *input signal*. The number of units that it can store is comparatively small and the time that it will retain them is short. This is the short persistence memory of what we intend to say next. We may think of this device as a tape recorder in which instructions are stored. Its tape drive is alternately started and stopped, and when the tape is stationary a given unit of instruction is repeatedly reproduced by a moving scanning head.

A stored unit of instruction, or input, corresponds to a unit of output. Each such unit furnishes what is termed a *control point*, sometimes

181

called *set point*. The control points are the unit goals of the output. The input signal corresponding to a control point goes simultaneously from the storage component to the controller's other two components, a *comparator* and a *mixer*. The comparator also receives the feedback signals, as stated earlier. With the input and feedback signals it performs a calculation, essentially subtraction, in which it determines the difference between the two. At any given time it thus yields a measure of the amount by which the control point has not yet been reached by the output, or a measure of the non-accomplishment of the control point. This measure is termed the *error signal*. In the act of speaking, the error signal, at the time in question, is the amount by which the intended speech unit, then displayed in the storage device, has not yet been produced by the effector.

The error signal will equal zero when the control point has been achieved by the effector. At such a time as it does not equal zero, the error signal provides data which cause the effector to modify its operation in such a manner as to bring the error signal closer to zero. It continues with time to modify the operation of the effector progressively so that the error signal approaches and finally reaches zero.

To bring this about the error signal is continuously fed into the mixer, the function of which is to combine error signal and input signal into the *effective driving signal*. The latter furnishes specific instructions to the effector. It alters the effector's operation, causing its output, relayed back to the comparator in the form of feedback signal, more nearly to equal the input signal and thus reduce the error signal. The reduced error signal is then fed into the mixer, modifies

the effective driving signal accordingly, and so on around the loop until the error signal equals zero.

At such a time the first unit has been completed and the system is ready for new instruction. The information that that is the state of the system is given, we repeat, by the fact of zero error signal. In the model you will note that the error signal is fed into the storage component as well as into the mixer. In the storage component, however, it acts in simple all-or-none fashion to trigger display of the next control point when it equals zero, or to retain a given control point when it does not equal zero. In the tape recorder that we imagined earlier as the storage device, it would start and stop the tape drive.

This triggering device has an important refinement of that basic operation. Since the time constants of the live speaking system are relatively long in comparison to the durations of steady states in the output, analogous time constants are assumed for the model. This being the case, the system would have a low ceiling on its rate of output, if advancement of instructions were permitted only at times of zero error signal. The comparator includes, therefore, a predicting device. By plotting the error signal as a function of time during production of a given unit, this device continuously predicts by extrapolation the future time at which the error signal will equal zero. Thus advancement of the storage component to the next control point is not necessarily delayed until the actual moment when a condition of zero error signal obtains. It may be triggered in advance of that time by an amount, let us say, equal to the relevant time constants. By this means, over suitable channels, a new input can be started on its way toward the effector before the previous control point has been reached so that it will arrive there at an appropriate anticipated time.

It may have been observed that, when the model starts operation from the inactive state, the effective driving signal is not at the outset modified by the error signal, there being as yet no error signal. Under such conditions the output is uncontrolled for an amount of time equal to the time constant of the entire system. This is inherent in a feedback-controlled system unless the time constant is negligible. In the live system it is suggested either that the excitation of the effector is highly generalized, resulting in an initial output that is undifferentiated until it comes under control, or that the effector's operation during this initial period is mediated by subtle programing of sequences not dependent upon sensory feedbacks.

The system has another important undiagramed characteristic. In the mixer the rate of change of the effective driving signal is caused to vary with the magnitude of the error signal. When the error signal is large, as at the start of a unit, the corrective change is rapid. It becomes progressively slower as the error signal is reduced. An advantage of this feature is reduction of overshoot.

Numerous times we have used the term *unit* in the sense of unit of control. Such a control unit should not be identified with any of the conventional units such as the phoneme, the syllable, the word, or the word group. There is no time to develop this idea for the live speaking system beyond saying, first, that it is not theoretically necessary that the unit of control be any presently identified phonetic unit, and, second, that we have evidence from several experiments suggesting that it is something

else. It might be ventured tentatively that the unit of control is a semi-periodic, relatively long, articulatory cycle, with a correlated cycle of output. It is more satisfactory at present, however, merely to propose the existence of a hypothetical unit of speech control, as yet unspecified and unnamed, whose characteristics are dimly coming to be seen.

The idea of building a mechanical model of the speaking system that we have discussed is appealing. Comparatively simple effector and sensor components which can process recognizable speech signal are within the art. We hope shortly to begin construction of a simple controller, based on a relay network, that works on paper. Although to validate the theory it is not necessary that the machine talk, it seems possible that a first approximation to connected speech can be realized.

One evident feature of the model, as well as of the live system, is that it contains many components in a complicated arrangement and readily becomes disordered. One type of disorder is part failure. In that case, unless the part can be replaced or repaired, the change in output must either be compensated or tolerated. A part disorder is also a system disorder. The model can be caused to repeat, prolong and hesitate by several different manipulations, one of which is feedback delay. By manipulations that are revealingly similar it can be caused to make other kinds of mistakes, such as substitutions, distortions and omissions. All such disorders are demonstrably caused by component deficiencies. In the model *organic* and *functional* are one.

Since the dynamic events of connected speech have become conveniently accessible through the X-ray motion picture and the acoustic spectrogram, students of speech perception have been giving considerable attention to the psychophysical significance of spectral changes in the speech signal. Although this subject is outside the scope of the present paper, a brief comment seems worthwhile.

Phoneticians have long recognized that the elements of speech are not produced in step-wise fashion like the notes of a piano, but by continuous modulation as a function of time. Certain of the elements, such as the diphthongs, involve characteristic changes during their durations, losing their entities if they do not so change. Other elements, such as the vowels, may be prolonged indefinitely in the steady state and change is not considered to be a defining feature. During production of elements of the latter type in connected speech, however, changes occur. Movements to and from articulatory positions result in acoustic transitions to and from steady states in the output.

In the model we have seen how a transition is used for purposes of control and prediction. From it is derived a changing error signal. The model's objective is to reduce this error signal to zero, and at such a time as that has been accomplished the control point will have been reached. In the case of the production of elements of speech that involve steady states, the control points and error signals correspond, respectively, to steady states and acoustic transitions in the output. It is to be emphasized that the steady states are the primary objectives, the targets. The transitions are useful incidents on the way to the targets. The roles of both are probably very analogous when the dynamic speech output is perceived by an independent listener.

References

1. BOTT, E. A. (Indirect personal communication.)
2. DAVIS, H. Auditory communication. *JSHD*, 16, 1951, 3-8.
3. MacCOLL, L. A. *Fundamental Theory of Servomechanisms*. New York: D. Van Nostrand, 1945.
4. PETERSON, G. E. Basic physical systems for communication between two individuals. *JSHD*, 18, 1953, 116-120.
5. SCRIPTURE, E. W. Der Mechanismus der Sprachsysteme. Z. *Experimentalphonetik*, 1, 1931, 85-90.
6. SHANNON, C. E. and W. WEAVER. *The Mathematical Theory of Communication*. Urbana: Univ. of Ill. Press, 1949.
7. TRIMMER, J. D. The basis for a science of instrumentology. *Science*, 118, 1953, 461-465.
8. ————. *Response of Physical Systems*. New York: Wiley, 1950.
9. WIENER, N. *Cybernetics*. New York: Wiley, 1948.
10. ————. *The Human Use of Human Beings*. Boston: Houghton Mifflin, 1950.

SOME EFFECTS OF TACTILE AND AUDITORY
ALTERATIONS ON SPEECH OUTPUT

ROBERT L. RINGEL

M. D. STEER

This investigation studied the effects on articulation, duration, average peak level, and fundamental frequency of speech demonstrated by normal subjects when oral region tactile and/or auditory sensory information is altered. Thirteen female subjects read a standard passage under the following six conditions: (a) control; (b) binaural masking; (c) topical anesthetization of the oral region by application of Xylocaine HCl 4%; (d) local anesthetization of the oral region by bilateral mandibular and infra-orbital nerve block techniques employing Xylocaine HCL 2%; (e) simultaneous administration of conditions b and c; (f) simultaneous administration of conditions b and d. Recorded speech samples for all conditions were subjected to analysis by use of a high speed level recorder, a phonation timer, and an oscillographic technique. The speech samples were also analyzed for articulatory deviations by a panel of judges. Statistical analysis of the data indicated that significant alterations in average peak level, articulation, and rate variability occur under conditions of altered tactile sensation. Similar trends were also noted for the mean syllable duration and phonation/time ratio variables. In addition it was found that the effects of multiple sensory disturbances are cumulative in nature for certain speech output variables.

The principal source of information concerning the relation between sensory alterations and speech performance has been the study of the effects of temporally delayed auditory feedback on speech output. It has been reported that under such conditions the articulation, speech sound duration, fundamental frequency, and sound pressure level characteristics of speech output are modified (Fairbanks, 1955).

Although research efforts concerned with systematic alterations of auditory feedback have been extensive, relatively little research has been conducted to assess the contribution of taction or the interaction of taction and audition upon the speech monitoring process. McCroskey (1958) attempted to clarify the role of tactile feedback in speech by eliminating the tactile cues in and around the oral region by local anesthesia. In general, he found that tactile disturbances resulted in decreased levels of articulatory accuracy.

The scarcity of research in this area may be attributed to the specialized skills required in using techniques which alter the tactile sense. Techniques such as anesthetization, while common in the physiologist's laboratory, do not

JOURNAL OF SPEECH AND HEARING RESEARCH, 1963, vol. 6, 369-378.

185

appear to have been used widely by speech scientists in their investigations of the speech mechanism. The present study was designed to determine the effects on such speech output variables as average peak level, fundamental frequency, speech duration, and articulation when auditory and oral region tactile sensory information is altered experimentally.

METHOD

Subjects. Thirteen females majoring in speech pathology and audiology served as subjects in this investigation. The age range of this group was 18-29 years, with a mean age of 20.1 years. The following criteria were met by all subjects: (a) normal hearing, as indicated by a pure tone audiometric test; (b) no previous adverse reaction to use of dental anesthesia; and, (c) willingness to submit to a series of intra-oral hypodermic injections by a qualified professional person.

Procedure. Oral region anesthetization was performed by a dental surgeon. Upon completion of the anesthetization procedures, each subject was seated in a dental chair located in an anechoic chamber. The headrest was adjusted so that the subject's mouth was directly in front of and 12 inches away from a microphone (Altec Model 29-A). The microphone and power supply (Altec Model 525-A) were used in conjunction with a tape recorder (Ampex Model 601) to record each subject's oral reading of a standard passage, under six experimental conditions.

Each subject was required to return to the laboratories on separate days for administration of one of each of the following six randomly assigned conditions: (1) control (absence of either anesthesia or experimentally introduced noise); (2) binaural white masking noise (94dB re:0.0002 dyne/cm²); (3) topical anesthetization of the oral region by application of Xylocaine HCl 4%; (4) local anesthetization of the oral region by bilateral mandibular and infra-orbital nerve block techniques as described by McCroskey (1958), employing Xylocaine HCl 2%; (5) simultaneous use of binaural masking noise and anesthetization of the oral region by topical application of Xylocaine HCl 4%; (6) simultaneous use of binaural masking noise and local anesthetization of the oral region by bilateral mandibular and infra-orbital nerve block technique, employing Xylocaine HCl 2%.

It was hypothesized that data obtained for these six experimental conditions provided information regarding speech output performance under the following feedback states: (a) absence of experimentally introduced feedback disturbances (condition one), (b) disturbed auditory feedback (condition two), (c) minimal interference in the tactile feedback channel (condition three), (d) severe alterations within the tactile feedback channel (condition four), and (e) simultaneous disturbances within the auditory and tactile feedback systems (conditions five and six).

Since the extent and speed of drug diffusion throughout the oral region is not known, statements regarding the effect of the drugs used must be guarded.

However, based on available anatomical information (Grant, 1956), results of pilot investigations dealing with tests of diadochocinesis under drug conditions (Ringel, 1962), and similar use of Xylocaine in other anatomical regions (Provins, 1955; Weidling, 1959, pp. 30-46), it seems tenable that the administration of Xylocaine to the oral region by either the topical or nerve blocking technique used in this investigation resulted in tactile sense deprivation.

Measurements and Instrumentation. Measurements of average peak level and fundamental frequency output were made upon the following sample sentence (Sentence No. 3) which was selected at random from the six-sentence passage previously mentioned: "Years later boilers and engines were invented and sailors could strike their enemies at will."

The recorded sample sentences were coupled from the tape recorder on which they were originally recorded to a high speed level recorder (Bruel and Kjaer, Model 2304), and average peak level measures were obtained from the resultant graphic recordings. The average, or mean, peak level was determined by a "peak counting" method which consisted essentially of measuring the amplitude of energy peaks above a pre-set reference base line (in the present investigation a 50 dB potentiometer was used and the base line was set at 60 dB SPL). Only those peaks which represented a difference of at least 5 dB from the preceding peak were counted. Mean fundamental frequency values were determined through analysis of photographic tracings taken from an oscilloscope (DuMont Dual Beam Oscilloscope, Model 322A, and Fairchild Oscillo-Record Camera, Model 246A). The photographic tracings of sound wave patterns were analyzed in segments of 1/26th of a second in a manner similar to that used for the analysis of photophonophenellograms (Hanley, 1951).

The measures of phonation/time ratio, mean syllable duration, and overall word-per-minute rate were made on the entire experimental reading passage through the use of the tape recorder and the Purdue Speech Timer. In addition, the word-per-minute rate for three sentences taken at random from the passage was also determined. In this analysis of sentences one, four, and six (S1, S4 and S6), the tape recorder and speech timer were also used. Inasmuch as the principles underlying the function of this timer have been described previously (Travis, 1957, p. 217) it is sufficient here to note that the timer was set to measure signals above a pre-set reference level of 48 dB SPL. As in the case of the speech duration measures, judgments of the subjects' articulation performance were made upon the entire reading passage. The recorded speech samples were reproduced for articulation judgments on the tape recorder and were monitored through matched sets of earphones (Telephonics TDH-39). The articulation judgments were made by a panel of four judges, each of whom has had extensive experience in evaluating articulatory proficiency in continuous speech. The judges were instructed to evaluate the recordings with respect to articulation as critically as possible and to indicate the number of articulatory deviations present in each recording on a prepared evaluation sheet, in accordance with the criteria suggested by Van Riper (1954, p. 165).

The means and standard deviations for each speech output variable for the 13 subjects are shown in Table 1. It is seen that, in general, the values associated with both the control and masking noise conditions are consistent with previously summarized research findings (Ham, 1957; Schwartz, 1957). Table 1 also shows that the presence of feedback disturbances is generally associated with speech output variable alterations.

TABLE 1. Summary of means and standard deviations for selected speech output variables.

Speech Output Variables			Experimental Conditions					
			$C°$	N	TA	NB	TAN	NBN
Average Peak Level (in dB		Mean	72.7	83.8	80.8	81.8	87.7	91.0
re: 0.0002 dyne/cm²)		SD	2.4	4.1	4.0	3.6	3.3	4.8
Fundamental Frequency		Mean	228.8	249.0	225.8	226.5	240.5	248.3
(in cps)		SD	16.8	25.3	20.8	22.5	15.3	14.8
Phonation/Time Ratios		Mean	.561	.712	.570	.600	.661	.683
(in sec)		SD	.050	.063	.096	.108	.086	.081
Word Per Min. Rate		Mean	172.6	160.0	170.6	161.4	161.5	152.9
		SD	17.9	19.1	17.6	18.2	21.5	24.9
	S1°°	Mean	211.4	202.4	216.4	193.6	204.5	182.7
		SD	25.9	27.0	24.8	31.3	32.0	27.1
Selected Sentence Word	S4	Mean	188.2	176.5	190.0	177.4	177.0	165.4
Per Min. Rate		SD	22.2	21.4	19.0	19.1	26.4	17.9
	S6	Mean	199.4	176.1	205.1	183.7	186.0	170.7
		SD	24.5	18.8	16.5	22.0	24.9	30.7
Mean Syllable Duration		Mean	.153	.202	.155	.172	.192	.207
(in sec)		SD	.022	.022	.026	.028	.022	.030
Articulation Error Scores		Mean	4.7	6.9	6.5	23.1	10.5	24.4
		SD	2.3	3.3	4.2	7.0	4.9	9.6

°Key: C = Control
N = Binaural Masking Noise
TA = Topical Anesthesia
NB = Nerve Block Anesthesia
TAN = Topical Anesthesia and Binaural Masking Noise
NBN = Nerve Block Anesthesia and Binaural Masking Noise
°°S1, S4, S6, refer to sentences 1, 4, 6, respectively

To determine the significance of the above noted alterations, the data were subjected to analysis of variance statistical procedures. The results of these analyses, summarized in Table 2, indicate that significantly large variance ratios exist when experimental conditions are compared relative to the average peak level, phonation/time ratio, mean syllable duration and articulation proficiency variables, and for fundamental frequency data ($p = .05$). In addition, Table 2

TABLE 2. Summary of analyses of variance tests for selected speech output variables.

Speech Output Variables	Source	df	ms	F	F.05°
Average Peak Level	Between Conditions	5	517.9	36.7[1]	2.39
	Within Conditions	72	14.2		
Fundamental Frequency	Between Conditions	5	60.8	3.9	2.39
	Within Conditions	72	15.5		
Phonation/Time Ratio	Between Conditions	5	.513	7.59	2.39
	Within Conditions	72	.068		
Mean Syllable Duration	Between Conditions	5	.727	10.9	2.39
	Within Conditions	72	.066		
Articulation Error Scores	Between Conditions	5	4058	12.9	2.21
	Within Conditions	306	314		
Word Per Min. Rate	Between Conditions	5	684.1	1.7	2.39
	Within Conditions	72	401.7		
Selected Sentence Word Per Min. Rate C	Between Sentences	2	1 762.8	3.4	3.26
	Within Sentences	36	518.5		
N	Between Sentences	2	2 961.3	5.8	3.26
	Within Sentences	36	514.5		
TA	Between Sentences	2	2 273.9	5.4	3.26
	Within Sentences	36	418.4		
NB	Between Sentences	2	867.1	1.4	3.26
	Within Sentences	36	611.2		
TAN	Between Sentences	2	2 544.6	3.3	3.26
	Within Sentences	36	782.9		
NBN	Between Sentences	2	1 029.9	1.5	3.26
	Within Sentences	36	667.7		

[1]Since the between-subject variance was not removed from the error term the F ratios shown above are spuriously low.
°F.05 for nearest tabled df values.

reveals that, although significant variability does not exist in relation to the overall word-per-minute rate, instances of significant rate variability are noted in relation to the selected sentence output variable for the control condition, and for those conditions which did not involve the use of nerve block anesthesia ($p = .05$). In view of these general statistical findings, further analysis of the data through the application of the Student-Newman-Keuls test (Steel and Torrie, p. 110) was conducted. The results of this multiple range test are summarized in Table 3. Briefly, the function of this test is to determine for each variable at a specified level of confidence which mean values, within a group of such values, differ significantly one from another. The findings for each of the speech output variables studied follow.

TABLE 3. Summary of results of Student-Newman-Keuls' tests for significance of differences between mean values for selected speech output variables.[*]

Speech Output Variables	Mean Values					
Average Peak Level	C 72.7	TA 80.8	NB 81.8	N 83.8	TAN 87.7	NBN 91.0
Fundamental Frequency	TA 225.8	NB 226.5	C 228.8	TAN 240.5	NBN 248.3	N 249.0
Phonation/Time Ratio	C .561	TA .570	NB .600	TAN .661	NBN .683	N .712
Mean Syllable Duration	C .153	TA .155	NB .172	TAN .192	N .202	NBN .207
Articulation Error Scores	C 4.7	TA 6.5	N 6.9	TAN 10.5	NB 23.1	NBN 24.4

[*]Any two means not underscored by the same line are significantly different at the 5% probability level.

Average Peak Level

Inspection of Table 3 reveals that under conditions involving the presence of masking noise, topical anesthesia, or block anesthesia, the average peak level of speech increases significantly in relation to the level obtained under the control condition ($p = .05$). Furthermore, the condition in which nerve block anesthesia and masking noise are used simultaneously results in a significantly higher average peak level than those levels obtained with injection and topical anesthesia alone, masking noise alone, or topical anesthesia in conjunction with masking noise ($p = .05$). In addition, Table 3 shows that the condition characterized by the simultaneous use of topical anesthesia and binaural masking results in an average peak level that is substantially greater than that obtained for either condition of anesthesia or noise separately. This increment, while relatively large, was not significant at the .05 probability level, however.

As noted in Table 1, an average peak level value of 72.7 dB is found during the control condition and an increment of about 10 dB occurs in the presence of high level masking noise. These findings are consistent with those previously reported (Miller, 1951, p. 32; Silverstein, 1953). The observed tendency toward increased amplitude of performance under tactile alteration conditions also agrees with the numerous reports of speech signal amplitude increments in the presence of delayed auditory feedback (Atkinson, 1952; Black, 1951; Fairbanks, 1955) and with Smith, McCrary, and Smith's (1960) report of amplitude disturbances on writing and drawing tasks under conditions of delayed visual feedback.

Fundamental Frequency

The results of the Student-Newman-Keuls test also revealed that a significant increase in the mean fundamental frequency of speech output is associated with the presence of high level masking noise ($p = .05$). However, anesthetization of the oral region by either topical or nerve block techniques alone does not result in mean fundamental frequency values which are significantly different from those obtained under the control condition.

Both the mean value of 228.8 cps obtained for the female subjects under the control condition and the rise in fundamental frequency in the presence of high level masking noise are consistent with previously noted observations (Curry, 1940; Silverstein, 1953). The failure to find statistically significant alterations in fundamental frequency which might be attributed to disturbances within the tactile feedback channels, however, does not agree generally with findings reported for alterations within the auditory feedback system. Lee (1950), Black (1955), and Fairbanks (1955) have reported that a common response to delayed auditory sidetone is a rise in pitch.

Speech Duration

The data in Table 3 reveal that the presence of high level masking noise is associated with a significantly increased phonation/time ratio ($p = .05$). It is also indicated that a similar tendency toward increased phonation/time ratio exists for the nerve block anesthesia condition.

Significant increments in mean syllable duration are shown in the comparisons between the control condition and those conditions involving the use of masking noise ($p = .05$). When conditions involving the use of anesthesia by itself are compared with conditions involving the use of masking noise by itself or in conjunction with anesthesia, significant differences in syllable length occur ($p = .05$). Finally, statistically unsignificant, but relatively large differences in mean syllable duration occur when the nerve block anesthesia condition is compared with the control and topical anesthesia condition.

As indicated in Table 2, the overall word-per-minute rate is not significantly altered under any of the experimental conditions. Attention should be directed, however, to the selected sentence word-per-minute data. As stated earlier, this data was derived from three sentences drawn at random from the entire passage and analyzed for rate. Table 1 contains the mean values determined for each of the three sentences. Table 2 contains the results of comparisons made among sentences one, four and six (S1, S4, and S6) for each condition. These data indicate the presence of significant variability of rate from sentence to sentence for the control condition, and for each of the other experimental conditions, except those involving the use the nerve block anesthetization ($p = .05$).

As in the instances previously noted, the results obtained in this investigation for the four speech duration variables are in general agreement with the findings reported by other investigators. The observation that phonation/time ratios increase in the presence of high level masking noise has been reported previously by Draegert (1951) and Hanley and Draegert (1949). Whereas the effects of nerve block anesthesia on phonation/time ratio were not as marked as those of masking noise, a trend was noted in the direction of an increase. Failure to find significant alterations for this variable have also been reported in delayed auditory sidetone research. Ham (1957) noted negligible phonation/time ratio changes under altered auditory feedback conditions, and Fairbanks (1955) stated that, while the average phonation time clearly increased under delayed sidetone, the pause time also increased in a proportionate manner. He concluded that the phonation/time ratio does not give a true picture of the effects of altered auditory feedback.

Retardation of speaking rate is generally considered a common sequel of altered auditory feedback (Atkinson, 1952; Hanley and Steer, 1949). In the present investigation, however, while the overall speaking rate was reduced under certain circumstances, it was not significantly retarded under any experimental condition. Variability of rate from sentence to sentence was found to exist under all conditions except those involving the use of injection anesthesia. These observations are consistent with those made by Kelly and Steer (1949) that the overall rate of speech is not a sensitive estimate of a speaker's performance. They noted that gross measures of overall rate do not indicate normal rate variability. Implied in the findings of Kelly and Steer and others (Murray and Tiffin, 1934) is the fact that normal speech rate is variable. Hence, the observation that only conditions involving the use of nerve block anesthesia did not show rate variability takes on increased significance.

The results of the mean syllable duration analysis conducted in this investigation revealed that the presence of significant syllable prolongations was associated with those conditions involving masking noise and the condition in which nerve block anesthesia was used alone. The presence of prolonged syllables in voice performance under noise had been reported earlier by Hanley and Steer (1949). In addition, the effects of tactile alterations on syllable length are in agreement with the results reported by Fairbanks (1955), McCroskey (1958), and Ham (1957) for the effects of delayed sidetone on syllable duration.

Articulation

Perhaps the speech output variable most severely affected by oral region anesthetization was articulation. It is noted from the Table 3 data that the presence of nerve block anesthesia is associated with significantly more articulatory errors than are found under any of the other experimental conditions ($p =$ .05). It is also observed that while the sole use of topical anesthesia or masking noise does not significantly impair articulation, their simultaneous use does result in a trend toward a significantly adverse effect on the level of articulatory proficiency demonstrated in the control, masking noise, or topical anesthesia conditions. It should be noted, however, that this effect is not as severe as that resulting from the injection of anesthesia into the oral region.

The presence of a significantly increased number of articulation errors under nerve block induced tactile feedback alteration conditions has also been reported by McCroskey (1958). Further support for the finding that errors of performance accuracy result from input alterations is demonstrated in the results of research on the auditory and visual sensory channels. Black (1955), Lee (1950), Fairbanks (1955), and Atkinson (1952) have described speech under delayed auditory feedback as being characterized by general articulatory inaccuracy while Smith, McCrary and Smith (1960), in describing visual and drawing performance under delayed visual feedback circumstances, noted seriously impaired performances and presented illustrations of generally inaccurate writing patterns.

SUMMARY

An investigation was conducted to determine the effects on speech output when oral region tactile and auditory sensory information is altered. Each subject was recorded during a reading of a standard passage under a series of experimental conditions involving two types of oral region anesthatization and/or binaural masking noise. Speech samples were analyzed for average peak level, fundamental frequency, speech duration and articulatory alterations.

The effects of binaural masking noise upon speech output were found to be consistent with those previously reported. Unique to this investigation, however, was the study of the effects on speech performance of oral region tactile alterations by themselves or in interaction with auditory disturbances. It is reported that, in general, under conditions of nerve block anesthesia, speech is characterized by significant increments in amplitude of performance, lack of rate variability, and articulatory inaccuracy. Finally, it is reported that for certain speech output variables the effects of multiple sensory disturbances are cumulative in nature.

The authors wish to acknowledge with appreciation the support given to this research by the Purdue Research Foundation and the American Speech and Hearing Foundation. This paper is based upon a doctoral dissertation completed by Robert L. Ringel at Purdue University under the direction of M. D. Steer.

REFERENCES

ATKINSON, C., Vocal responses during controlled aural stimulation. *J. Speech Hearing Dis.,* 17, 419-426 (1952).

BLACK, J., The effects of delayed sidetone upon vocal rate and intensity. *J. Speech Hearing Dis.,* 16, 56-60 (1951).

BLACK, J., The persistence of the effects of delayed sidetone. *J. Speech Hearing Dis.,* 20, 65-68 (1955).

CURRY, E., The pitch characteristics of the adolescent male voice. *Speech Monogr.,* 7, 48-62 (1940).

DRAEGERT, G., Relationships between voice variables and speech intelligibility in high level noise. *Speech Monogr.,* 18, 272-278 (1951).

FAIRBANKS, G., Selected vocal effects of delayed auditory feedback. *J. Speech Hearing Dis.,* 20, 333-336 (1955).

GRANT, J., *An Atlas of Anatomy* (4th Ed.). Baltimore: Williams & Wilkins (1956).

HAM, R., Certain effects of speech alternations in the auditory feedback of speech defectives and normals. Ph.D. dissertation, Purdue Univ. (1957).

HANLEY, T., An analysis of vocal frequency and duration characteristics of selected samples of speech from three American dialect regions. *Speech Monogr.,* 18, 78-93 (1951).

HANLEY, T., and DRAEGERT, G., Effects of level of distracting noise upon speaking rate, duration and intensity. Tech. Report SDC 104-2-14. Contract N 60 ri 104. T.C. II, 1949.

HANLEY, T., and STEER, M., Effects of level of distracting noise upon speaking rate, duration and intensity. *J. Speech Hearing Dis.*, 14, 363-368 (1949).

KELLY, J., and STEER, M., Revised concept of rate. *J. Speech Hearing Dis.*, 14, 222-226 (1949).

LEE, B., Effects of delayed speech feedback. *J. acoust. Soc. Amer.*, 22, 824-826 (1950).

McCROSKEY, R., The relative contributions of auditory and tactile cues to certain aspects of speech. *Southern Speech J.*, 24, 84-90 (1958).

MILLER, G., *Language and Communication*. New York: McGraw-Hill (1951).

MURRAY, E., and TIFFIN, J., An analysis of some basic aspects of effective speech. *Arch. of Speech*, 1, 61-83 (1934).

PROVINS, K., The role of receptors in muscle and tendon in controlling the application of finger pressure in man. *J. Physiol. (London)*, 128, 55-56 (1955).

RINGEL, R. L., Some effects of tactile and auditory alterations on speech output. Ph.D. dissertation, Purdue Univ. (1962).

SCHWARTZ, R., Vocal responses to delayed auditory feedback in congenitally blind adults. Ph.D. dissertation, Purdue Univ. (1957).

SILVERSTEIN, B., Auditorily induced changes in the vocal attributes of voice defectives. Ph.D. dissertation, Purdue Univ. (1953).

SMITH, W., McCRARY, J., and SMITH, K., Delayed visual feedback and behavior. *Science*, 132, 1013-1014 (1960).

SPILKA, B., A study of relationships existing between certain aspects of personality and some vocal effects of delayed speech feedback. Ph.D. dissertation, Purdue Univ. (1952).

STEEL, R., and TORRIE, J., *Principles and Procedures of Statistics*. New York: McGraw-Hill (1960).

TRAVIS, L. (Ed.), *Handbook of Speech Pathology*. New York: Appleton-Century-Crofts (1957).

VAN RIPER, C., *Speech Correction: Principles and Methods*. New Jersey: Prentice-Hall (1954).

WIELDLING, S., *Xylocaine, The Pharmacological Basis of Its Clinical Use*. Stockholm: Almqvist and Wiksells Boktryckeri AB. (1959).

EFFECTIVENESS OF CERTAIN PROCEDURES FOR ALTERATION OF AUDITORY AND ORAL TACTILE SENSATION FOR SPEECH[1]

HERBERT F. SCHLIESSER   AND   RALPH O. COLEMAN

Summary.—To determine the effectiveness of auditory masking and intra-oral anesthetics on speech, certain motor and sensory tests were administered under 4 conditions: (1) auditory masking and oral anesthesia, (2) oral anesthesia alone, (3) auditory masking alone, and (4) normal. These speech samples were compared with a sample judged to be of "moderate" defectiveness by clinical standards. Within the limitations of the study, 3 conclusions appear justified. (1) One's own auditory feedback can be effectively eliminated by a combination of white and sawtooth noise. (2) Tactile sensation can be eliminated from the oral cavity without significantly interfering with motor innervation. (3) Speech that is intelligible and exhibits a degree of defectiveness which is less than that of a clinically "moderate" speech problem can be produced without oral tactile and auditory feedback.

While considerable study has been given the effects upon speech of alterations of auditory sidetone, relatively little has been reported regarding alterations of oral tactile sensation or combined auditory and oral tactile changes. These sensory modalities are regarded as important feedback mechanisms which enable a speaker to monitor his speech output. In the reported work (McCroskey, 1958; McCroskey, Corley, & Jackson, 1959; Ringel & Steer, 1963), there is consistent agreement that interference with normal oral tactile sensory information only or in combination with altered air-borne auditory sidetone results in greater speech disturbance than under the condition wherein auditory sidetone alone is changed. These findings suggest insufficient attention has been given the contributions provided by oral tactile cues for normal speech production. As a preliminary step to a broad investigation of the effect on speech of alterations in sensory feedback, an effort has been made to validate the effectiveness of certain procedures to alter such feedback.

Interference with air-borne auditory feedback traditionally has been accomplished by introducing various amplified delay times and by the use of masking noise. The effect on speech of delayed/amplified auditory sidetone is well known. The efficiency with which one's own voice can be masked, however, has not been well described. It has been the authors' experience that complete masking is difficult to achieve using either a white or sawtooth noise. White noise is an inefficient masker for low frequencies and sawtooth noise is inefficient for the high ones. Also, the "Lombard Effect" causes speakers to increase vocal intensity and it is possible to override a masking noise that is presented at maximum tolerance levels.

[1]Supported by Grant G4171-14, University of Nebraska Research Council, Lincoln, Nebraska.

PERCEPTUAL AND MOTOR SKILLS, 1968, vol. 26, 275-281.

Changes in oral tactile sensation have been effected by means of topical and nerve-block anesthesia. In both cases, the elimination or reduction of oral tactile cues was assumed to have occurred, with no subsequent interference of motor pathways. This position seems justified, in view of the fact that the nerves under anesthesia were all branches of the trigeminal nerve which is, for the most part, sensory in the oral region (Grant, 1956). However, if speech under anesthesia is to be studied, it is necessary to ascertain the degree of reduction of oral tactile sensation and whether, in fact, the innervation of motor pathways is disturbed. To investigate the extent to which auditory and oral sensory feedback can be eliminated, an experiment designed to answer these questions was carried out: (1) Can tactile and positional sense within the mouth be eliminated by the anesthetic? (2) Is the motility of the oral structures affected by the anesthetic? (3) Can an auditory masking noise be effective in eliminating one's own auditory feedback? A description of some speech samples obtained under the four experimental conditions is also provided.

METHOD

Five normal-hearing male Ss, between the ages of 20 and 44, recorded 42 sentences taken from a standard reference (Fairbanks, 1960) under each of four speaking conditions. These conditions were: (1) oral anesthesia and bilateral air-borne auditory masking, (2) oral anesthesia alone, (3) bilateral air-borne auditory masking alone, and (4) no interference of sensory feedback mechanisms. Oral anesthetization was performed only once and the speaking conditions including it were systematically rotated with successive Ss. The other conditions were presented on days before or after those involving anesthesia. Thus, conditions were not randomized but their order of occurrence was reasonably well controlled.

Anesthesia

An orthodontist on the staff of the College of Dentistry, University of Nebraska, performed the anesthetization of the oral areas of each S. A bilateral mandibular nerve block and a nerve block in the area of the incisive foramen of the anterior hard palate were administered employing Xylocaine HOL 2%. A topical anesthetic was applied to the entire surface of the hard palate.

Auditory Masking

The masking noise was prepared by mixing white and sawtooth noise recorded from a Grason-Stadler, Model 162 speech audiometer. These noise spectrums were chosen because of the preponderance of low frequency energy in sawtooth noise and the equal distribution of energy in white noise. Each was recorded on a separate channel of an Ampex, Model PR-10 two-channel tape recorder, combined and presented to the listener through Sharpe Model HA-10 earphones.

The intensity relationship between the two noises was controlled at the output of each tape recorder channel and the "mix" producing the optimal masking effect determined by trial and error. Subsequent verification of the relative intensity of the two signals indicated that the sawtooth noise was 10 db more intense than the white noise. The combined noise was then dubbed to a second tape recorder to provide a permanent noise of 30-min. duration.

It was found that without exceeding tolerance levels, it was possible to eliminate S's hearing his own voice at all levels but a loud shout. The amplifier setting which produced noise at the most effective levels was then marked for future use for each S.

During the experiment, Ss were found to vary in their noise tolerance and the previously established maximum noise levels could not be sustained for all Ss. To prevent Ss from increasing their vocal intensity in response to the noise and possibly overriding the masking, a control over speaker out-put was established. This control consisted of visually monitoring a VU meter set to the level of each speaker's "comfort level." Under these conditions all Ss reported complete absence of auditory feedback without discomfort.

Oral Stereognosis

The degree of reduction of tactile sensation by the anesthesia was tested by oral stereognosis. Ten plastic objects of geometric design, .5 in. in diameter and .25 in. in thickness, were used. They ranged in difficulty from simple forms, such as a square and a circle, to items such as a cube, a rounded cube, and a circle with a hole in it. Each sterilized object was placed in S's mouth and he was instructed to identify it by palpating it with his tongue. Identification was made by pointing to an object of a corresponding set of items in a tray. Stereognostic testing was conducted during Condition 4, when no interference of sensory feedback mechanisms was used and under anesthesia at the conclusion of the second of the two conditions involving interference with oral tactile sensation.

Restricted Motility of Speech Musculatures

Mean rates of repetitive speech and nonspeech activities have been used to determine the degree of restricted motility of the speech musculatures of neuromuscularly handicapped youngsters (Hixon & Hardy, 1964; Heltman & Peacher, 1943) and relate quite well with measures of their speech problems. These have long been used diagnostically by speech pathologists when there is some belief that a speech-handicapped individual may have a neuromuscularly involved speech mechanism. For this reason, the use of the mean rates of such activities may be a means of determining whether and to what degree motor pathway efficiency may be affected by anesthesia.

Ss were asked to repeat accurately /mʌ/, /dʌ/, /gʌ/, and /pʌtʌkʌ/ as fast as possible for three trials of 10 sec. each. They were asked to repeat this procedure with tongue lateralization, a nonspeech activity requiring that the tongue

197

be moved from one side of the mouth and back again as rapidly as possible while still maintaining accuracy of movement. The mean of the three trials for each of the speech activities and for the nonspeech activity comprised the criterion measure for restricted motility of the speech musculatures. This testing, too, was conducted during Condition 4 under normal sensory feedback circumstances and under anesthesia at the conclusion of the second of the two conditions involving interference with oral tactile sensation.

Speech Samples

The 42 sentences from Fairbanks comprising the speech material were read by each S under each experimental condition and recorded on an Ampex Model PR-10 tape recorder at approximately equal intensities. Ss were instructed to read as naturally as possible and to begin each new sentence immediately after completing the present one.

These sentences have long been used to assess articulation skills of individuals with reading ability. Each sentence can be used to test a specific phoneme in an initial, medial, and final position of words included in it for that purpose. The sentences are also sufficiently representative, however, of the variety and incidence of phonemes in connected speech to be usable as an initial means for studying over-all speech changes under the experimental conditions.

A 15-sec. segment of speech was randomly selected from the recorded sentences of each S for each condition. These segments were randomized and spliced onto a listening tape. This tape was then presented in a sound-treated room to a panel of 12 graduate students and professional workers in speech pathology who listened to the speech samples and judged them for speech defectiveness by the method of direct magnitude estimation described by Prather (1960).

The panel rated the samples for speech defectiveness by assigning them numbers proportional to the given value of a 15-sec. *standard* speech sample. The latter was selected from the listening tape by two speech pathologists, other than the authors, who were assigned to choose a *standard* on the criterion that it would be representative of a "moderate" speech problem by clinical standards. A sample which had been recorded under the condition of masking noise and anesthesia was chosen the *standard* and a copy was spliced onto the listening tape after every fifth speech sample prior to the listening task. This *standard* was assigned an arbitrary value of 100 and each 15-sec. sample of speech was judged by the listening panel relative to this value. If a sample were deemed to be twice as defective as the standard, the listener was instructed to assign it the number 200; if it were deemed to be half as defective as the sample the number 50 was assigned, etc. The mean of the ratings assigned each sample comprised the measure of relative speech defectiveness of that sample.

The panel was instructed to consider those characteristics commonly associated by speech pathologists with speech defectiveness, i.e., articulatory deviations, voice quality deviations, and undesirable aspects of pitch and loudness usage. No other definition of speech defectiveness was provided.

RESULTS AND DISCUSSION

Oral Stereognosis

Stereognostic testing was conducted at the conclusion of the second of the two speaking conditions involving anesthesia, or approximately 8 to 10 min. after anesthetization was performed. There were five correct identifications and 45 instances of incorrect responses. The total number of items tested per *S* was ten.

Since the number of correct responses was essentially what would be expected to result from guessing, virtually total intra-oral tactile insensitivity can be assumed. All *S*s correctly identified all objects in the unanesthetized condition.

An additional test of anesthetization consisted of manipulation of the tongue with forceps. *S*s, with eyes closed, were instructed to identify the type of movement and the static tongue position. It was possible to draw the tongue from the mouth, twist it one-quarter turn, and roll it back without *S*'s being able to identify either the motion or the tongue position. At extremes of any of the above positions *S*s reported feelings of tension in the musculature of the pharynx and neck although not in the body of the tongue.

Restricted Motility of Speech Musculatures

Mean rates of the repetitive speech activities and the repetitive nonspeech activity (tongue lateralization) were used to compute a grand mean for the group for the condition of normal speaking (no anesthesia or masking noise) and for the condition of anesthetization. Correlated *t* tests were employed to determine whether significant differences existed between the grand means for those conditions for each of the activities. The results are presented in Table 1.

None of the group-mean rate differences were statistically significant and all of these rates are within clinically judged normal limits for such repetitive activities as well as being in agreement with previous findings for very similar ac-

TABLE 1

GROUP MEAN RATE DIFFERENCES BETWEEN CONDITIONS OF NORMAL SPEAKING AND ANESTHETIZATION FOR REPETITIVE SPEECH ACTIVITIES AND REPETITIVE NONSPEECH ACTIVITY

Activity	Normal Speaking	Anesthetization	t^*
$/m_\Lambda/$	65.0	62.2	.95
$/d_\Lambda/$	67.8	65.2	.78
$/g_\Lambda/$	59.2	54.8	1.59
$/p_\Lambda t_\Lambda k_\Lambda/$	25.0	21.8	1.64
tongue lateralization	23.8	19.2	1.37

$^*t = 2.78, p < .05.$

tivities for physically normal adults (Canter, 1965). It seems that very little interference, if any, of motor innervation to the speech musculatures occurred from the anesthesia procedure used in this study.

Speech Defectiveness Ratings

Interobserver reliability of the mean scale values of the speech defectiveness ratings was obtained by using Ebel's (1951) intraclass correlation technique. The obtained intraclass correlation coefficient of .96 indicates that the panel of listeners judged the speech defectiveness of the Ss with a high degree of reliability under the experimental conditions.

The mean scale values of the ratings of speech defectiveness obtained under each of the four speaking conditions of anesthesia and masking, anesthesia alone, masking alone, and unaltered (normal) were 95.7, 37.9, 33.9, and 12.6, respectively. These values may be compared with the 100.0 assigned the *standard*, which was considered to represent a "moderate" speech problem.

Speech was judged to be markedly less adequate under the condition when auditory masking and anesthesia were both present than in any of the other conditions. It should be noted, however, that the speech under this condition was judged to be less defective than a "moderate" speech problem in the clinical sense. It was also the subjective impression of the investigators that the intelligibility of the Ss' speech did not deteriorate. In view of the stress placed by current speech control theory upon the importance of auditory and tactile feedback, the presence of understandable speech is provocative.

That practically total elimination of tactile sensitivity in the oral mechanism occurred from the anesthesia while motor innervation to the speech musculatures remained essentially intact was demonstrated as possible for the Ss of this study. Auditory masking was provided optimum control by a mixture of sawtooth and white noise and by having Ss monitor their speech by means of a VU meter so they could avoid overriding the masking stimulus. It is apparent that an individual is able to maintain a degree of accuracy in articulation, rate of speaking, and inflection that is not very far from acceptable limits in the absence of auditory or oral tactile sensation. Possibly an individual utilizes well-learned motor patterns with a high degree of accuracy so that no sensory monitoring is required at least for the short term.

REFERENCES

CANTER, G. Speech characteristics of patients with Parkinson's disease: III. Articulation, diadochokinesis, and over-all speech adequacy. *Journal of Speech and Hearing Disorders*, 1965, 30, 217-223.

EBEL, R. Estimation of the reliability of ratings. *Psychometrika*, 1951, 16, 407-424.

FAIRBANKS, G. *Voice and articulation drillbook.* (2nd ed.) New York: Harper, 1960.

GRANT, J. *An atlas of anatomy.* (4th ed.) Baltimore: Williams & Wilkins, 1956.

HELTMAN, H., & PEACHER, G. Misarticulation and diadochokinesis in the spastic paralytic. *Journal of Speech Disorders*, 1943, 8, 137-145.

HIXON, T., & HARDY, J. Restricted motility of the speech articulators in cerebral palsy. *Journal of Speech and Hearing Disorders*, 1964, 29, 293-306.

MCCROSKEY, R. The relative contributions of auditory and tactile cues to certain aspects of speech. *Southern Speech Journal*, 1958, 24, 84-90.

MCCROSKEY, R., CORLEY, N., & JACKSON, G. Some effects of disrupted tactile cues upon the production of consonants. *Southern Speech Journal*, 1959, 25, 55-60.

PRATHER, E. Seeking defectiveness of articulation by direct magnitude estimation. *Journal of Speech and Hearing Research*, 1960, 3, 380-392.

RINGEL, R., & STEER, M. Some effects of tactile and auditory alterations of speech output. *Journal of Speech and Hearing Research*, 1963, 6, 369-377.

A METHODOLOGICAL CONSIDERATION IN KINESTHETIC FEEDBACK RESEARCH

John L. Locke

In the last fifteen years there have been several attempts to define the role of kinesthetic feedback in articulation. Investigators have attempted to reduce kinesthetic cues experimentally, reasoning that articulation impairment under such conditions would support the importance of kinesthetic feedback in monitoring articulation. Guttman (1954), McCroskey (1958), Weber (1961), and Ringel and Steer (1963) all found that articulation deteriorated significantly when subjects had been given intra-oral nerve block injections. These investigators concluded that kinesthetic cue reduction impairs articulation and, therefore, kinesthetic feedback is essential to normal articulation.

A recent study by Locke (1967) suggests that the methodology employed in kinesthetic feedback studies may be questionable. In this investigation nine young adults with normal speech and hearing were given an intra-oral topical anesthetic which reduced tactile sensitivity and an intra-oral local anesthetic which nearly eliminated tactile and kinesthetic sensitivity in the articulatory organs and structures. The procedures and their effects closely parallel those reported by McCroskey (1958).

In order to determine whether the injections had produced any motor impairment, in addition to anesthesia, subjects were instructed to produce each of five CV syllables as rapidly as possible for five seconds. This task was performed (1) under no anesthesia, (2) under topical anesthesia, and (3) under local anesthesia. Figure 1 shows an obvious slowing of repetitive articulatory movements under local anesthesia, especially of the tongue tip contacts in [dʌ] production. Of course some reduction in diadochokinetic rate may also be attributable to insufficient sensory reporting, suggesting a limitation of

diadochokinesis testing as a method of assessing motor function.

In the administration of intra-oral hypodermic injections, the dentist intends to

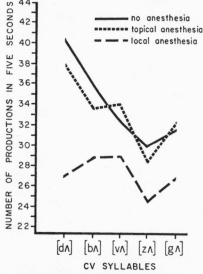

CV SYLLABLES

FIGURE 1. Mean number of productions of five CV syllables in five seconds. Subjects were nine young adults who articulated under conditions of no anesthesia, topical anesthesia, and local anesthesia.

block only the sensory nerves. However, according to the cooperating dentist, the proximity of sensory and motor nerves is such that individual differences among subjects, human error, and/or drug diffusion could lead to motor impairment as well (Cuckler, 1967, personal communication).

JOURNAL OF SPEECH AND HEARING RESEARCH, 1968, vol. 11, no. 3, 668-669.

The studies cited above failed to test specifically for muscular disturbance. Unless one tests specifically for motor interference, however, articulatory alterations under these conditions cannot safely be attributed to insufficient sensory feedback. Many statements concerning the contribution of kinesthetic cues in articulation monitoring may be based on inappropriate evidence. Fortunately, future experimental research may profit from the recent observation (Schliesser and Coleman, 1968) that partial oral-cavity anesthetization does not seem to impair motor processes significantly.

REFERENCES

GUTTMAN, N., Experimental studies of the speech control system. Doctoral thesis, Univ. of Illinois (1954).

LOCKE, J. L., An investigation into the effect or reduced auditory, tactile and kines- thetic feedback on the articulation of selected speech sounds. Unpublished manuscript (1967).

McCROSKEY, R., The relative contributions of auditory and tactile cues to certain aspects of speech. S. Speech J., 24, 84-90 (1958).

RINGEL, R., and STEER, M., Some effects of tactile and auditory alterations on speech output. J. Speech Hearing Res., 6, 369-378 (1963).

SCHLIESSER, H. F., and COLEMAN, R. O., Effectiveness of certain procedures for alteration of auditory and oral tactile sensation for speech. Percept. Motor Skills, 26, 275-281 (1968).

WEBER, B., Effect of high level masking and anesthetization of oral structures upon articulatory proficiency and voice characteristics of normal speakers. Master's thesis, Pennsylvania State Univ. (1961).

ARTICULATION AND STRESS/JUNCTURE PRODUCTION UNDER ORAL ANESTHETIZATION AND MASKING

SYLVIA A. GAMMON, PHILIP J. SMITH, RAYMOND G. DANILOFF, and CHIN W. KIM

Eight subjects, half of them naive and the other half aware of the purpose of the experiment, spoke 30 pairs of sentences involving the production of intricate stress/juncture patterns along with a passage containing all major consonant phonemes in English in various intraword positions. All subjects spoke all materials under: ¯(1) normal conditions, (2) 110 dB re: 0.0002 ubar white noise masking, (3) extensive local anesthesia of the oral cavity, and (4) masking and anesthesia combined. Stress and juncture patterns were correctly produced despite all feedback disruption, and there was no difference between naive and aware subjects. Noise masking produced a decline in speech quality and a disruption of normal rhythm, both of which were even more seriously affected by anesthesia and anesthesia plus masking. There were no significant vowel misarticulations under any condition, but there was nearly a 20% rate of consonant misarticulation under anesthesia and anesthesia and noise. Misarticulation was most severe for fricatives and affricates in the labial and alveolar regions, presumably because these productions demand a high degree of precision of articulate shape and location and hence, intact feedback. Results are discussed in terms of feedback-control mechanisms for speech production.

Attempts have been made to assess the relative importance of auditory, tactile, and kinesthetic feedback during speech production. Various combinations of oral topical and local anesthesia and auditory masking have been used to disrupt such feedback during speech. McCroskey (1958) (using delayed auditory feedback), Weber (1961), Ladefoged (1967), Ringel and Steer (1963), and Schliesser and Coleman (1968), all using auditory masking, have observed that rate of articulation, voice pitch and intensity, and vowel quality are significantly and adversely affected by disrupted auditory feedback. They found that oral anesthetization (of varying kinds and extents) produced increased misarticulation, especially when a local rather than topical (Ringel and Steer, 1963) anesthetic was used. Anesthesia also produced some decline in speech quality as well. However, Ladefoged (1967) and Schliesser and Coleman (1968) observed that speech remained highly intelligible under all combinations of anesthesia and noise, suggesting that articulation depends most heavily on the relatively intact kinesthetic feedback. In general, all experimenters agree that articulatory integrity and speech quality are increasingly disrupted as feedback disruption increases.

JOURNAL OF SPEECH AND HEARING RESEARCH, 1971, vol. 14, no. 2, 271-282.

In one short experiment dealing with auditory feedback, Kozhevnikov and Chistovich (1966) considered the possibility that afferent impulsations occurring at the first syllable of a word "triggered" the pronunciation of the subsequent syllables. The experiment consisted of a single subject, who read a phrase 14 times soundlessly. The durational characteristics of the same phrase spoken normally coincided with its duration spoken soundlessly. This led them to hypothesize that the rhythmic features of speech are not dependent upon intact auditory feedback, contra McCroskey (1958).

Statement of Problem

In this experiment, we sought to measure the degree to which auditory and supra-glottal tactile feedback are important to another type of articulatory task, the production of stress and juncture in English. Present linguistic research suggests a possibility that a unit of articulation, once programmed through learning, becomes relatively self-perpetuating (Kozhevnikov and Chistovich, 1966). If this is the case, then this unit would be to some extent independent of any feedback system.

Most previous studies called for a subjective judgment as to the "normalcy" of speech produced under the various conditions of reduced feedback. In this study we proposed to obtain more exacting and more readily quantifiable data on the speech produced. To this end, a set of stimulus sentences were devised which involved intricate stress and juncture differences and which were also subjected to an extensive phonemic analysis.

The ability of the speaker to produce the specifiable junctural and stress patterns in the sentences was measured during: (1) complete auditory and tactile feedback (control), (2) auditory masking, (3) tactile anesthetization of the oral region, and (4) auditory masking and tactile anesthetization (both).

A specialized reading passage[1] was chosen for the phonemic evaluation of articulatory integrity because it was devised to permit analyses of all English phonemes in a number of word positions. The voice quality and rhythm of the sentences spoken were measured by a panel of judges, using an equal-appearing intervals scaling technique.

GENERAL METHOD

The subjects in the experiment served in the control condition as well as in all three of the experimental conditions. Eight college students, all native speakers of American English, were chosen, four naive of the task required and four aware of the objectives of the experiment. It was assumed that awareness of the task would enable the speakers to perform more successfully. Partial support for this assumption is provided by Weber (1961). He suggested that the speakers of his study who were aware of the task may have performed

---

[1]Hultzén, L. Private materials, prose passage, "Grip the rat." Champaign, Illinois (1965).

with higher articulatory proficiency under certain conditions as opposed to less sophisticated speakers.

Materials

Thirty paired sentences were constructed involving the pronunciation of stress and juncture differences in compound and cognate words. The first 15 sentences involved compounds of the type: *redcoat/red coat*. Example: *The boy's life was saved by the warmth of the Redcoat/red coat.*

The correct pronunciation of these words involves an intricate, highly structured set of stress rules, as described by Chomsky and Halle (1968).

Another set of experimental sentences involved stress differences of the kind: *impact* (verb) vs *impact* (noun). To assign stress contours correctly to this type of words, again, Chomsky and Halle (1968) have set forth a series of stress assignment rules whose "apparent" complexity, by assumption, can be construed to mean that correct stress assignment by the speaker is an intricate task.

It is reasonable to expect that the compound and cognate word stress contours require the use of all possible sources of feedback on the part of the speaker for successful production. Consequently, any deterioration in the monitored feedback should be evident quite early in the production of these sentences. The compound words used were very familiar to the subjects and listeners.

One restriction on sentence design involved the elimination of certain allophonic cues to the existence of juncture differences in the paired compound words. Lehiste (1961) and Potter (1961) have shown that many compound words are identified primarily, not through stress variations, but through the allophonic cues present in certain juncture situations. For instance, in the pair *plum pie* and *plump eye*, there is likely to be a glottal attack on /ai/ in *eye*, whereas in the /aɪ/ of *pie* there will not. Such cues were minimized where possible to restrict the study more closely to difference in juncture or stress alone.

In addition to reading the 30 specially constructed sentences, the speakers read a prose passage that contained each of the phonemes and clusters of American English. A recording of their rendition of this prose passage provided the basis for detailed phonetic analysis of the talker's speech.

Reliability

All phonetic transcriptions, error counts, and analyses of stress-juncture patterns were made by an experienced phonetician. To assess the reliability of the analysis produced, a second experienced observer was used. The second observer listened to 10% of productions of the "prose" passage, and mean percentage discrepancies were computed for interjudge reliability.

For judgment of stress and juncture, the two judges concurred in 97% of all cases. For the segmental phonemic analysis, 84% agreement was achieved concerning the identity of the error committed. We consider both of these to be adequate for the purpose of this study.

EXPERIMENTAL PROCEDURE

Each subject read the stimulus sentences under four conditions:

A. with normal feedback systems (N),
B. under 110 dB SPL (re 0.0002 ubar) white noise, binaural auditory masking (M),
C. with oral anesthetization (A), and
D. with auditory masking and oral anesthetization (A + M).

The subjects were seated in an IAC sound-proofed booth containing a window through which the experimenter monitored each task. All sentences were recorded through a Grason-Stadler model 162 speech audiometer and microphone into a Berlant-Concertone tape recorder with a frequency response of ±3 dB, 40 to 10,000 Hz at 7½ ips. The audiometer microphone was placed approximately 12 inches in front of the speaker's mouth. The subject's vocal intensity level was monitored by means of a VU meter. When the production exceeded 70 dB SPL, a voice-operated level detector (laboratory constructed) flashed a light in the booth, informing the subject that he should reread the previous sentence at a lower level.

During the control situation, the subjects read the sentences at a conversational pitch and effort level. This was carefully monitored because speaking at a much greater level required the use of too intense a masking noise during the noise masking condition.

In Condition B, 110 dB of earphone-limited Gaussian noise produced by the speech audiometer was delivered to the subject through TDH-39 earphones. Care was taken to insure that no more than 10-12 dB of temporary threshold shift occurred in the speech frequencies during the experimental condition not involving masking.

In Condition C, the tactile feedback of the subject was minimized by means of the following series of dental injections administered by an oral surgeon (D.D.S.).

Bilateral Infra-Orbital blocks, affecting the anterior and middle superior alveolar nerves, anesthetizing the upper lip, alveolar ridge, and anterior maxillary teeth.
Bilateral inferior alveolar blocks, affecting the inferior alveolar nerve and to some extent the lingual nerve, anesthetizing the anterior two-thirds of the tongue and the lower alveolar ridge, teeth, and lip.
One Nasopalatine block, affecting the nasopalatine nerve, anesthetizing the anterior one-third of the palate.
Bilateral Posterior Palatine blocks, affecting the middle palatine nerve, and the posterior two-thirds of the palate, see Sicher (1960).

A solution of 2% xylocaine was used in all the above injections with the oral surgeon remaining in attendance during Conditions C and D to handle any difficulties which might have arisen. The anesthetic took effect almost immedi-

207

ately and remained at full strength for about one hour. All subjects performed a series of diadochokinetic tasks before and well after oral anesthetization. No differences were observed. In addition, each produced [pʌ, tʌ, kʌ] as fast as possible; speed of production was also unaffected by anesthetization.

Rating Procedures

For measures of voice quality and speech rhythm changes under each experimental condition, the first five and last five sentences spoken by each subject under each condition (B,C,D) were selected and spliced at random in pairs into a master tape. The tape consisted of sentence pairs, the first being the sentence produced under control (normal condition), and the second, the same sentence produced under one of the experimental conditions. The order of presentation of sentences was completely randomized over conditions and subjects, each subject's normal speech serving as his own standard.

Voice quality was, for purposes of instruction, broken into subconstituents such as hoarseness, nasality, breathiness, etc. The experimenter prepared a training tape in which four examples of each aspect of quality were presented. For example, normal (rated 1), moderately normal (rated 3), nasal (rated 5), and very nasal (rated 7) speech samples were spoken and presented by tape to each judge.

For rhythm, actual examples of normal (1), moderately disrupted (3), disrupted (5), and very disrupted (7) speech were selected and presented to judges. Only after hearing the training tape and discussing aspects of quality and rhythm was judging commenced.

Eleven judges in the quality study and fourteen in the rhythm study listened to the master tapes. Judges were instructed to consider the normal sentence of each pair to have a value of one, and were to assign values of 1 to 7 to the second sentence, according to whether it was normal or extremely disrupted or poor in terms of rhythm and/or voice quality. Judges were repeatedly cautioned to ignore the misarticulations occurring in the second sentence of each pair in forming their judgments.

RESULTS

Data Analysis

All the sentences produced under all conditions were analysed for stress and juncture, and phonetic evaluation of the prose passage was made by the phonetician. Each of the passages under each of the conditions was analyzed for misarticulations in voicing, place, and manner of phoneme production. The number of omissions involved was also noted. Because subject naivete produced no observable differences in experimental performance, the data were pooled for analysis.

Stress and Juncture

The single most significant finding of this study is that neither noise, nor anesthesia, nor both, reduced the ability of the speakers to produce the proper stress and juncture. In Table 1, the average number of errors (for 30 sentences) is tabulated. These results exhibit no differences between any of the conditions. Stress and juncture, at least for short term feedback disruption, are governed by feedback and/or control not affected by noise masking or oral anesthesia. Note also that Subject Two, perhaps the most experienced subject and well aware of the experiment's purpose, produced the highest overall error rate.

Misarticulations

A phonetic analysis of the prose passage yielded marked differences between the speakers' performance under the experimental conditions. Each of the speakers' misarticulations was analyzed in terms of voicing, place, manner, and total omissions. The tables for phonetic analysis contain consonant errors only because the number of vowel errors was negligible.

Figure 1 presents the overall articulation errors (in percent form) listed in Tables 2 and 3. The majority of place misarticulations occur at the front of the oral cavity, specifically in the bilabial and labio-dental regions. We assume that the precision of articulatory contact needed for correct pronunciation (and hence the need for much intact tactile feedback) of bilabial and labio-dental consonants is greater than that needed for alveolar, palatal, or velar consonant production.

Except for bilabials, anesthesia and masking produced more errors than anesthesia alone, but only marginally so. Hence, reduction of auditory feedback doesn't seem to be crucial to consonant production in the immediate sense.

The anesthesia used in this experiment did not affect the glottal region, nor do glottals, e.g. [h], demand articulator contact, hence the lack of errors is quite understandable.

TABLE 1. Errors in stress and juncture for various kinds of feedback disruption based upon eight subjects speaking 30 sentence pairs each.

Subject	Conditions			
	Control	Masking	Anesthetization	Combined
1	2	1	1	1
2	5	3	5	3
3	2	1	4	2
4	2	1	0	0
5	3	2	0	1
6	0	1	2	3
7	1	0	0	1
8	1	0	1	0
Mean	2.000	1.125	1.625	1.375

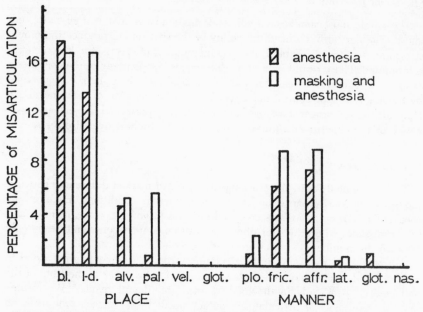

FIGURE 1. Percentage of misarticulations for place and manner of production. Based on eight subjects speaking the prose passage under oral anesthesia and/or masking.

Fricative and affricate manner of production errors greatly outnumber those for plosive, lateral, glide, and nasal manner errors. Fricatives and affricates require production of a precise opening for air turbulence, whereas plosives require a simpler open/closed mechanism, which requires much less articulatory precision and feedback (Peterson and Shoup, 1966). In addition one may

TABLE 2. Frequency of occurrence of misarticulations for consonants grouped according to place of articulation, based on eight subjects reading the prose passage. A means anesthetization; A&N mean anesthetization plus masking noise.

Phonemes Intended		Total Spoken	Bilabial	Labio-dental	Alveolar	Palatal	Velar	Glottal
Bilabial	A	–	–	162	8	1	–	–
	A&N	968	–	157	2	–	–	–
Labiodental	A	–	–	3	124	6	–	–
	A&N	1008	–	7	156	–	–	–
Alveolar	A	–	48	32	–	9	–	67
	A&N	3824	17	35	–	31	1	99
Palatal	A	–	–	4	–	–	–	–
	A&N	3411	7	3	–	9	–	–
Velar	A	–	–	–	–	–	–	–
	A&N	1008	–	–	–	–	–	–
Glottal	A	–	–	–	–	–	–	–
	A&N	368	–	–	–	–	–	–

210

TABLE 3. Frequency of occurrence of misarticulations for consonants grouped according to manner of articulation, based on eight subjects reading the prose passage. A means anesthetization; A&N mean anesthetization plus masking noise.

Phonemes Intended		Total Spoken	Plosive	Fricative	Affricate	Lateral	Glide	Nasal
Plos.	A	–	–	19	1	–	2	–
	A&N	2296	–	48	–	–	2	3
Fric.	A	–	136	–	5	–	2	6
	A&N	2394	198	–	4	–	10	4
Aff.	A	–	–	9	–	–	–	1
	A&N	136	6	4	–	–	1	1
Lat.	A	–	–	–	–	–	1	–
	A&N	416	–	–	–	–	3	–
Gli.	A	–	–	4	1	2	–	–
	A&N	840	–	–	–	–	–	1
Nas.	A	–	1	–	–	–	–	–
	A&N	1488	–	–	–	–	1	–

need more careful monitoring of auditory feedback for fricatives and affricates as well as tactile, hence the sizeable increase in error for both when masking is added to anesthesia. The small percentage of glide and lateral errors may relate to their vowel-like nature. As such, the feedback for /l, r, w, j/ may be governed by the kinesthesia utilized in vowel production. Nasals, the last manner category, may be resistant to misarticulation because they, like plosives, require only the binary open/closed response of the velum and simple closing of lips or tongue raising.

Table 4 presents the pooled data on misarticulation for manner, place, voicing, and omission errors. The number of place errors under anesthesia and masking are approximately 23% greater than those under anesthesia alone. Similarly with manner errors, the differential is 15% for anesthesia and masking. The total number of omissions under anesthesia and masking is much larger, having 615 to the 484 omissions under anesthesia alone, a 27% difference. The total number of errors under anesthesia and masking is about 19% greater than under anesthesia alone (1443-1188). The number of place and

TABLE 4. Overall articulation errors for various feedback deprivations based on eight subjects reading the prose text.

Errors	Anesthesia		Anesthesia Plus Masking		Total No.
	No.	%	No.	%	
Place	424	35.7	524	36.4	948
Manner	191	16.1	221	15.4	412
Voicing	91	7.6	83	5.4	174
Omiss.	482	40.6	615	42.8	1097
Total	1188	48.9	1443	51.1	2631

211

manner errors differ because quite a number of articulation errors were multiple errors, e.g., of place and manner both.

Examination of Tables 2 and 3 reveals the error trends in the data. The most frequent error is the substitution of plosives for fricatives (occurs in all but 32 of the 334 fricative errors). The plosive closure would be produced when the speaker is no longer capable of the fine tactile control needed to produce the fricative slit. The next most frequent error is a substitution of labio-dental for bilabial articulation (occurs in 319 of 330 bilabial errors). Since the speakers' lips were so completely anesthetized, a misarticulation such as this is quite understandable.

A reversal of the first major error, seen when 67 plosives became fricatives, would be understandable when one considers that almost all bilabials became labio-dentals. A slight disalignment of two lips would make the articulation a labio-dental, and obstruant labio-dentals are in nature fricatives (i.e., there is no labio-dental stop). In this sense, these are not true counter-examples to the trend from fricative to stop.

One of the most interesting results is the fact that the majority of mistakes, except bilabial stops becoming labio-dental fricatives, occur as a result of changes from one manner or place to another rather than across such classes. There is a general trend for place errors to be a result of backward movement (i.e. labio-dental to alveolar) and for manner errors to go from open to closed (i.e. fricatives and affricatives to plosives). These trends were found to be approximately the same under both the anesthesia and combined conditions.

Voice Quality and Rhythm

Figure 2 presents the median scaled values and semi-interquartile ranges of vocal quality and speech rhythm. Each additional feedback disruption yielded increasing loss of normal rhythm and quality. A Friedman 2-way non-

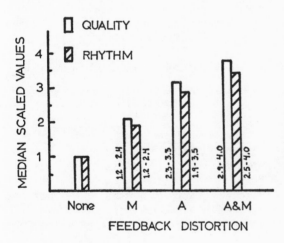

FIGURE 2. Median scaled values of vocal quality and vocal rhythm and mean semi-interquartile range for eight speakers as assessed by 11 judges for quality and 14 for rhythm under oral anesthesia alone or with anesthesia and masking.

parametric analysis of variance of the scaled values of rhythm and quality showed that their values were significantly different from each other (p 0.0001). The results must be tempered, however, by the fact that the listeners' judgments (although instructed otherwise) may have been influenced to some degree by the misarticulations occurring in the passages. However, this would not explain the fact that masking noise did affect quality and rhythm but had no effect upon misarticulations.

It is possible that the kinesthetic feedback (which was not much affected) yields information which allows for sufficiently accurate tongue placement to produce proper phonemic vowel quality, but auditory and tactile feedback are needed to yield the fine adjustments of tongue shape and location needed for good phonetic quality as well. This is in addition to the laryngeal-tone contributions to vocal quality.

DISCUSSION

Stress and Juncture

The stress/juncture production tasks were not disrupted by blocking auditory and tactile feedback. Therefore the projection of stress/juncture rules upon the articulatory mechanism probably occurs at a high level in the decoding process (Kozhevnikov and Chistovich, 1966) and is largely feedback free, just as an instruction to separate or close the fingers will not be disrupted by numb fingers. Also, the apparent complexity of linguistic rules (for the assignment of stress and juncture) may have little or no relation to the complexities of articulation behavior. Alternatively, stress and juncture may be produced and governed at a laryngeal (Netsell, 1969) or sublaryngeal level (Fonagy, 1966; Lebrun, 1966; Stetson, 1951; Ladegfoged, Draper, and Whitteridge, 1958; Lieberman, 1967).

Articulation

Articulation of consonants suffered most from tactile deprivation; auditory deprivation affected consonant production only slightly. Vowel production was literally unaffected by either or both forms of feedback deprivation, in agreement with McCroskey (1958), Weber (1961), and Ringel and Steer (1963). Tongue positioning for vowel production can be done with kinesthetic feedback alone over the short run; in addition, there is probably more freedom in perceptual space for vowel than for consonant production—that is, tongue position and configuration can vary considerably before there is a change of phonemic class for the produced vowel.

Tactile feedback, information concerning articulator shape, area of contact, pressure of contact, etc., is very important to consonant production whereas auditory feedback deprivation elicits few short-term effects. Kinesthetic feedback alone is insufficient for good consonant articulation. Figure 1 and Tables

2 and 3 show the relationship between precision of articulator contact needed and degree of misarticulation. Fricatives, which require production of a precise opening for air turbulence, were more often misarticulated than plosives, which as a class require less precision of articulator shape and placement. Laterals and glides were relatively successfully produced, hence kinesthetic feedback alone (as with vowels) may be sufficient for correct production. Despite massive feedback disruption, more than 80% of all consonants were correctly articulated, testifying to the integrity and relative independence of the articulatory system when faced with temporary feedback deprivation.

Voice Quality

Under the auditory masking, vocal quality declines because of inability to monitor vocal output. Fine adjustments of vocal fold tension and mechanical operating characteristics affecting things such as minute fundamental frequency variations, sentence intonation, and source harmonic spectrum might be difficult to produce and maintain when auditory feedback is diminished.

Anesthesia deprived the speaker of tactile feedback from his articulators; the decrease in vocal quality is greater than that for noise alone. Precision of articulator placement and shape which is difficult under loss of tactile sensation must contribute heavily to vocal quality. Combined masking and anesthesia yielded poorest articulation and poorest voice quality. Acceptable voice quality demands intact auditory, tactile, and kinesthetic feedback, even in the short-term sense.

Vocal Rhythm

Rhythm can be considered to be the product of successive variations in syllable stress. In this study, stress and juncture were unaffected by feed-back deprivation, but rhythm was. Therefore, there must be factors involved in rhythm not previously considered in studies relating stress to rhythm. Close study of the master tapes indicated that the rhythm irregularities were largely a result of the intrusion of pauses within the sentences. Lenneberg (1967), Kozhevnikov and Chistovich (1966), and Zinkin (1968) suggest that the physiological events involved in the production of rhythm correlate well with observed rhythm in brain activity, as if there were a central rhythm generator.

The maintenance of speech rhythm may depend upon auditory and/or tactile feedback. This does not limit the speaker to a single rate of speech since it is possible that a train of syllables can be distributed over centrally-generated rhythmic pulses in a number of days. It is this effective distribution of syllables (rather than the rhythmic pulses themselves) which is most likely affected by a deterioration of feedback channels, explaining why rhythm was affected while stress remained intact. The unrhythmic aspect of the sentences resulted from the intrusion of pauses between syllables rather than within, leaving intact the durational characteristics of the syllable itself, and preserving the stress relationship. Goldman-Eisler (1967) noted that intrusive pauses are natural to fluent speech, are well integrated into the syntactic structure, and fall at predictable points such as at clause junctures. The points at which pauses become intrusive (interrupt the rhythmic flow of speech) under masking conditions are yet to be determined.

ACKNOWLEDGMENT

This research was supported in part by Public Health Service Research Grant NB-07346 from the National Institute of Mental Health to the Children's Research Center. S. A. Gammon's current address is Department of Speech, Adelphi College, Garden City, New York. P. J. Smith is also at the Carle Clinic in Champaign/Urbana, Illinois. R. G. Daniloff is at the Children's Research Center and Speech Research Laboratory, and C. W. Kim is at the Department of Linguistics of the University of Illinois.

REFERENCES

CHOMSKY, N., and HALLE, M., *The Sound Pattern of English.* New York: Harper & Row (1968).

FONAGY, I., Electrophysiological and acoustic correlates of stress and stress perception. *J. Speech,* 10, 122-130 (1967).

GOLDMAN-EISLER, F., Sequential temporal patterns and cognitive processes in speech. *Lang. Speech,* 10, 122-130 (1967).

KOZHEVNIKOV, V. A., and CHISTOVICH, L. A., Speech: articulation and perception. Washington: Joint Publications Research Service, U. S. Bureau of Commerce, 30, 543 (1966).

LADEFOGED, P., DRAPER, M. H., and WHITTERIDGE, D., Syllables and stress. *Miscellanea Phonetica,* III, London: International Phonetic Assn. (1958).

LADEFOGED, P., *Three Areas of Experimental Phonetics.* London: Oxford Univ. Press (1967).

LEBRUN, Y., *Linguistic Research in Belgium.* Belgium: Universa Wetteren (1966).

LEHISTE, I., Acoustic studies in boundary signals, *Proc. Fourth Internat. Cong. Phonet. Sci.,* Helsinki, Finland: Mouton (1961).

LENNEBERG, E. H., *The Biological Foundations of Language.* New York: Wiley (1967).

LIEBERMAN, P., *Intonation, Perception and Language.* Research Monograph No. 38, Cambridge: M.I.T. Press (1967).

McCROSKEY, R., The relative contributions of auditory and tactile cues to certain aspects of speech. *Southern Speech J.,* 24, 84-90 (1958).

NETSELL, R., *Underlying physiological mechanisms of syllable stress.* Paper presented to the 78th meeting of the Acoustical Society of America, November 4-7, San Diego (1969).

PETERSON, G. E., and SHOUP, J. E., A physiological theory of phonetics. *J. Speech Hearing Res.,* 9, 5-67 (1966).

POTTER, S., Syllabic juncture. *Proc. Fourth Internat. Cong. of Phonet. Sci.,* Helsinki, Finland: Mouton (1961).

RINGEL, R. L., and STEER, M.D., Some effects of tactile and auditory alterations on speech output. *J. Speech Hearing Res.,* 369-378 (1963).

SCHLIESSER, H. F., and COLEMAN, R., Effectiveness of certain procedures for alteration of auditory and oral tactile sensation for speech. *Percept. motor skills,* 26, 275 (1968).

SICHER, H., *Oral Anatomy.* St. Louis: C. V. Mosby (1960).

STETSON, R. H., *Motor Phonetics; A Study of Speech Movements in Action.* Amsterdam: North-Holland (1951).

WEBER, B. A., Effect of high level masking and anesthetization of oral structures upon articulatory proficiency and voice characteristics of normal speakers. Unpublished Master's thesis, Pennsylvania State (1961).

ZINKIN, N. I., *Mechanisms of Speech.* The Hague, Netherlands: Mouton (1968).

COMMENT ON "ARTICULATION AND STRESS/JUNCTURE PRODUCTION UNDER ORAL ANESTHETIZATION AND MASKING"

Ralph O. Coleman

Herbert F. Schliesser

In an article appearing in the June, 1971 issue of the *Journal of Speech and Hearing Research*, Gammon, Smith, Daniloff, and Kim indicated that the articulatory success they observed in subjects speaking under conditions of auditory masking and oral anesthesia was the result of "kinesthetic" feedback in the tongue. Our experience (Schliesser and Coleman, 1968) with similar experimental conditions does not support the concept of an intact kinesthetic. or positional sense, in the tongue following bilateral blocking of the mandibular branch of the trigeminal nerve. Their finding that reasonably good speech can be produced under conditions of auditory masking and oral anesthesia is similar to ours; where we differ is in the role assigned to kinesthesis in the tongue in maintaining this articulatory accuracy. We reported a simple experiment with our anesthetized subjects (p. 279) as follows:

> An additional test of anesthetization consisted of manipulation of the tongue with forceps. S's, with eyes closed, were instructed to identify the type of movement and the static tongue position. It was possible to draw the tongue from the mouth, twist it one-quarter turn, and roll it back without S's being able to identify either the motion or the tongue position. At extremes of any of the above positions S's reported feelings of tension in the musculature of the pharynx and the neck but not in the body of the tongue.

Since we were both subjects in this study, the experience described here is a first-hand one. Any sense of where one's tongue was in space was simply not there.

This would seem to make sense neurologically. According to Gray (1959), the lingual branch of the trigeminal nerve forms the nerve of "ordinary sensibility" for the anterior two-thirds of the tongue, and the lingual branch of the glossopharyngeal nerve

JOURNAL OF SPEECH AND HEARING RESEARCH, 1972, vol. 15, no. 3, 669-670.

216

is distributed to the mucous membrane at the base and sides of the tongue. Bilateral anesthetization of the inferior branch of the trigeminal nerve would in all likelihood involve the lingual branch as well, thereby blocking that sensory pathway or at least reducing its effectiveness. This eventuality is recognized by Gammon et al. (1971, p. 274) when they state that their anesthetic involved, to some extent, the lingual nerve. In our case the involvement appears to have been essentially total and in the absence of reports to the contrary, it might be hypothesized that similar anesthesiological procedures affected their subjects in the same way as ours. Innervation by the unanesthetized glossopharyngeal nerve may have accounted for the sensations accompanying extreme movements that we experienced.

The whole question of a position sense in the tongue is controversial. In recent articles by Ringel (1970) and Shelton (1971) the entire concept is questioned. Shelton (1971), for example, states flatly that "there does not appear to be a physiological mechanism for kinesthesis in unjointed structures such as eyes, palate, lips, or tongue." He goes on to state that motor learning may be attributable to touch receptors with which the tongue is liberally endowed. Gardner, Gray, and O'Rahilly (1963, p. 911) on the other hand has summarized a series of anatomical studies as follows:

> The sense of position of the tongue depends largely on an intact innervation from the mucous membrane. Neuromuscular spindles, however, have been found in both the extrinsic and intrinsic muscles of the tongue, and it has been suggested that the lingual nerve, owing to its plexiform communications with the hypoglossal nerve, may provide a proprioceptive pathway from the muscles.

Descriptions provided by Crosby, Humphrey, and Lauer (1962) tend to confirm Gardner's summary, and the interconnection between the lingual branch of the trigeminal and hypoglossal nerves can be easily seen in an illustration appearing in Gray (1959, p. 1009). The importance of this interconnection for sensations arising from the deep muscles of the tongue, however, is not discussed by these authors, and our experience would not be helpful since the lingual branch of the trigeminal was presumably anesthetized and therefore unable to transmit sensory information.

In any event a reliance on kinesthesia or some positional sense in the tongue to explain articulatory accuracy under the experimental conditions referred to earlier seems unnecessary. An attractive alternative hypothesis is provided by Gammon et al. (1971) who refer to a statement by Koshevnikov and Chistovich to the effect that a unit of articulation, once programmed through learning, may become relatively self-perpetuating. Gammon et al. go on to conclude that if this is the case, then this unit would be to some extent independent of any feedback system.

Clearly more research on the presence or absence of kinesthesia in the tongue and its contribution to articulatory accuracy is indicated. Our experience is based on only a few subjects ($N = 5$) and different results might be obtained in a study involving a larger population or following different procedures.

REFERENCES

CROSBY, E. C., HUMPHREY, T., and LAUER, E. W., Correlative Neuroanatomy of the Nervous System. New York: Macmillan (1962).

GAMMON, S. A., SMITH, P. J., DANILOFF, R. G., and KIM, C. W., Articulation and stress/juncture production under oral anesthetization and masking. J. Speech Hearing Res., 14, 271-282 (1971).

GARDNER, E., GRAY, D. J., and O'RAHILLY, R., Anatomy: A Regional Study of Human Structure. Philadelphia: Saunders (1963).

GRAY, H., Anatomy of the Human Body (27th ed.). Philadelphia: Lea and Febiger (1959).

RINGEL, R. L., Oral sensation and perception: A selected review. In Speech and the Dentofacial Complex: The State of the Art, ASHA Reports 5. Washington, D.C.: American Speech and Hearing Association (1970).

SHELTON, R. L., Oral sensory function in speech production. In W. C. Grabb, S. W. Rosenstein, and K. R. Bzoch (Eds.), Cleft Lip and Palate. Boston: Little, Brown (1971).

SCHLIESSER, H. F., and COLEMAN, R. O., Effectiveness of certain procedures for alteration of auditory and oral tactile sensation for speech. Percept. mot. Skills, 26, 275-281 (1968).

A REPLY TO COLEMAN AND SCHLIESSER'S "COMMENT ON ARTICULATION AND STRESS/JUNCTURE PRODUCTION UNDER ORAL ANESTHETIZATION AND MASKING"

S. A. Gammon   P. J. Smith   R. G. Daniloff   C. W. Kim

Coleman and Schliesser remark that when anesthetized "with similar experimental conditions," as in our study, Gammon, Smith, Daniloff, and Kim (1971), neither Schliesser nor Coleman could discern where his anesthetized tongue tip was when "manipulated" with a forceps.

First, we are unsure that the Schliesser and Coleman (1968) experiment involved the same kind of anesthetic, the same extent of anesthetization, and the same depth of anesthetization as in our study. Second, it is untrue that mechanical manipulation of a passive tongue is identical to tongue movements initiated by the speaker's own muscles in terms of resulting proprioception. The first author of our study (who also served as a subject) was well aware of her tongue location; she remarked that she was aware of holding her tongue more rearward than usual to avoid biting her tongue tip accidentally. Third, the experience of the second author with oral anesthetization has been that under anesthetic such as used in our study, talkers are usually not deprived of all sense of tongue position despite deep anesthetization.

Our use of the term *kinesthesis* to describe position sense for the tongue during anesthesia may not be warranted since kinesthesis is, as Coleman and Schliesser say, reserved for sensation evoked from sensory receptors located in ligaments and tendons at the joints. However, there is recent evidence (Granit, personal communication; and Goodwin, McCloskey, and Matthews, 1972) that neuromuscular spindles within such muscles as those of the tongue may have neural projections to thalamic and higher brain centers such that subjects are aware of muscle stretch and length at a less than fully conscious level. Under appropriate conditions (Goodwin et al., 1972), subjects are consciously aware of the feedback from such muscle spindles.

An excellent discussion of the difference between conscious and unconscious sensation arising from the oral region and the potential role of such sensations in the control of speech and in the mediation of responses to standard tests of oral sensitivity is contained in the work of Ringel (1970) and Hardy (1970).

Until the extent and import of such neuromuscular spindle feedback is determined and until there is further evidence concerning the effect of anesthetic upon such different neuronal pathways, one cannot rule out proprioceptive sensation in the maintenance of articulation control under anesthetization.

REFERENCES

GAMMON, S. A., SMITH, P. J., DANILOFF, R. G., and KIM, C. W., Articulation and stress/juncture production under oral anesthetization and masking. *J. Speech Hearing Res.*, 14, 271-282 (1971).

GOODWIN, C. M., McCLOSKEY, D. I., and MATTHEWS, P. C. B., Proprioceptive illusions induced by muscle vibration: Contribution by muscle spindle to perception? *Science*, 175, 1382-1384 (1972).

HARDY, J. C., Development of neuromuscular systems underlying speech production. In *Speech and the Dentofacial Complex: The State of the Art, ASHA Reports 5.* Washington, D.C.: American Speech and Hearing Association (1970).

RINGEL, R. L., Oral sensation and perception: A selected review. In *Speech and the Dentofacial Complex: The State of the Art, ASHA Reports 5.* Washington, D.C.: American Speech and Hearing Association (1970).

SCHLIESSER, H. F., and COLEMAN, R. O., Effectiveness of certain procedures for alteration of auditory and oral tactile sensation for speech. *Percept. mot. Skills*, 26, 275-281 (1968).

218

ARTICULATION WITHOUT
ORAL SENSORY CONTROL

CHERYL M. SCOTT *and* R. L. RINGEL

Oral sensory deprivation was induced in two subjects by nerve block injections, and the effect on articulation was investigated. Twenty-four bisyllabic words produced under control and nerve block conditions were phonetically transcribed according to a close transcription scheme. Wide-band spectrograms provided acoustic information which was helpful in clarifying certain articulatory events. Articulatory changes caused by deprivation were largely nonphonemic in nature and included the loss of retroflexion and liprounding gestures, less close fricative constrictions, and retracted place of articulation. Results were interpreted to suggest that speech control involves a closed-loop component which is operative for certain types of articulatory events and not for others.

Previous investigators have attempted to delineate the role of oral sensation in the speech control process by noting the effect of oral sensory deprivation (generally achieved through nerve block procedures) on selected speech output variables such as rate, sound pressure level, fundamental frequency, and articulation (McCroskey, 1958; Ringel and Steer, 1963). Of the effects reported, perhaps the most interesting was articulatory inaccuracy. Articulation analysis usually took the form of phoneme error counts which permitted the demonstration of statistically significant increases in the deprivation condition. Having once established that oral sensory deprivation results in disordered articulation, most researchers attempted to describe the nature of the misarticulations.

In general, errors were classified according to a conventional substitution, omission, addition, and distortion scheme. McCroskey, Corely, and Jackson (1959) reported that stop and fricative substitutions and distortions accounted for most of the observed misarticulations. A majority of consonant errors were classified as distortions in the Ringel and Steer investigation (1963); Thompson (1969) mentioned that errors consisted largely of sibilant distortions and omissions. While these descriptions provide information about the phoneme classes most likely to be disturbed by oral sensory deprivation, they provide little insight into the real nature of peripheral articulatory events responsible for misarticulations. The question naturally arises as to what phonemes are substituted for one another and why some phonemes sound different from an accepted standard.

JOURNAL OF SPEECH AND HEARING RESEARCH, 1971, vol. 14, no. 4, 804-818.

Gammon, Smith, Daniloff, and Kim (1971) attempted to deal with such questions in their treatment of oral sensory deprived speech samples. Errors made during a nerve block condition were classified according to voicing, manner, and place of articulation features. Results were then presented in production confusion matrices where, for example, manner errors were tallied in a matrix plotting manner-intended against manner-produced. The most common manner change was the production of intended fricatives as stops; with respect to place of articulation, bilabials often become labiodentals. While this approach represents a neat way of quantifying and categorizing phonemic articulatory changes, it does not provide a means of recording nonphonemic changes. Indeed, the conclusion of Gammon et al. that the majority of errors occur as a result of changes from one manner or place to another rather than within such classes is the only possible one, considering that errors were tallied on a matrix with discrete manner and place categories. Preliminary work during the present investigation suggested that the articulary effects of oral sensory deprivation are largely nonphonemic in nature; for example, an intended fricative produced in the deprivation condition may differ in a definable way from a control fricative production, but it is, nevertheless, a fricative.

The present investigation sought a more detailed phonetic description of the effects of oral sensory deprivation on speech production. Phonetic and acoustic analyses of material spoken under control and nerve block conditions provided the data for the study. Results are discussed in relation to current speech control theory.

PROCEDURE

Subjects

Two adult males, age 24 and 29, served as speakers. Both subjects spoke a Midwestern dialect of American English. They had normal speech and hearing, normal oral-structural relationships, and reported no present or past sensory or motor disturbances.

Conditions

The study involved two experimental conditions: (1) control and (2) induced oral sensory deprivation through the use of nerve block anesthesia (hereafter referred to as control and block conditions, respectively). A state of oral sensory deprivation was achieved through a series of bilateral mandibular, infraorbital, posterior palatine, and medial nasopalatine nerve block injections of Xylocaine (2%, with epinephrine). The injection series resulted in the elimination of sensation from surface receptors in all supraglottal structures with the exception of the pharynx and posterior third of the tongue.

The extent to which the injections interfered with proprioceptive impulses from receptors such as muscle spindles cannot be stated with certainty. Considerable controversy surrounds the issue of the course of afferent projections

220

from muscle spindles in the human lip and tongue. If, as Hosokawa (1961) believes, the facial nerve serves as the afferent pathway from spindles in facial muscles, lip proprioception would not be commonly affected by the infraorbital injection used in this study. Afferent projections from spindles in the tongue have been attributed variously to the hypoglossal nerve itself (Langworthy, 1924), the lingual nerve, and the cervical dorsal roots (Bowman and Combs, 1969). The mandibular injection would interfere with lingual proprioception only if the lingual nerve serves as the afferent pathway.

At present, the practical possibility of obtaining a purely sensory nerve block to the oral structures is still in question. The mylohyoid nerve, supplying motor innervation to the mylohyoid muscle and the anterior belly of the digastric muscle, branches from the inferior alveolar nerve in the vicinity of the mandibular foramen. It is possible that motor innervation to these two muscles may be blocked as a result of the mandibular injection. This contention is supported by the preliminary work of Harris (1970) who was unable to detect electromyographic potentials in the mylohyoid muscle following mandibular injection. It is difficult, however, to state with certainty the consequences of isolated mylohyoid and digastric paralysis since these muscles work in synergy with other suprahyoid muscles. We suspect that the effect on speech would be minimal.

Recording and Materials

The speakers recorded a list of 24 bisyllabic words from the spondee word list (C.I.D. Auditory Test W-1), pausing for approximately four seconds between words. They were instructed to produce the words in as natural a manner as possible—the matter of syllable stress being left to their own discretion. The 24 words contain a fairly representative sample of the consonants of American English in syllable-initial and syllable-final positions and in clusters; however, the voiced fricatives /vðzʒ/ and the velar nasal /ŋ/ sounds are not included in the material. All vowels are represented at least once. The 24 spondee words used are as follows:

nutmeg	northwest	earthquake
backbone	birthday	whitewash
oatmeal	duckpond	footstool
headlight	sundown	hardware
hotdog	schoolboy	woodwork
toothbrush	airplane	drawbridge
shipwreck	eggplant	mushroom
hedgehog	scarecrow	woodchuck

The original choice of the 24 words was governed by the fact that phonetic and acoustic data on the same words produced by dysarthric speakers have

221

been published (Lehiste, 1965). Since dysarthria is generally viewed as a motor neuropathology, we wondered whether articulatory differences could be demonstrated between dysarthric and sensory deprived speakers. Such differences, if found, would emphasize the unique contribution of oral sensory information in articulation (Scott and Ringel, 1971).

The words produced during control and block conditions were recorded on high-quality magnetic tape following standard recording procedures. The recording equipment consisted of a condenser microphone (Bruel and Kjaer 4131) and a tape recorder (Ampex 602) arranged conventionally between an anechoic chamber and a control room.

Analysis

The major data of the investigation were the phonetic transcriptions of control and block productions of 24 bisyllabic words. The tapes were spliced so that the control production was followed immediately by the block production; transcription was facilitated by repeated listening. The words were transcribed by one of the authors (CMS); the second author also listened to the tapes, and his observations served as a reliability check. As difficult phonetic decisions arose, we consulted with various persons of phonetic sophistication and asked them on occasion to listen to particular productions. In most cases the perceptual observations of such persons agreed with ours. Transcription reliability, although handled informally, was considered to be good.

The nonphonemic nature of articulatory changes brought about by deprivation required the adoption of a close transcription scheme. Employing a classification system outlined by Peterson and Shoup (1966), secondary articulatory parameters such as air release, laryngeal action, apex shape, and lip shape were identified as well as primary manner and place parameters. In addition to the phonetic transcriptions, wide-band spectrograms were made of control and block words. The spectrograms were helpful in clarifying certain articulatory events and were used in making comparative measurements of formant frequency and segment durations (for example, stop closure, stop release, syllable nuclei).

RESULTS

This section identifies the types of articulatory changes observed during the nerve block condition with reference to the control condition. The results presented are data based on phonetic transcriptions and are organized according to stop, fricative, sonorant, nasal, and vowel manner categories.

Stop Production

The effects of deprivation on the articulation of stop consonants are identified and listed in Table 1. The number of occurrences (NO) of each type of articula-

222

tory change is listed separately for both speakers. An indication of the prominence of a particular feature is obtained by comparing the number of occurrences with the number of potential occurrences (NPO).

Table 1 shows that very few stop deviations involved clear-cut manner substitutions. Under conditions of oral sensory deprivation, both speakers almost always produced stops when stops were called for in the material. The produc-

TABLE 1. Articulatory changes during block productions of stop consonants.

Articulatory Changes in Comparison with Control	Speaker 1		Speaker 2		Specification of NPO in Material
	NO°	NPO°	NO	NPO	
Manner substitution—stop becomes fricative or affricate.	3	44	2	44	All stops in all positions
Place of tongue closure is retracted.	25	34	10	34	/tdkg/ in all positions
Place of closure for bilabial stops is labiodental.	0	10	4	10	/pb/ in all positions
Unilabial stops—lower lip against motionless upper lip.	6	10	3	10	/pb/ in all positions
Air release—intended aspirated stop is produced with affricated release.	4	6	1	6	/ptk/ in syllable-initial positions

°NO = number of occurrences; NPO = number of potential occurrences

tion of the bilabial fricative [β] for intended syllable-initial /b/ or /d/ accounted for four of the five stop-manner substitutions.

Alveolar and velar stops were frequently produced with a closure that was retracted from the place of closure for control productions. Retraction was particularly prominent for the velar stops, which Speaker 1 produced as uvular stops [qɢ] in every possible case. The relative lowering of F_2 seen in the release of [q] in the block production of *shipwreck* (illustrated spectrographically in Figure 1) is consistent with a retracted place of articulation (Fant, 1960). Similarly, the alveolar stops /td/ were produced with a retracted closure in the prepalatal or palatal area where contact was made with a relatively large surface area of the tongue including part of the blade as well as the apex.

In typical bilabial stop production, the upper lip flattens and lowers slightly against the teeth, thereby facilitating closure. In approximately half of the potential instances, however, intended bilabial stops were produced with a closure formed almost entirely by the upward movement of the lower lip against a motionless upper lip. This particular type of stop deviation is recorded in Table 1 as unilabial stop production. The phonetic observation of unilabial stops was strengthened by our visual recollection of block /pb/ articulation indicating that the upper lip was completely inactive and the lower lip was particularly passive, appearing to be carried along by the upward movement of the mandible. In addition, motion pictures taken during bilabial articulation in two different speakers deprived of lip sensation (Butt, 1970) seem to support

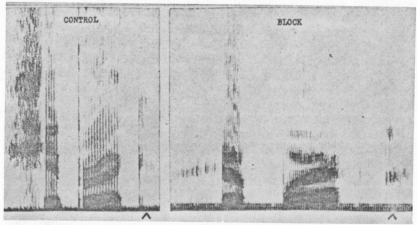

FIGURE 1. Spectrograms of control and block productions of the word *shipwreck*. Arrows refer to syllable-final /k/ segments.

this observation. The tendency of Speaker 2 to produce /p/ and /b/ with a labiodental closure is, perhaps, also connected with the observed upper lip inactivity. If the upper lip is inactive, it would conceivably be easy for the lower lip to make contact with the upper teeth in the course of its upward movement.

The release characteristics of voiceless stops in syllable-initial positions were often altered in block productions. In American English, such stops are characterized by aspiration. During the block condition, however, /p/ and /t/ were sometimes released in an affricated (protracted) manner. Spectrograms of initial /t/ in *toothbrush* produced by Speaker 1 are reproduced in Figure 2.

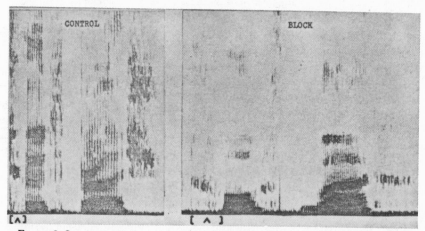

FIGURE 2. Spectrograms of control and block productions of the word *toothbrush*. Arrows refer to syllable-initial /t/-segment durations which are defined by brackets.

Whereas the control release in this example is 60 msec, the block release is 120 msec.

The fortis-lenis distinction between stops was always maintained during block articulation. That is, intended fortis stops /ptk/ were never produced as lenis stops /bdg/ and vice versa. It was our belief that both fortis and lenis stops were produced with less overall supraglottal energy—an observation which seemed to correlate on an acoustic level with spectrographic evidence of diminished spike amplitude in block stops as compared to control stops.

In summary, the articulation of stop consonants during oral sensory deprivation was characterized by (1) retracted place of closure for /tdkg/, (2) upper lip inactivity for /pb/, and (3) the affricated release of voiceless syllable-initial stops.

Fricative Production

Fricatives produced by both speakers during the block condition always retained their characteristic fricative manner of production. The tendency for fricatives to become stops reported by Gammon et al. (1971) was never observed in the present investigation.

Table 2 is organized in a manner similar to Table 1 and shows the type and frequency of articulatory changes noted during block productions of sibilants /s/ and /ʃ/. As indicated in Table 2, /s/ and /ʃ/ were almost always produced with a less close constriction involving the loss or reduction of the fine apex and blade constriction adjustments characteristic of sibilants. In addition, sibilants produced by Speaker 1 were characterized by a retracted place of constriction.

TABLE 2. Articulatory changes during block productions of sibilants /s/ and /ʃ/.

Articulatory Changes in Comparison with Control	Speaker 1		Speaker 2	
	NO	NPO	NO	NPO
/s/ primary constriction is retracted.	3	5	0	5
/s/ primary constriction is less close.	4	5	3	5
/ʃ/ primary constriction is retracted.	4	4	0	4
/ʃ/ primary constriction is less close.	4	4	4	4

Comparison of the spectrograms of control and block productions of /ʃ/ in the word *shipwreck* (reproduced in Figure 1) illustrates the acoustic result of sibilant articulatory changes. Initial /ʃ/ in the block condition was produced as the less close palatal fricative [çʸ]. The high-frequency energy of the control /ʃ/ segment is considerably diminished in the block spectrogram where an energy band representing the second formant of the entire vocal tract appears. The larger opening in the case of the block fricative contributes toward em-

225

phasizing formants (in this case the second) which depend on the entire vocal tract rather than only those in front of and in the area of the constriction.

The production of /θ/ during the block condition was retracted in two of three potential occurrences by both speakers. The labiodental fricative /f/ occurred only once in the material; there were no apparent changes from control productions.

Sonorant Production

The types of articulatory changes associated with block consonant /r/ articulation are summarized in Table 3. Block productions of /r/ by Speaker 1 were characterized by a reduction or total loss of the retroflex articulatory gesture.

TABLE 3. Articulatory changes during block productions of consonant /r/.

Articulatory Changes in Comparison with Control	Speaker 1 NO	Speaker 1 NPO	Speaker 2 NO	Speaker 2 NPO
Nonretroflexion	5	9	1	9
Omitted with labialization of contiguous vowel	2	9	1	9
Omitted	1	9	2	9

On an acoustic level, retroflexion is correlated with an F_3 position which is low and in close proximity to F_2 (Fant, 1960). Spectrograms of the word *drawbridge* produced by Speaker 1 are reproduced in Figure 3, where the lack of F_3–F_2 proximity during the /r/ segments is obvious in the block production. Consonant /r/ in the first syllable of the block version of *drawbridge* was completely omitted with strong labialization of the contiguous vowel; /r/ in the

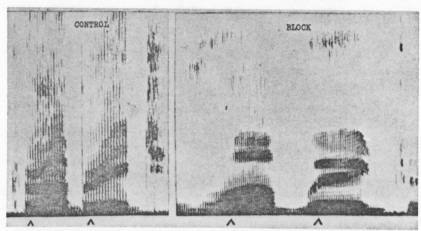

FIGURE 3. Spectrograms of control and block productions of the word *drawbridge*. Arrows refer to consonant /r/ segments.

226

second syllable was produced with a reduced degree of retroflexion. Similar acoustic effects can be observed by comparing control and block /r/ segments in the spectrograms of *shipwreck* and *toothbrush* (Figures 1 and 2, respectively).

Consonant /r/ was omitted entirely three times by each speaker. In a few of these instances, the adjacent vowel was produced with strong labialization, perhaps representing a compensatory gesture. Speaker 1 articulated two of three block productions of vocalic /ər/ with a loss of retroflexion.

Block productions of the sonorant /w/ were characterized by delabialization, or a lip configuration which was less close and less protruded (in three out of seven cases by Speaker 1 and in six of seven cases by Speaker 2). There were no apparent differences between control and block productions of the lateral /l/.

In summary, block productions of sibilants /s/ and /ʃ/ were frequently articulated with a less close and retracted constriction. The apical retroflexion gesture during consonant /r/ was occasionally lost or reduced in the block condition. Finally, block productions of the sonorant /w/ were characterized by delabialization.

Nasal Production

In general, the production of nasal consonants was not affected in any important way by the loss of oral sensation. On two (out of 11 possible) occasions, Speaker 1 replaced nasal consonants with a strongly nasalized version of the contiguous vowel. Both speakers retracted block productions of the alveolar nasal /n/ in two of eight possible cases. There were no apparent articulatory changes during block productions of the bilabial nasal /m/. The ability to form a bilabial closure for /m/ might be unexpected, in light of data presented earlier concerning block articulation of bilabial stops; however, there is some reason to believe that labial closing and opening dynamics for /m/ are different from those for /p/ and /b/, since /m/ closure does not require the containment of an oral overpressure (Fujimura, 1961).

Vowel Production

Like consonants, vowels which call for labial articulatory adjustments were often altered during oral sensory deprivation. Block productions by both speakers of the back vowel series /ɔouu/ were less rounded than control productions in over half of the potential cases. A second type of alteration was the occasional production of a less close version of high front and high back vowels.

It is highly probable that vowels were sometimes produced with a retracted place of articulation. Recalling the strong tendency for block productions of stops and fricatives to be retracted, it seems naive to think that vowels in the vicinity of such consonants were not retracted as well. While a slight degree of tongue retraction would result in a phonetically (perceptually) observable

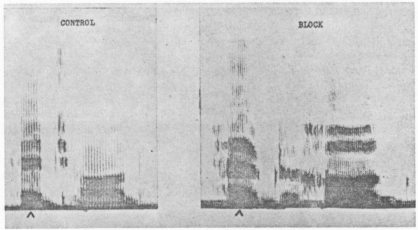

CONTROL | BLOCK

FIGURE 4. Spectrograms of control and block productions of the word *hedgehog*. Arrows refer to syllable nucleus /ɛ/.

change in a fricative, the same amount of retraction during vowel production might not cause any perceptible phonetic shift.

Measurements of the first and second formant center frequencies for vowels tend to support the contention that vowels were produced with retracted and less close, or more neutral articulatory configurations. Spectrograms of the word *hedgehog* (reproduced in Figure 4) represent an example of considerable second formant lowering in the front vowel /ɛ/. The center frequency of F_2 in the control version is 1850 Hz, while F_2 in the block example is 1600 Hz. Close comparison of syllable nuclei in other spectrograms presented thus far reveals similar cases of downward formant shift. Changes in fundamental frequency were also noted in some instances. These effects were thought to be of a secondary nature, since there is no reason to believe that oral anesthesia would have an effect on laryngeal function.

With the exception of the examples discussed, the majority of vowels in the block condition sounded much like the corresponding control productions. Formant frequency measurements, however, support the view that articulatory changes do, in fact, occur, but may not be significant in a perceptual sense. In light of the foregoing discussion, the statements made by previous researchers to the effect that vowels are unaffected by deprivation calls for reexamination. Also in need of reevaluation is the assertion that vowels are monitored, therefore, by channels presumed to be undisturbed by the nerve block—such as a kinesthetic channel (Gammon et al., 1971) or the auditory channel (Ladefoged, 1967).

DISCUSSION

The results of earlier deprivation studies were, for the most part, interpreted to support Fairbanks's servo-mechanistic theory of speech control (1954). According to Fairbanks, speech output (in the form of auditory and oral sensory feedback) is continually sampled and compared to the input signal. The system calculates the difference between the output and input signals; the resulting error signal serves to modify the original driving signal to form an effective driving signal for the production system. The important point to be made is that all driving signals received by the articulatory structures are signals that have been processed, or altered in accordance with information from peripheral receptors.

Previous investigators reasoned that the demonstration of articulatory error in a nerve block condition offered direct support for a servomechanistic, or closed-loop speech control system. Such an interpretation ignores the fact that, in spite of some subtle (nonphonemic) articulatory changes, speech remains highly intelligible under conditions of oral sensory deprivation. A theory based entirely on closed-loop control, such as Fairbanks's, would seem to predict a severe level of artiulatory breakdown in the absence of peripheral oral sensory information. One might argue that the elimination of oral sensory information would never produce a major articulatory breakdown because the auditory system takes on additional control responsibilities. Speech is also highly intelligible, however, following simultaneous oral sensory and auditory deprivation (Ringel and Steer, 1963). Schliesser and Coleman (1968) reported that the misarticulations brought about by deprivation constitute a mild degree of articulatory dysfunction. We could agree with Schliesser and Coleman that "in view of the stress placed by current speech control theory upon the importance of auditory and tactile feedback, the presence of understandable speech is provocative."

An alternative point of view is that speech control is largely open-loop in nature—that is, speech is controlled autonomously in the absence of peripheral oral sensory feedback. The essence of an open-loop control mechanism, according to MacNeilage (1970), is that "it would not have to wait for information associated with actually reaching the previous location in order to control the following movement appropriately." If speech control were entirely open-loop in nature, however, we would expect no articulatory changes during a condition of oral sensory deprivation.

An additional consideration that elicits concern is that acceptance of an open-loop system would require the prestoring and ready recall of perhaps as many as 100,000 unique allophonic motor patterns (MacNeilage, 1970). While the storage of such a number of motor patterns is certainly conceivable, investigators have been bothered intuitively by the apparent inefficiency of a system functioning in that manner.

The attempt to accommodate such considerations has led several investigators to hypothesize open- and closed-loop control in speech and to search for specific examples in support of either possibility. For example, MacNeilage, Krones, and Hanson (1970) have reported data on jaw movement which were interpreted to suggest closed-loop control in the initiation of speech. Summarizing the data, MacNeilage (1970) stated:

> ... although the amount of opening of the jaw varies over a range of several milli-
> meters under nonspeech conditions, the jaw position adopted for a given initial seg-
> ment shows very little variation (1-2 mm) with repetitions of the same utterance.
> For this to be so, the production mechanism must take into account the pre-speech
> position of the jaw, and make a speech-initial jaw movement contingent upon the
> pre-speech position. (p. 192)

Data which would appear to support the view of closed-loop control in on-going speech has been reported by Ohman (1965). Despite the obvious articulatory differences involved in producing the stop /d/ in /idi/ and /ada/ contexts, Ohman found that vowel-consonant and consonant-vowel formant transition durations were almost identical. If the acoustic measures reflect a corresponding difference in articulatory transition duration, Ohman suggests that a closed-loop mechanism operates to accelerate the gesture in the /ada/ context. Further evidence of closed-loop control is found in the work of Kozhevnikov and Chistovich (1965), who reported that the velocity of the lower lip closure in bilabial consonants is directly proportional to the amount of lip opening for the preceding vowel.

It seems important to point out that many of the recent discussions concerning open- versus closed-loop control have been stimulated by the problem of motor equivalence in speech production. That is, by what means do the articulators achieve a relatively constant target from a variety of initial positions? The investigations mentioned above were designed to deal with this question. Our study deals with a fundamentally different question, namely, are all types of articulatory events necessarily controlled in the same manner? Solutions to both types of problems will undoubtedly have implications for speech control theory.

The data presented here do not allow us to postulate an open or closed-loop system, but rather lead us to support the view that articulatory activity is dependent upon both open- and closed-loop components. The lack of phonemic change in the deprivation condition is evidence that speakers were able to execute basic manner gestures such as (1) palatal opening and closing, (2) complete vocal tract closures, (3) close vocal tract constrictions, and (4) vocal tract configurations appropriate for vowels. This brief review of articulatory activities which were accomplished in spite of almost total lack of information from peripheral receptors supports the view of a speech mechanism which operates in response to autonomous motor commands (or target specifications) which are largely manner types of instructions. Having issued such instructions, however, the speech mechanism calls for certain closed-loop refinements which are particularly prominent for phonemes involving precise types of apical and blade configurations, such as sibilants and the consonant /r/. Information from oral receptors appears to be a necessity for the successful execution of certain labial, apical, and blade refinements which are more important for some phonemes than for others.

The results of this study are consistent with ideas reported by Liberman et al. (1967) concerning the nature of motor commands:

These instructions might be of two types, "on-off" or "go to," even in a maximally simple model. In the one case, the affected muscle would contract or not with little regard for its current state (or the position of the articulator it moves): in the other, the instruction would operate via the γ-efferent system to determine the degree of contraction (hence, the final position of the articulator, whatever its initial position). (p. 447)

The authors state further that the "go to" instructions may operate in articulatory gestures that are relatively precise. While it is not known with certainty whether information from muscle spindles (contributing to the gamma-efferent system) was interrupted during the block condition, the tongue tip is particularly well supplied with specialized tactile and pressure receptors which might operate in a functionally similar manner (Rose and Mountcastle, 1959).

Seen in this light, articulatory gestures which were unaffected by deprivation, such as palatal opening and closing and lingual closure for stops, may respond to "on-off" types of instruction which are primarily open-loop in nature.

The "on-off" type of instruction does not necessarily imply a corresponding binary type of articulatory gesture at the peripheral level. In fact, palatal positioning has been found to vary considerably as a function of phone type, duration, and context. Moll and Shriner (1967) hypothesize that the variable (nonbinary) nature of palatal activity can be attributed to anatomical interconnections with other structures and that the underlying neuromuscular activity is binary, or high-level versus low-level. Lubker (1968), on the other hand, has reported palatal electromyographic data which are at variance with the hypothesis of binary neuromuscular instructions.

Conversely, "go to" instructions which are dependent upon peripheral sensory information for their realization are sent to articulatory structures such as the intrinsic tongue muscles, which are responsible for refinements applied to the more basic manner gestures. The elimination of peripheral sensation has the apparent result of reducing the ability of the articulators to approximate the target specifications inherent in the "go to" instructions. Hence, as the results of this study show, the articulators are characterized by a generalized "undershoot," or reduced articulatory amplitude in the form of (1) less close sibilant constrictions, (2) reduced degrees of retroflexion and lip rounding, and (3) a slight tendency toward a more neutral vocal tract configuration during vowel production.

In the design of an articulatory model of speech production for computer simulation, Henke (1967) raises the question of the relation between oral sensory feedback and temporal characteristics of speech. More specifically, his model is designed so that the timing or rate of progression of events is made contingent upon the response of the model articulators. As an example, Henke describes the production of a stop in which on-going articulation waits until contact between articulators (closure) is attained, and then uses the awareness of this happening, presumably through proprioceptive feedback, as a trigger for further articulator activity. The model thus predicts that in the absence of peripheral information, the temporal characteristics of speech may become disorganized. Duration measurements of stop-consonant production in the present investigation are suggestive of a possible connection between peripheral feedback and timing of instructions to articulators. The reader will recall that the release phase of voiceless stops was considerably prolonged in the block condition and that voicing for the contiguous vowel was, in such cases, delayed in comparison to control examples. Whether the voicing delay is the passive result of slower supraglottal pressure release, or whether the timing of the glottal instruction for voicing is delayed in light of incomplete information concerning stop closure is unanswerable at present.

The results of this investigation do not have a direct bearing on the advisability or inadvisability of utilizing the oral sensory channel in retraining articulation in the clinical setting. In our opinion, the finding of articulatory changes following oral sensory deprivation has been mistakenly interpreted by some researchers to imply that the oral sensory channel is more important than the auditory channel and should be stressed in retraining procedures. We believe that the neurological mechanisms underlying the use of sensory information for conscious introspection in the clinical setting are very different from those which operate at a highly automatic level in normal speech. It is hoped, of course, that accumulating knowledge and understanding of sensory control in speech will eventually lead to improved training techniques in the clinic.

ACKNOWLEDGMENT

This investigation was supported in part by Public Health Service Awards 1 KO3 DE 32614-03 and 1 RO1 DE 02815-02 from the National Institute of Dental Research and by the Purdue Research Foundation. Requests for reprints should be addressed to R. L. Ringel, Department of Audiology and Speech Sciences, Purdue University, Lafayette, Indiana 47907.

REFERENCES

BOWMAN, J. P., and COMBS, C. M., The cerebrocortical projection of hypoglossal afferents. *Exp. Neurol.*, 23, 291-301 (1969).

BUTT, ANNE H., Some observations of lip articulation during labial sensory deprivation. Master's thesis, Purdue Univ. (1970).

FAIRBANKS, G., Systematic research in experimental phonetics. I. A theory of the speech mechanism as a servosystem. *J. Speech Hearing Dis.*, 19, 133-140 (1954).

FANT, G., *Acoustic Theory of Speech Production*. The Hague: Mouton (1960).

FUJIMURA, O., Bilabial stop and nasal consonants; a motion picture study and its acoustical implications. *J. Speech Hearing Res.*, 4, 233-247 (1961).

GAMMON, SYLVIA A., SMITH, P., DANILOFF, R., and KIM, C., Articulation and stress/juncture production under oral anesthetization and masking. *J. Speech Hearing Res.*, 14, 271-282 (1971).

HARRIS, KATHERINE S., Physiological measures of speech movements: EMG and fiberoptic studies. In *Proceedings of the Workshop Speech and the Dentofacial Complex: The State of the Art. ASHA Reports Number 5*, 271-282 (October 1970).

HENKE, W., Preliminaries to speech synthesis based upon an articulatory model. Paper presented at the Conference on Speech Communications and Processing, Cambridge, Mass. (1967).

HOSOKAWA, H., Proprioceptive innervation of striated muscle in the territory of the cranial nerves. *Tex. Rep. Biol. Med.*, 19, 405-464 (1961).

KOZHEVNIKOV, W. A., and CHISTOVICH, L., *Rech: Artikulyatsiya i Vospriyatiye* (Speech: articulation and perception). Moscow-Leningrad: Nauka (1965). (Translation avaliable from the Joint Publications Research Service, U. S. Dept. Commerce, Washington, D. C., No. 30, 543.)

LADEFOGED, P., *Three Areas of Experimental Phonetics*. London: Oxford Univ. (1967).

LANGWORTHY, O. R., A study of the innervation of the tongue musculature with particular reference to the proprioceptive mechanism. *J. comp. Neurol.*, 36, 273-298 (1924).

LEHISTE, ILSE, Some acoustic characteristics of dysarthric speech. *Bibl. phone.*, Fasc. 2, New York: S. Karger (1965).

LIBERMAN, A. M., Cooper, F. S., Shankweiler, D. P., and Studdert-Kennedy, M., Perception of the speech code. *Psychol. Rev.*, 74, 431-463 (1967).

LUBKER, J. F., An electromyographic-cinefluorographic investigation of velar function during normal speech production. *Cleft Pal. J.*, 5, 1-17 (1968).

MacNEILAGE, P. F., Motor control of serial ordering of speech. *Psychol. Rev.*, 77, 182-196 (1970).

MacNEILAGE, P. F., KRONES, R., and HANSON, R., Closed-loop control of the initiation of jaw movement for speech. *J. acoust. Soc. Amer.*, 47, 104 (1970).

McCROSKEY, R., The relative contributions of auditory and tactile cues to certain aspects of speech. *South. Speech J.*, 24, 84-90 (1958).

McCROSKEY, R., CORELY, N., and JACKSON, G., Some effects of disrupted tactile cues upon the production of consonants. *South. Speech J.*, 25, 55-60 (1959).

MOLL, K. L., and SHRINER, T., Preliminary investigation of a new concept of velar activity during speech. *Cleft Pal. J.*, 4, 58-69 (1967).

OHMAN, S. E. G., Durations of formant frequency transitions. Stockholm, Sweden: Royal Institute of Technology, STL-QPSR, 10-13 (1/1965).

PETERSON, G. E., and SHOUP, JUNE, A physiological theory of phonetics. *J. Speech Hearing Res.*, 9, 5-67 (1966).

RINGEL, R. L., and STEER, M. D., Some effects of tactile and auditory alterations on speech output. *J. Speech Hearing Res.*, 6, 369-378 (1963).

ROSE, J. E., and MOUNTCASTLE, V. B., Touch and kinesthesis. In J. Field, H. W. Magoun, and V. E. Hall (Eds.), *Neurophysiology*. Vol I. Washington, D. C.: American Physiological Society (1959).

SCHLIESSER, H. F., and COLEMAN, R., Effectiveness of certain procedures for alteration of auditory and oral tactile sensation for speech. *Percept. mot. Skills*, 26, 271-281 (1968).

SCOTT, CHERYL M., and RINGEL, R. L., The effects of motor and sensory disruptions on speech: A description of articulation. *J. Speech Hearing Res.*, 14, 819-828 (1971).

THOMPSON, R. C., The effects of oral sensory disruption upon oral stereognosis and articulation. Paper presented at the 45th Annual Convention of the American Speech and Hearing Association, Chicago (1969).

233

THE EFFECTS OF MOTOR AND SENSORY
DISRUPTIONS ON SPEECH:
A DESCRIPTION OF ARTICULATION

CHERYL M. SCOTT and R. L. RINGEL

Eleven spondee words produced by six dysarthric and two sensory-deprived speakers were phonetically transcribed in order to determine whether motor and sensory dysfunctions result in distinctive articulatory patterns. In general, the types of articulatory deviations produced by dysarthric speakers were different from those produced by speakers deprived of oral sensation. Stop and fricative error patterns in particular appear to differentiate the two groups of speakers. The results serve to emphasize the unique contribution of information from peripheral oral receptors in the control of ongoing speech.

Criticism of research that has attempted to study the role of the oral sensory system in speech control through nerve-block anesthetization procedures has focused on the potential motor effects of the intended sensory blocks. Tests which assess the integrity of the motor system in isolation (that is, without interaction with sensory control mechanisms) are difficult to conceive, and evidence to support the view that "sensory-deprived" speech is purely that, is not available. One approach to resolving the controversy would seem to be the description of the effects on speech production of known motor disorders (dysarthric speech) and the comparison of such a pattern to that observed during the hypothesized state of sensory deprivation. While the difficulty of making definitive statements about the level of speech disturbance based solely upon the acoustic and perceptual analyses of such speech is recognized, it is expected that if sensory block procedures do not produce a motor paralysis, then sensory and motor disabilities should be associated with unique patterns of speech. Such comparisons might also be expected to shed light upon the respective roles of the sensory and motor systems in the control of normal speech activities. With this framework in mind, a study was conducted in which speech samples obtained from persons with motor disabilities were compared to those obtained from persons who were deprived of normal sensation in the mouth.

METHOD

The data in this investigation are phonetic transcriptions of eleven spondee words (Table 1) produced by six adult dysarthric speakers and two speakers

JOURNAL OF SPEECH AND HEARING RESEARCH, 1971, vol. 14, no. 4, 819-828.

TABLE 1. Eleven spondee words produced by dysarthric and sensory-deprived speakers.

toothbrush	schoolboy
shipwreck	airplane
northwest	eggplant
birthday	drawbridge
duckpond	mushroom
sundown	

deprived of oral sensation. The six dysarthric speakers were part of a larger dysarthric group studied extensively by Tikofsky and Tikofsky (1964) and Lehiste (1965). Pertinent biographical information concerning the dysarthric speakers was originally reported by Tikofsky and Tikofsky and is reproduced in Table 2.

The sensory-deprived speakers were two adult males with normal speech and hearing who were subjected to a series of nerve-block injections· designed to eliminate sensation in the oral region. All subjects were speakers of a midwestern dialect of American English. The speech samples produced by the dysarthric and sensory-deprived subjects were transcribed phonetically according to a close transcription scheme in which articulatory parameters such as lip shape, apex shape, and air release as well as place, manner, and voicing were identified (Peterson and Shoup, 1966). Wide band spectrograms of dysarthric productions were made and were helpful in clarifying certain articulatory events. A more detailed account of the analysis procedure and injection series has been presented in an earlier communication (Scott and Ringel, 1971).

RESULTS

Table 3 lists the major types of articulatory aberrations observed during the production of stops, fricatives, and sonorants as well as the number of occurrences (NO) of each for both speaker groups. In order to gain perspective as to the prominence of a particular type of deviation, the number of potential occurrences (NPO) of each misarticulation in the total speech sample is also shown in Table 3.

Stop Production

As indicated by inspection of Table 3, stop consonant deviations produced by dysarthric and sensory-deprived speakers were overwhelmingly changes within the stop manner category. In other words, both groups almost always produced stops when stops were called for in the speech material. In general, dysarthric stop deviations involved changes in one or more of the features of voicing and aspiration.

Devoicing of intended voiced syllable-initial stops was the most common

235

TABLE 2. Biographical information for dysarthric speakers.

Biographical Factors	Subjects					
	1	2	3	4	5	6
Age	38	35	42	38	25	52
Education	3 years college	10th grade	M.D.	High school diploma	2⅔ years college	B.A.
Neurological diagnosis	Closed head injury	Post-encephalitic brain deficit	Post-traumatic brain and cerebellar deficit	Fredrick's ataxia	Post-traumatic brain stem damage	CVA
Etiology	Auto accident	Acute encephalitis	Auto accident	Unknown	Auto accident	CVA
Judgment of speech severity	Mild-moderate	Severe	Moderate	Moderate	Moderate	Severe
Amount of speech therapy	2 weeks	None	2 months	None	1½ years	3 years

TABLE 3. Type and number of articulatory deviations in the production of stops, fricatives, and sonorants by dysarthric and sensory-deprived speakers. NO means number of occurrences of a deviant feature; NPO, number of potential occurrences of a deviant feature in the material (11 spondee words) × number of speakers.

Deviations	Dysarthric		Sensory-Deprived	
	NO	NPO	NO	NPO
Stops				
Interclass manner changes (e.g., substitution of a fricative for a stop)	2	120	3	40
Intraclass manner changes				
Devoicing of intended voiced initial stops	20	48	1	16
Deaspiration of intended voiceless initial stops	8	24	0	8
Affricative release of intended voiceless initial stops	0	24	5	8
Place changes				
Place of lingual closure for /tdkg/ is retracted	2	72	12	24
Unilabial stops—lower lip against motionless upper lip	0	48	6	16
Omission of final or cluster stops	4	48	0	16
Fricatives				
Voicing of intended voiceless fricatives	4	54	0	18
Substitution of dental stop for syllable-final /θ/	6	18	0	6
Omission of syllable-final /θ/	3	18	0	6
Substitution of one American English fricative for another	5	54	0	18
Constriction for /s/ is retracted	0	18	1	6
Constriction for /s/ is less close	0	18	3	6
Constriction for /ʃ/ is retracted	0	18	3	6
Constriction for /ʃ/ is less close	1	18	6	6
Constriction for /θ/ is retracted	0	18	4	6
Sonorants				
Nonretroflexion of consonant /r/	11	42	4	14
Omission of consonant /r/	5	42	6	14
Omission of /l/	4	18	0	6

stop deviation in the dysarthric group. Forty-two percent (20/48) of the intended voiced initial stops were devoiced by this group. An acoustic illustration of devoicing is provided in Figure 1 which shows the spectrogram of the word *schoolboy* produced by a dysarthric speaker. In this example, voicing of the contiguous vowel following the release of syllable-initial /b/ was delayed by approximately 35 msec. Acoustic measures of voicing lag in devoiced stops produced by dysarthric speakers always exceeded 20 msec. This value should be viewed in light of voicing onset measurements reported by Lisker and Abramson (1964) for /b/ and/d/ as produced by

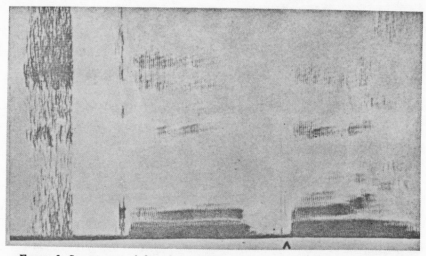

FIGURE 1. Spectrogram of dysarthric production of the word *schoolboy* which provides an acoustic illustration of the devoicing of syllable-initial /b/. The arrow refers to the stop release segment.

normal speakers of American English. In their investigation, voicing either preceded the stop release or began no later than 5 msec, on the average, following the stop release. As Table 3 indicates, devoicing was not characteristic of stops produced by sensory-deprived speakers.

Voiceless syllable-initial stops with expected aspiration were deaspirated eight times, or in approximately one-third of the potential instances, by dysarthric speakers. Figure 2 illustrates acoustically the deaspiration of /p/ in *duckpond* where the aspiration interval duration was 20 msec. This value is considerably less than the average aspiration duration of about 60 msec for /p/ reported by Lisker and Abramson (1964). Deaspiration was never observed in stops produced by sensory-deprived speakers. Rather, the release phase was lengthened in time, resulting in an affricated release.

Intended alveolar and velar stops produced by sensory-deprived speakers were retracted in half of the potential cases. In addition, intended bilabial stops were often articulated in a unilabial manner in which the upper lip was completely inactive. Neither of these articulatory patterns was characteristic of stops produced by dysarthric speakers.

In general, the comparison of dysarthric and sensory-deprived stop deviations revealed that each group made unique kinds of articulatory errors.

Fricative Production

As shown in Table 3, the fricative error pattern differed considerably between the two groups of speakers. Syllable-final /θ/ in the words *tooth-*

238

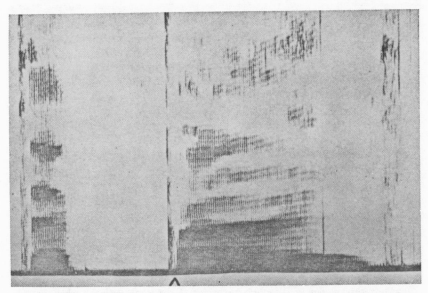

FIGURE 2. Spectrogram of dysarthric production of the word *duckpond* which provides an acoustic illustration of the deaspiration of syllable-initial /p/. The arrow refers to the stop release segment.

brush, northwest, and *birthday* was either omitted or produced as a dental stop nine times, or in half the potential instances, by the dysarthrics. The spectrogram of a dysarthric speaker's production of *northwest,* reproduced in Figure 3, clearly illustrates the production of intended /θ/ as a dental stop [t̪]. Other fricative errors produced by the dysarthrics include the substitution of one American English fricative for another, and the occasional voicing of intended voiceless fricatives. Sensory-deprived speakers, on the other hand, showed none of the same types of difficulties in producing fricatives. The very consistent trend in the production of fricatives by sensory-deprived speakers was that of less close and retracted versions of sibilants /s/ and /ʃ/. It is apparent that fricative articulatory patterns differ considerably between the sensory- and motor-disturbed speakers.

Sonorant and Vowel Production

Both groups had difficulty articulating phonetically acceptable productions of consonant /r/. Thirty-eight percent of /r/ occurrences were either omitted or produced with less retroflexion by dysarthric speakers; the same was true of 71% of potential /r/ occurrences produced by the sensory-deprived speakers. Dysarthric speakers occasionally omitted the lateral /l/ as well as /r/. Neither group had difficulty producing phonetically acceptable vowels, although the dysarthric group occasionally produced syllable nuclei which involved a type of diphthongization of normally nondiphthongized vowels.

239

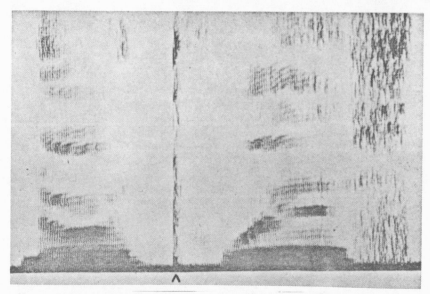

FIGURE 3. Spectrogram of dysarthric production of the word *northwest* which provides an acoustic illustration of the production of syllable-final /θ/ as a dental stop [t̪]. The arrow refers to the stop release.

Deviations at the Laryngeal and Velar Levels

Table 4 lists the type and number of laryngeal and velar deviations observed as well as the number of potential occurrences of each deviation. The most prominent deviation at the laryngeal level produced by the dysarthric speakers involved a type of laryngealization characterized by slow and

TABLE 4. Articulatory deviations at the laryngeal and velar levels.

Deviations	Dysarthric		Sensory-Deprived	
	NO	NPO	NO	NPO
Laryngeal Level				
Laryngealization	22	•	3	•
Breathy phonation	6	•	0	•
Devoicing of sonorants	3	66	0	22
Velar Level				
Audible nasal air release in syllable final position	10	132	0	44
Denasalization of initial nasals	2	12	0	4
Nasalization of syllable nuclei				
Compensatory	5	48	2	16
Assimilation	11	48	1	16

* These features can occur essentially anywhere in the spondee words.

irregular vocal fold vibration. Laryngealization appears in spectrograms as widely spaced, or biphasic vertical striations and is illustrated in Figure 4 during the word *shipwreck* as spoken by a dysarthric subject. The dysarthrics occasionally produced syllable nuclei characterized by breathy phonation and sonorants which were devoiced. The lack of deviation at the laryngeal level in words produced by sensory-deprived speakers was expected since the injection series did not inferfere with laryngeal sensation.

As shown in Table 4, nasal airflow was clearly audible in syllable-final

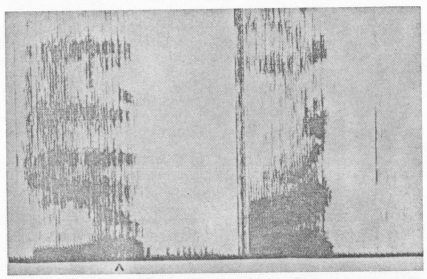

FIGURE 4. Spectrogram of dysarthric production of the word *shipwreck* which provides an acoustic illustration of laryngealization during the syllable nucleus /ɪ/. The arrow refers to the laryngealized syllable nucleus.

positions in 10 instances for the dysarthric group. Another deviant velar feature was the denasalization of initial /n/ in the word *northwest* which resulted in the production of the devoiced lenis alveolar stop [d̥]. Examples of compensatory and assimilation nasalization of syllable nuclei were found in both dysarthric and sensory-deprived speech; however, assimilation nasality was considerably more prominent in words produced by the dysarthrics.

DISCUSSION

Within the limitations of the small subject group size and material analyzed, the results of this investigation indicate that speakers whose articulatory difficulties arise from damage to motor pathways can be distinguished from those with sensory-based problems on the basis of close phonetic analysis of consonant misarticulations. Stop and fricative error patterns, in particular, appear to differentiate dysarthric and sensory-deprived speakers. The view that various disturbances in nervous system integrity are reflected in unique patterns of articulation is consistent with the research of Darley, Aronson, and Brown (1969). While their investigation demonstrated that specific types of dysarthrias (such as Parkinsons, bulbar palsy) are distinguishable on the basis of articulatory characteristics, our study would seem to indicate that "the dysarthric" articulatory pattern can be distinguished from patterns of speech demonstrated by persons with sensory-based difficulties.

Careful study of Table 2 which lists pertinent biographical factors concerning the six dysarthric speakers reveals that the group was heterogeneous with regard to etiology and diagnosed neuropathology. The reader might question, consequently, whether this group represents "pure" dysarthria; indeed, he may suspect that factors in addition to dysarthria such as dyspraxia or perhaps even a sensory deficit contribute to the articulatory patterns described here. We would point out, however, that no single dysarthric speaker presented an articulation pattern approximating that of the sensory-deprived speakers. We believe that the heterogeneity of the dysarthric group can be interpreted as strengthening the validity of our view that the loss of peripheral sensory information normally used in the control of speech results in a unique constellation of articulatory deviations.

Although dysarthric speakers in this investigation had sustained motor difficulties for relatively long periods of time, the drug-induced sensory deprivation experience was, of course, temporary, lasting approximately two hours. In addition, the injection series induced a bilateral, peripheral sensory lesion, the extent of which is seldom, if ever, observed clinically. From a clinical standpoint, it is interesting to ask whether the articulatory differences noted here would be seen in a sensory-deprived group whose loss was long-standing, like that of the dysarthrics. We know of only one published account dealing with the articulatory characteristics of a speaker with diagnosed chronic oral sensory neuropathology. MacNeilage, Rootes, and Chase (1967) discussed the results of a phonological, electromyographic, and cinefluorographic examination of a 17-year-old female with a generalized congenital oral sensory deficit. While her articulatory difficulties were apparently more severe than that of the sensory-deprived speakers we studied, many of the cinefluorographic patterns observed by MacNeilage, Rootes, and Chase seem to correspond with phonetic observations noted in our study. Articulatory patterns common to their subject and sensory-deprived speakers include retracted velar and alveolar stop production as well as the inability to selectively shape the apex of the tongue. Such similarities suggest that articulatory differences reported here between sensory-deprived and dysarthric speakers may generalize for a group of speakers with long-standing oral sensory pathology.

As stated earlier, this investigation was in part motivated by controversy dealing with the potential motor effects of oral region nerve block pro-

242

cedures. The validity of observations drawn from such studies rests with the assumption that nerve-block injections are selectively sensory. Electromyographic evidence suggesting that sensory blocks may result in motor artifacts has been reported recently by Harris (1970), who found mylohyoid paralysis following mandibular nerve block. While her data may represent a specific exception, observations reported here based upon the careful analysis of speech would encourage the view that sensory deprivation in the oral region does not produce concurrent generalized motor effects.

ACKNOWLEDGMENTS

This investigation was supported in part by Public Health Service Awards 1 K03 DE 32614-03 and 1 R01 DE 02815-02 from the National Institute of Dental Research and by the Purdue Research Foundation. We requested and received tape recordings of spondee words produced by the dysarthric subjects from Ronald S. Tikofsky. His cooperation is acknowledged and appreciated.

REFERENCES

DARLEY, F. L., ARONSON, A. E., and BROWN, J. E., Differential diagnostic patterns of dysarthria. *J. Speech Hearing Res.*, 12, 246-269 (1969).

HARRIS, KATHERINE S., Physiological measures of speech movements: EMG and fiberoptic studies. *Speech and the Dentofacial Complex: The State of the Art. Asha Reports No. 5*, 271-282 (1970).

LEHISTE, ILSE, Some acoustic characteristics of dysarthric speech. *Bibl. phonet.*, Fasc. 2 (1965).

LISKER, L., and ABRAMSON, A. S., A cross-language study of voicing in initial stops: Acoustical measurements. *Word*, 20, 384-422 (1964).

MACNEILAGE, P. F., ROOTES, T. P., and CHASE, R. A., Speech production and perception in a patient with severe impairment of somesthetic perception and motor control. *J. Speech Hearing Res.*, 10, 449-467 (1967).

PETERSON, G. E., and SHOUP, JUNE, A physiological theory of phonetics. *J. Speech Hearing Res.*, 9, 5-67 (1966).

SCOTT, CHERYL, and Ringel, R. L., Articulation without oral sensory control. *J. Speech Hearing Res.*, 14, 804-818 (1971).

TIKOFSKY, R. S., and TIKOFSKY, RITA, Intelligibility measures of dysarthric speech. *J. Speech Hearing Res.*, 7, 325-333 (1964).

SOME OBSERVATIONS OF ARTICULATION
DURING LABIAL SENSORY DEPRIVATION

ANNE H. B. PUTNAM and ROBERT L. RINGEL

Photographic measurement techniques were used to study labial movement under normal speaking conditions and when sensory feedback from the lips was reduced by trigeminal nerve-block anesthesia. Lip activity was photographed as a subject spoke monosyllabic words initiated by /p/, /b/, or /m/. Qualitative observations were made of general articulatory characteristics, and frame-by-frame quantitative analyses were performed on the release phase of each bilabial consonant. The labial sensory deprivation condition resulted primarily in phonetic articulatory changes due to an overall reduction in the normal rate, accuracy, and extent of lip movement. The data were discussed in terms of the differential effects of reduced labial sensory feedback on the bilabial consonants and interpreted with respect to open- and closed-loop control of articulation.

Patterns of articulatory movements are of interest in the study of speech production. An understanding of these movement patterns necessarily involves the collection of descriptive information about the functional components of the system (motor and sensory), and the relative contribution of each component to accurate articulation. The current trend in theories of speech production is to emphasize sensory experience as a necessary entity of the neuromotor system effecting finely coordinated speech movements. Specifically, the consideration of oral sensory feedback has stimulated research aimed at demonstrating the relative importance of this sensory channel to adequate articulation. One experimental technique useful to the study of oral sensory mechanisms in speech involves a temporary reduction of oral sensory acuity in normal talkers via nerve-block anesthesia. Such was the technique employed in this investigation.

The lips constitute a readily accessible set of articulators. Their normal movement characteristics during speech have been studied indirectly by acoustic and electromyographic means, and directly by photographic methods. In a lengthy study of the acoustic manifestation of coarticulation in VCV utterances, Ohman (1966) distinguished two classes of lip movement for speech production: one for consonants (closing and opening) and one for vowels (rounding and spreading). He hypothesized that labial stop consonant gestures are superimposed on the underlying lip gesture for a neighboring vowel. Electromyographic researchers at the Haskins Laboratories (Lysaught, Rosov, and Harris, 1963; Cooper, 1965; and Harris, Lysaught, and Schvey,

JOURNAL OF SPEECH AND HEARING RESEARCH, 1972, vol. 15, 529-542.

1965) reported that muscle activity in the lips during the articulation of /p/, /b/, and /m/ showed no significant differences among the durations and intensities of muscle gestures for those phonemes. These findings of electromyographic invariance were later contradicted by Fromkin (1965), who recorded electromyographic potentials in the orbicularis oris muscle during the production of /p/ and /b/. She found significant differences in the lip muscle gestures for the cognates, both between them and among the positionally distinct allophones of each. Ohman's EMG data (1967) on the labial gestures for /p/ and /b/ also distinguished between these consonants on the basis of strength-of-onset and -release commands.

Direct photography of the lips has been effective in resolving the ambiguity and inconsistencies found in the electromyographic data on labial articulatory gestures. Fromkin (1964) used still photography and lateral x-rays to study lip positions during vowel production. Fujimura (1961) employed high-speed stroboscopic photography to study the labial articulatory dynamics of /p/, /b/, and /m/ in CVC syllables. The film records which he obtained displayed distinct, measurable spatial differences in lip activity for each of the consonants in their closure, hold, and release gestures across time. His data also revealed characteristic lip activity for the bilabials in each of the phonetic contexts under study. The present investigation sought to provide, by means of photographic measurement techniques similar to those of Fujimura, a description of some aspects of lip movement under normal speaking conditions and when sensory feedback from the lips was reduced by nerve-block anesthesia. The lips lend themselves well to this type of study since they may be desensitized independently of the other articulators.

METHOD

Subject and Conditions

One adult female, age 24, served as the talker for this study. She spoke a western dialect of American English, had normal speech and hearing, exhibited normal oral structures, and reported no history of sensory or motor problems. The experimental condition in which she spoke with her normal oral sensory feedback was considered the control condition. The condition in which the usual tactile and pressure sensitivity of her lips had been reduced by nerve-block anesthesia was designated the block condition.

Labial desensitization was induced via bilateral infraorbital and mandibular injections of Xylocaine (2% with epinephrine). The anesthetic was administered by a dentist to those trigeminal nerve branches which are known to serve as afferent pathways for sensations of touch, pressure, pain, and temperature in the lips, that is, the infraorbital nerves (upper lip) and the inferior alveolar nerves (lower lip). These nerve-block procedures profoundly reduced the pain, pressure, and tactile sensitivity of the subject's lip tissue. Extreme care was taken to avoid possible involvement of the more superficial motor elements

245

of the facial nerve, as well as nearby motor branches of the trigeminal itself. For example, the mylohyoid nerve, a motor ramus which branches off the inferior alveolar nerve somewhat before the site of infiltration for lower lip desensitization, provides a potential site of difficulty. For further discussion of this problem, see Harris (1970) and Scott and Ringel (1971).

Even in light of careful injection procedures, the practicability of a purely sensory block is still questionable. Irrespective of direct motor involvement by mistake, it is conceivable that in the course of the experimental procedure, diffusion of the anesthetic could take place through the soft tissues of maxilla, mandible, and lips to involve nearby motor nerves, end plates, or muscle spindles. Whatever the extent of such possible localized infiltration and partial paralysis, its effects on speech might be difficult to predict or even recognize unequivocally. The only conclusion which can safely be made about the physiological affect of the labial nerve-block procedure used here is that touch and pressure sensation in the lips was reduced to a point which the subject described as substantially numb, while at the same time she was able to voluntarily purse her lips and move them in a relatively normal manner. It was under this condition that our block data were collected.

A 16-mm high-speed motion-picture camera was used to photograph the subject's lip movement. Exposures were made with a constant light source at 250 fps. Two lights, one driven by a timing-light generator and the other activated by a voice-operated relay, were adapted for use in the camera housing to provide time and voice-onset markers on the film. In addition, a metric reference was positioned below the subject's lips in the field of view. Simultaneous high-fidelity audio recordings were made of the subject's speech to supplement the photographic data.

The subject spoke the 21 words listed here. All of the utterances are meaningful English words with the exception of /pun/. This word sample was designed to include the bilabial consonants /p/, /b/, and /m/ in the monosyllable-initial position (as in /pit/), or in the intervocalic position preceded by an unstressed /ə/ (as in /ə 'pit/). The list also included the bilabials in initial

Word	IPA Equivalent	Word	IPA Equivalent
peat	/pit/	preen	/prin/
a peat	/ə 'pit/	breed	/brid/
pack	/pæk/	plead	/plid/
"poon"	/pun/	bleed	/blid/
beat	/bit/	speed	/spid/
a beat	/ə 'bit/	spree	/spri/
boon	/bun/	spleen	/splin/
meat	/mit/	prove	/pruv/
a meat	/ə 'mit/	spruce	/sprus/
mack	/mæk/	smack	/smæk/
moon	/mun/		

double- or triple-consonant clusters with /s/, /l/, or /r/. The vowel elements of monosyllables—/i/, /æ/, and /u/—were chosen to provide spread, wide, and rounded labial contexts, respectively, for the bilabial consonants. The final consonant elements were selected to require minimal transitory lip movements from the vowel posture. The subject was familiarized with the words prior to the photographic sessions. She spoke them in a normal manner, pausing about two seconds between each utterance.

Initially, qualitative observations were made of the filmstrips as they were projected at standard speed. The subject's lip movements under the block condition were described relative to their normal activity as recorded during the control condition. For more quantitative information, the films of lip activity were enlarged and projected frame by frame. A series of tracings was made from the films of lip movement for each word. Each trace was an outline of the inner perimeter of the lip opening visible in a frame. A tracing series for a word began where an opening between the lips was first noticeable on the bilabial consonant release, and included the next 96 msec (24 frames) of lip release activity. A trace was also made of that frame which represented the maximum lip opening for the vowel gesture in the word. The traces resembled ellipses although they were typically asymmetrical, especially early in the release gesture. Each trace was digitized into a number of discrete points, and the area within the points was determined by computer. A series of such areas for one word provided data on the rate of lip opening for the bilabial consonant gesture in that particular phonetic context.

Fujimura, in his study of lip movement on bilabial consonants (1961), calculated the area of lip opening by using the standard formula for the area of an ellipse, assuming the horizontal and vertical dimensions of a lip opening to be the major and minor axes of the ellipse. Fujimura considered this method to be accurate to within 10% of the real area values (calculated with a planimeter) except in the rounded vowel context. Since the outlines of lip opening obtained in the present study were typically quite irregular, especially under the block condition, it was felt that the interlip areas could be more accurately determined using a digitized series of points which represented the outline of a lip opening. For several utterances in this study, area values obtained by the method reported here and those obtained by Fujimura's method were compared with values calculated with a polar planimeter. It was found that the more time-consuming and involved digitizer process was nonetheless the more accurate, since it agreed more closely with the planimeter results.

Photographic Data: Qualitative Analysis

The following descriptions were derived from observations of the data films projected at 24 fps.

Control. Normally, the subject's lips appeared to assume a slightly spread preparatory posture just prior to the onset of articulatory movement. Similar lip activity has been documented and described by Ohman (1967) as an underlying tonic posture, effected by the superior labial levator muscles and the inferior labial depressor muscle, on which specific labial articulatory movements are superimposed. Specific lip articulatory postures observed in the present study seemed to be of four general types: wide open, with large horizontal and vertical dimensions (as in /æ/); spread, with more narrow vertical separation (as in /i/); close and rounded, with small horizontal and vertical dimensions (as in /u/ or /r/); and closed (as in the hold phase of /p/, /b/, and /m/).

Figure 1 shows some sample photographic frames of the subject's normal lip activity on articulation of the words /pit/, /pæk/, and /pun/. Both lips normally participated actively in the closing and opening gestures for the bilabial consonants and consistently achieved complete closure during the hold phases. Right-to-left assimilatory influences on lip activity were apparent: for instance, when /p/ or /b/ was followed by /l/, the release of the bilabial was consistently characterized by a lip opening which began to one side of the midline of the mouth (that is, a unilateral release). Bilabial consonants were released with pursed labial postures when followed by /r/ or /u/.

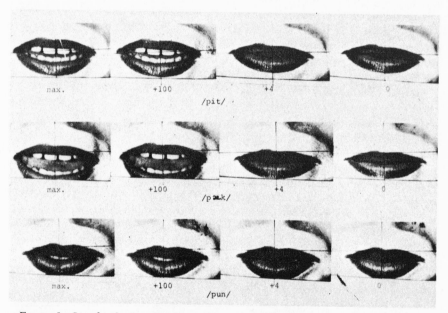

FIGURE 1. Sample photographic frames of the subject's normal lip activity on the production of /pit/, /pæk/, and /pun/. Time proceeds from right to left. The first frame at the right of each row (0) shows the lips closed in the final stages of the hold phase for /p/. The second frame from the right (+4) is 4 msec later than the first and shows the initial lip-opening area for the /p/ release phase. The interlip openings in the +4 msec samples are extremely small and difficult to see. Note, however, that evidence of lip spreading or rounding is already apparent in the lip release posture. The third frame from the right (+100) shows the lip opening after 100 msec of the /p/ release. The left-most frame (max.) in each row represents the maximum lip opening achieved for each word.

Block. Compared to their activity in the control condition, the subject's lip movements during speech in the block condition appeared to be less accurate and less extensive. For example, the lips tended to assume an exaggerated, spread-close posture at rest or during articulatory movements. This speech posture might well have been an uninhibited extension of the tonic labial posture which had normally appeared only between periods of dynamic speech activity. All of the bilabial consonants produced in the block condition appeared to be articulated unilabially. That is, the lower lip was elevated to attempt closure against a relatively immobile upper lip. Perhaps partly as a result of this minimal upper lip movement, the stop portions of all six /sp/ clusters called for in the test words were made with incomplete closure of the oral cavity. A tiny, slit-like opening remained between the lips during the subject's attempt to produce these /p/ phonemes. Finally, there was a consistent alteration in mouth opening dimensions for vowels following a unilabial consonant release: in every case, normally lip-open gestures (as in /i/ or /æ/) were less open; normally rounded gestures (as in /r/ or /u/) were not round.

Graphic Data: Quantitative Analyses

Lip-opening activity in the first 100 msec of a bilabial consonant release and a maximum mouth opening value for the vowel in each test word, under both conditions, were plotted for quantitative comparisons. A sample graphic display for /pit/ is described in the legend of Figure 2a.

Control. The graphic data for lip activity in the control condition can be summarized as follows. In every case, increase in the horizontal distance between the corners of the lips during the bilabial consonant release contributed more to growth in interlip area than the vertical separation between the lips. Maximum values for the vertical dimension usually came to only 15 or 25% of the horizontal distance. The lips achieved widest opening values for /æ/ and least for /u/. Growth on the horizontal dimension was most noticeable for /i/.

In single-initial forms of /p/, /b/, and /m/, the rate of initial lip opening was fastest for /p/ and slowest for /m/. (This distinction was not made, however, in the intervocalic production of these consonants; that is, /ə 'pit/, /ə 'bit/, and /ə 'mit/.) Differences in the speed of lip opening among the single-initial forms may be related to the fact that the greater intrabuccal air pressure usually associated with the hold phase of /p/ (Fujimura, 1961; Ohman, 1967; Malecot, 1970) effectively parts the lips more rapidly during the initial release phase. As an interesting tangent to this discussion, the slopes of lip separation for /m/ were in general smoother than those for /p/ or /b/. Fujimura (1961) noted this phenomenon in his data, too, and suggested that the discrepancy might be explained by the presence of lip vibrations he observed in the oral stop releases, but not in the nasal releases. Presumably, since /m/ initially has a nasal release of the breath stream, air pressure at the lips during its oral release is smaller than that for /p/ or /b/, and insufficient to blow the lips apart as rapidly ini-

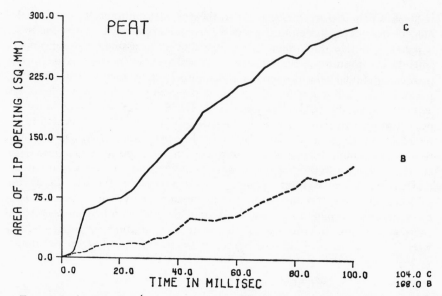

FIGURES 2a, b. Time functions for lip-opening activity during the release phase of /p/ in the words *peat* (/pit/, 2a) and *speed* (/spid/, 2b). The continuous curves represent the control condition (normal articulation); the broken curves represent the block condition (reduced labial sensitivity). The functions of time show the area of the opening between the upper and lower lips. (See the text for further explanation of area measurements.) Each figure shows the performance of a single talker for the utterance indicated. Plotted at the right of each figure are the maximal interlip area values that occurred during the production of the test word. The times at which the maxima occurred are indicated below the plotted points; maxima occurring in the control condition are plotted as C, while maxima in the block condition are shown as B.

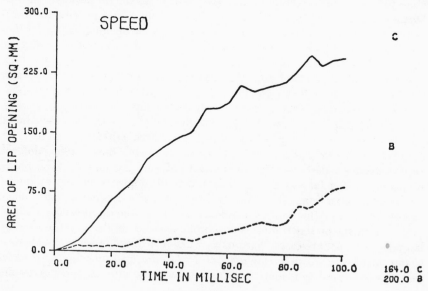

tially or set them into vibration. Although such slope differences were noticeable in the graphic data reported here, concrete evidence of regular labial oscillations during the /p/ or /b/ release was not consistently demonstrated.

Some interesting graphic data were collected about the consonant clusters involving bilabial consonants. Aerodynamically, it is known that when the fricative /s/ precedes /p/, a decrease in aspiration of the stop is expected. Fujimura (1961) noted such an influence of /s/ on the speed of the /p/ release in his photographic data. In the present study, the aspiration decrease was noticeable in the interlip area functions for the release of /p/ in all the test words beginning with an /sp/ cluster, and is exemplified in the graph for /spid/, in Figure 2b. Indications that the lips flew apart at a much slower rate than they had for single-initial /p/ can be seen by comparing the control graphs of Figures 2a, b. The slope for the /p/ release gesture in /spid/ is less steep than the slope for the release of /p/ in /pit/. The fricative element apparently reduced the effective implosion of intraoral air pressure during the hold phase of /p/. This diminished the force acting to part the lips during the release of the stop.

When /l/ followed /p/ or /b/ (as in /plid/ or /blid/), lip opening for the stop release was primarily on the horizontal dimension. This was quantitative evidence for the markedly lateralized releases observed in the filmstrips of these words. When /p/ or /b/ was followed by /r/ (as in /prin/ or /brid/), the regressive rounding influence of the /r/ apparently restricted the dimensions of mouth opening for the release of stops.

In the triple consonant clusters /spl/ and /spr/, release of the /p/ usually showed the assimilation effects of both neighboring consonants. For example, when the effects of both /s/ and /r/ influenced the release of /p/ in /spri/, the graph of lip-opening area appeared to be a combination of the rounded release posture of /pr/ with the slower release gesture effected by the sibilant in an /sp/ cluster. Similar assimilatory effects could be observed in lip opening for /p/ in /sprus/. The addition of the /u/ did not seem to exert any more regressive rounding influence on the /p/ release than the /r/ had already effected. The only apparent individual effect was that the /u/ probably kept the lips rounded longer into the syllable.

Block. The graphs of lip-opening activity in the block condition provided interesting comparisons with the control data. For example, maximum lip-opening areas for /æ/ and /i/ were reduced to about half their control values. Maximum areas for /u/, however, were increased to two or three times their control values, thus providing quantitative evidence for the lack of rounding which had been noticed in the block condition films for that vowel.

Lip separations for single-initial and intervocalic /p/, /b/, and /m/ were slower and less extensive. This reduction in rate was most noticeable for /p/; /m/ seemed least affected. Spectrograms revealed that the release of the single-initial /p/ phonemes had, in fact, been fricated, that is, lengthened, under anesthesia. Possibly this affrication was an expression of the subject's inability to accurately monitor the intrabuccal air pressure normally imploded during the hold phase of /p/. If that pressure were less than normal, the pressure stop-release characteristics of the consonant might conceivably have been reduced. Although there was no change in the manner of production, that is, stop, for the single-initial /p/ consonant under anesthesia, the intervocalic /p/ in /ə 'pit/ did undergo a phonemic change. It was produced as a bilabial fricative. Perhaps inadequate closure made a potentially less forceful production of /p/ even weaker under anesthesia, by impairing the implosion of intraoral air pressure. The block productions of intervocalic /b/ and /m/ did not exhibit such phonemic changes. The fact that /m/ seemed to be least affected by the anesthesia (that is, in release rate its block production differed only slightly from the control) suggests that the integrity of labial tactile and pressure sensitivity in the release phase of /m/ is less crucial to the normal production of the nasal than it is to the production of a stop.

Graphic displays of the double and triple consonant cluster data for the block condition were especially informative. In the films of the block condition, the subject did not achieve complete labial closure for /p/ in any of the test words initiated by an /sp/ cluster. Spectrographic analysis confirmed that these bilabial stops had,,in fact, been produced as fricatives /ɸ/. Graphs of an arbitrarily defined release for the bilabial fricatives indicated that the lips parted very slowly, as shown in the curves for /sɸid/, in Figure 2b. This /sɸ/ release behavior under labial anesthesia may be related to the effects of progressive assimilation when /s/ precedes /p/, or to the fact that a bilabial fricative release would be less forceful than a bilabial stop release, or to both. In closing the lips for /p/ from a spread posture for /s/, the subject may not have been able to adequately sense when full closure was achieved. Furthermore, inadequate labial sensitivity to intraoral pressure may have increased the possibility of an inadequate hold phase for a stop already rendered less aspirated by the preceding sibilant.

The effect of the anesthesia on the rounding influences of /r/ and /u/ could be inferred from the block condition data. The graphs for the /pr/ and /br/ gestures of /prin/ and /brid/ showed a lack of the anticipatory lip rounding for /r/ that was noticed in the control words. This corroborated the visual impression that the /r/ gesture was not rounded under labial anesthesia. However, the graphic data for /pruv/ and /sprus/ in the block condition were perhaps the most interesting. Graphs for /pruv/ showed that the rate of lip separation for /p/ was comparable to the control. The /r/ was also only slightly less rounded than usual. Possibly the regressive assimilatory influence of /u/ counteracted the lack of a rounding tendency seen heretofore in the block productions of rounded phonemes. In this case, however, the maximum area of lip opening for /u/ was also found to be comparable to normal, although the horizontal dimension values were considerably larger for the block production. Perhaps the regressive influence of the terminal labiodental consonant /v/ suppressed extensive lip opening and helped to maintain a closer, although not necessarily as rounded, labial coarticulation for /u/.

In /sɸrus/, the production of a bilabial fricative after the /s/, as well as the regressive assimilatory influence of /u/ combined to render the labial release activity of /ɸ/ slower and less extensive as compared to the control word. The right-to-left assimilatory effects of the /u/ seemed effective here in maintaining a more rounded labial posture for the /r/, but that influence was seemingly not as effective in the production of the vowel itself. The maximum lip excursion width achieved for the /u/ in this word under anesthesia was twice as large and hence less round than the control.

Discussion

A preparatory gesture of the lips prior to the onset of speech and the active participation of both lips in the production of bilabial consonants were characteristic of normal lip activity in this study. These labial activities were noticeably altered by lip anesthesia: the preparatory gesture was exaggerated, and bilabial movements became unilabial. The expected coarticulatory effects of combinatory phonetics on the spatial and temporal characteristics of normal lip opening for /p/, /b/, and /m/ were observed. The progressive influence of /s/ (Fujimura, 1961) was apparently exaggerated by labial anesthesia; the regressive influences of /r/ and /u/ (Fujimura, 1961; Daniloff and Moll, 1968) were differentially effected, depending on how they were reinforced by phonetic context.

This study presented evidence for distinctions between the homophenes /p/, /b/, and /m/, at least on the basis of initial lip-opening rates in the release phase. These data, like those of Fujimura (1961), show characteristic rates of lip opening for each of the bilabial consonants which seem to be logically related to factors of air pressure and articulatory effort. According to Malecot (1970), the accurate production of a stop is primarily dependent on a talker's ability to sense appropriate levels of intrabuccal air pressure. Since the voiceless stops are generally considered to be produced with greater intraoral air pressures than voiced stops or continuants, probably sensitivity to intrabuccal air pressure is more critical to the articulation of the voiceless stop. This assumption appears to have been substantiated by the results reported here. The /p/ phoneme was more drastically affected by reduced labial sensation than /b/ or /m/. Labial sensory deprivation seems to disrupt some feedback as to intraoral pressure levels necessary for an accurate production of /p/; apparently such feedback is not so crucial to the articulation of /b/ or /m/. These assumptions remain questionable, however, since intraoral pressure measurements were not taken along with the photographic data. Certainly intraoral pressure values would be an important complement to the results reported here, especially in light of recent data (Prosek, 1971) suggesting that feedback from intraoral pressures is not as crucial to the production of intelligible speech as has been hypothesized.

Consider these data in terms of the effect of a lip sensory nerve block on the motor control of lip articulation. The anesthetizing procedure used here was an attempt to profoundly reduce pressure and tactile sensation in the lips.

253

Such a deficit might reasonably account for several of the most noticeable changes in lip movement under the block condition. If the subject had lost tactile cues as to the state of lip apposition and separation, she might have moved the lips less confidently, hence less extensively, and probably would have failed to sense adequate closure.

In spite of labial sensory deprivation, however, the subject was able to produce intelligible speech with only minor changes in manner and place of articulation. The simple combination of a single-initial bilabial consonant and vowel was always produced with adequate lip closure and shape. The disruptive effects of the anesthesia on lip articulation became more noticeable as the phonetic content of the test words became more complex. In general, noticeable articulatory changes could be described as a loss of refinement in lip movements involving the production of complex consonant clusters, lip rounding, or extent of lip opening relative to normal.

The results of this study may be interpreted as qualitative evidence for the inclusion of both open- and closed-loop systems in the motor control of labial articulation. The term *open-loop control* as used here refers to the autonomous generation of neuromotor impulses from the central nervous system to the articulators, without reference to peripheral sensory feedback from the oral cavity. On the other hand, a closed-loop control system in this discussion is one which constantly adjusts its neuromotor output on the basis of peripheral feedback information. Several aspects of the present data could be interpreted as supportive of the hypothesis that autonomous open-loop controls seem to be operating in the initial portion of a word, during the vowel elements, and perhaps at the end of a single-word utterance, while a closed-loop system is operating via oral sensory feedback to refine ongoing articulation. The fact that the subject's speech remained clearly intelligible in the block condition logically argues for some open-loop operations which can carry on adequately when sensory feedback is deficient. Furthermore, in every case where a single /p/, /b/, or /m/ initiated a word, no major changes occurred in the manner of their production. Changes did occur within words, however, where peripheral sensory feedback might be important in monitoring and compensating for contextual constraints. For example, intervocalic /p/ and /p/ phonemes following /s/ underwent phonemic changes and were produced as fricatives, not stops; /r/ and /u/ were not often rounded; the rate and extent of lip movements were abnormal and inaccurate.

This discussion should not be carried too far, however, before its limitations with respect to the lips are noted. The concept of closed- and open-loop controls of lip movement in speech is necessarily complicated by the fact that the lip has two sources of dynamic input: a direct or active motor system and an indirect or passive one. In the active system, lip movement is effected by voluntary efforts of the labial and facial musculature. In the passive case, the lower lip is moved up to or down from the upper lip by movements of the mandible, and there is a slight time lag in the lip's passive "following" movement. Movements of the mandible are generally believed to be monitored by the temporomandibular joint, the sensory acuity of which was not thought to be affected by the anesthetic technique used in this study. MacNeilage (1970) has reported that closed-loop controls in speech have been best documented with respect to speech-initial jaw movements. To the extent, then, that the lower lip "rides" passively on the mandible, the closing and opening activity of the lips under labial anesthesia can still benefit from the intact sensory system operating to control jaw movement. Thus, for example, the fact that no major changes occurred in the manner of production of single-initial /p/, /b/, or /m/ under the anesthetic cannot be interpreted simply as demonstrative of speech-initial open-loop lip controls operating irrespective of labial sensory information. The passive effect of closed-loop speech-initial mandible activity may have sufficed to help the lips perform adequately (albeit more slowly, as the data show).

For the sake of argument, but with the aforementioned limitations in mind, the data of this study might be interpreted in terms of the model of speech production offered by Liberman et al. (1967). In this model, precise initial closure gestures for the single bilabial consonants are directed by open-loop, or "on-off" controls. These directions can operate independently of peripheral feedback from the lips and therefore are not compromised by labial sensory deprivation. Precise labial articulatory movements during the release of the initial consonant and the production of successive phonemes, however, require "go to" instructions. These can specify target positions for the lips only when feedback from the periphery supplies "from-where" information. When the latter feedback was drastically reduced by labial anesthesia, the "go to" instructions were rendered inadequate, and the lips undershot their targets to an abnormal extent. Open gestures were less open, rounded phonemes were less round, and closures were not achieved for /p/ within a word.

With particular respect to the effects of labial anesthesia on /p/, the present data can also be considered in terms of Henke's model (1967). He considered that the normal temporal progression of speech movements is largely dependent on peripheral sensory feedback for the completion of one gesture and readiness for the next. He suggested that articulation does not proceed after the production of a stop consonant until information that closure has been achieved is received centrally. When such peripheral information is blocked by anesthesia, the usual temporal progression from stop to succeeding phoneme is altered. This phenomenon was observed in the present study. Initial /p/ under anesthesia consistently exhibited a fricated release. A similar fricated release for /p/ was noted in a more extensive anesthetization procedure by Scott and Ringel (1971); they correlated this phonetic change in the stop release with delayed voice onset for the following vowel.

When oral somesthetic feedback is reduced, closed-loop control of speech is presumed to be carried out primarily by proprioceptive feedback from muscle spindles and tendon organs. Whether or not proprioception was interrupted by the labial anesthesia used in the present study is uncertain. However, it does seem reasonable that loss of tactile and pressure sensation in the labial mucosa would be somewhat crucial to labial articulation, especially in view of the high density of sensory endings in the lips. At any rate, in the absence of some aspects of peripheral sensory feedback, closed-loop control of lip movements in speech appears to be rendered less efficient. The lips are able to compensate for the mechano-inertial constraints of left-to-right assimilation less effectively. Hence, left-to-right influences, which are logically adjusted via a "go to" system, are exaggerated and haphazard. It is interesting to speculate, however, that right-to-left assimilatory influences, like that exerted by /u/ on lip opening gestures in the present data, are underlying "on-off" target instructions on which closed-loop refinements for specific phonemes are superimposed (Ohman, 1967). Perhaps the anticipatory effect on the lip musculature of open-loop instructions for /u/ managed to keep the lips closed for the production of the preceding consonants in /pun/ or /sɸrus/. The /u/ itself, however, was usually unrounded. Thus, although the underlying vowel command is present and operative, some closed-loop operation seems necessary to adjust its production relative to the specific constraints of its phonetic surroundings. To extend this discussion one step further, it would be of interest to determine whether or not final as well as initial articulatory targets in a single word utterance are under autonomous "on-off" control. The example which raises the question is the word /pruv/. The /r/ and the /u/ were produced with adequate labial closeness, although not necessarily normal labial protrusion and rounding. Perhaps the underlying influence of an open-loop instruction defining the labial coarticulation for the final /v/ as closed, exerted an influence on the lip musculature which was not confounded by reduced labial sensory information.

Certainly on the basis of the hypotheses presented and the questions raised previously, it cannot be denied that research into the relative importance of oral sensory feedback to speech has provided much information about the motor control of articulation and demands still more investigation.

In conclusion, the dynamics of lip articulation for the production of /p/, /b/, and /m/ were adequately recorded by the photographic method used in this study. High-speed photography is an excellent means of making detailed observations of the coarticulatory effects of assimilation on lip activity during single-word utterances and connected speech. In future studies it would be beneficial to perform a more detailed spectrographic analysis of speech under labial anesthesia and to include other phonemes besides /p/, /b/, and /m/ in the investigation (for example, /r/, /l/, and the vowels of the current study).

By the same token, some of the present data suggest motor involvement as well as sensory deprivation. It would behoove experimenters in the future to supplement their photographic and acoustic analyses of speech under oral sensory deprivation with electromyographic records of muscle activity to determine the symmetry and extent of motor involvement, if any (Harris, 1970). Certainly the combined techniques of photography, spectrography, and electromyography, when applied to the study of oral sensory deprived speech, will prove to be extremely useful in understanding the motor control of articulation.

ACKNOWLEDGMENT

This research was supported in part by National Science Foundation Traineeship Award GZ 1594, by Public Health Service Awards 1 K03 DE 32614-03 and 1 R01 DE 02815-02 from the National Institute of Dental Research, and by the Purdue Research Foundation.

REFERENCES

COOPER, SYBIL, Research techniques and instrumentation: Electromyography. In *Proceedings of the Conference: Communicative Problems in Cleft Palate, ASHA Reports 1.* Washington, D.C.: American Speech and Hearing Association, 153-168 (1965).

DANILOFF, R., and MOLL, K., Coarticulation of lip rounding. *J. Speech Hearing Res.*, 11, 707-721 (1968).

FROMKIN, VICTORIA, Parameters of lip position. *Work. Pap. Phonet.*, 1, Los Angeles: Univ. of California, 15-21 (1964).

FROMKIN, VICTORIA, Location of lip muscles by electromyography. *Work. Pap. Phonet.*, 2, Los Angeles: Univ. of California, 51-54 (1965).

FUJIMURA, O., Bilabial stop and nasal consonants: A motion picture study and its acoustical implications. *J. Speech Hearing Res.*, 4, 233-247 (1961).

HARRIS, KATHERINE S., Physiologic measures of speech movements: EMG and fiberoptic studies. In *Speech and the Dentofacial Complex: The State of the Art: Proceedings of a Workshop, ASHA Reports 5.* Washington, D.C.: American Speech and Hearing Association, 271-282 (1970).

HARRIS, KATHERINE, LYSAUGHT, G. F., and SCHVEY, M. M., Some aspects of the production of oral and nasal labial stops. *Lang. Speech*, 8, 135-147 (1965).

HENKE, W., Preliminaries to speech synthesis based upon an articulatory mode. Paper presented at the Conference on Speech Communications and Processing, Cambridge, Mass. (1967).

LIBERMAN, A. M., COOPER, F. S., SHANKWEILER, D. P., and STUDDERT-KENNEDY, M., Perception of the speech code. *Psychol. Rev.*, 74, 431-463 (1967).

LYSAUGHT, G., ROSOV, R. J., and HARRIS, KATHERINE, Electromyography as a speech research technique with an application to labial stops. *J. acoust. Soc. Amer.*, 33, 842 (1961).

MACNEILAGE, P. F., Motor control of serial ordering of speech. *Psychol. Rev.*, 77, 182-196 (1970).

MALECOT, A., The lenis-fortis opposition: Its physiological parameters. *J. acoust. Soc. Amer.*, 47, 1588-1592 (1970).

OHMAN, S. E. G., Coarticulation in VCV utterances: Spectrographic measurements. *J. acoust. Soc. Amer.*, 39, 151-168 (1966).

OHMAN, S. E. G., Peripheral motor commands in labial articulation. *STL-QPSR*, Royal Institute of Technology, Stockholm, Sweden, 4, 30-63 (1967).

PROSEK, R. A., An evaluation of the role of oral sensation in consonant production. Doctoral dissertation, Purdue University (1971).

SCOTT, CHERYL M., and RINGEL, R. L., Articulation without oral sensory control. *J. Speech and Hearing Res.*, 14, 804-818 (1971).

257

ACOUSTIC CHARACTERISTICS OF SPEECH
PRODUCED WITHOUT ORAL SENSATION

YOSHIYUKI HORII, ARTHUR S. HOUSE, KUNG-PU LI, and ROBERT L. RINGEL

The acoustic characteristics of continuous speech produced by an adult male talker with and without oral (nerve block) anesthesia were investigated using digital speech processing procedures. Vowel-to-consonant ratios, long-time and short-time spectra, fundamental frequency distributions, phonation-time ratios, and rate of utterances were calculated and compared for the normal and anesthetized conditions. The results showed that the speech produced without oral sensation was characterized by a reduction and shift of high-frequency energy, temporal disorganization primarily manifested as prolongation of utterance, and higher and more variable fundamental frequencies. The study also demonstrated applicability of computer techniques on general acoustic analysis of continuous speech.

A number of investigations have studied the effect of oral sensory deprivation upon speech as a means of delineating the role of oral sensation in the control of the speech mechanism. Such studies often have taken the form of phonetic and phonemic analyses with supplemental acoustic analyses (McCroskey, Corley, and Jackson, 1959; Ringel and Steer, 1963; Thompson, 1969; Gammon et al., 1971; Scott, 1970; Scott and Ringel, 1971; Prosek, 1971). Systematic acoustic analysis, however, may be helpful in providing new insights about production and perception of speech produced without oral sensation, and in interpreting the articulatory processes described by the phonetic and phonemic analyses. In addition, such detailed acoustic information might be expected to shed light on the continuing controversy revolving around sensory vs sensory-and-motor deactivation as a result of oral region anesthetization procedures commonly used. This report quantitatively describes the acoustic characteristics of continuous speech produced by a talker whose oral sensation was eliminated by nerve-block anesthesia. The study also attempts to demonstrate applicability of digital speech-processing procedures in general acoustic analysis of connected speech. The physical measures obtained by digital speech-processing procedures include intensity level, vowel-to-consonant ratio, long-time and short-time spectra, fundamental frequency, rate, and phonation-time ratio.

PROCEDURES

Speech Materials. The speech materials were recorded on a high-quality magnetic tape record-reproduce system. The passage was a short story (181

JOURNAL OF SPEECH AND HEARING RESEARCH, 1973, vol. 16, no. 1, 67-77.

258

words) used routinely in phonetic studies. The talker read the passage in a natural conversational style, using no external devices to monitor speech level or rate. The durations of the normal (control) and anesthetized (block) passages, including pauses, were approximately 85 seconds in each case.

The talker was a young adult male who spoke a midwestern dialect of American English, had normal oral-structural relationships, and no history of sensory or motor disturbances or speech and hearing problems. Sensation was eliminated through a series of nerve-block injections of Xylocaine (2% with epinephrine). Sensation was eliminated from surface receptors in all supra-glottal structures, with the exception of the pharynx and posterior one-third of the tongue. The procedures are described in detail and discussed by Scott (1970) and Scott and Ringel (1971).

Digital Speech Processing. The speech signals were reduced to digital form by means of a computer facility. The analog recording was played on a high-quality recorder-reproducer for presentation to a set of 35 bandpass filters. The center frequencies of the filters ranged from approximately 270 to 9.5 k Hz with 10% bandwidths. (This treatment of the speech sample obviously results in loss of some information below 250 Hz.) After rectification and smoothing, the filter outputs were scanned by a multiplexer at 10-msec intervals, linearly quantized and stored on magnetic tape. Thus, spectral information for each 10 msec was represented by a set of 35 values, each value representing the amplitude (in 1024 levels on a linear scale) of the energy passed through one of the 35 filters. In the following discussions, any set of 35 values obtained over a 10-msec interval constitutes a time sample. Finally, the acoustic characteristics of the speech were determined by a series of computer programs operating on the digital data. A more detailed description of the filter characteristics is given by Hughes and Hemdal (1965).

RESULTS

Intensity. The intensity level of a time sample in dB was estimated by taking the log of sum of squares of the filter outputs. Levels obtained from the spectral data in this manner were compared informally to theoretical values calculated from time-sampled data and were in good agreement. The effect of the high-pass condition (caused by the fact that the cut-off frequency of the lowest filter is about 250 Hz) on the intensity level measurements was also investigated using synthesized vowels with various fundamental frequencies (80 to 300 Hz). The results showed that error magnitude involved in estimating intensity level was about 1 dB for most of the vowels; a maximum difference of about 3 dB was observed for the vowel /i/ between F_0 = 80 Hz and 270 Hz.

The distributions of intensity levels of the normal speech (control) and the speech produced under nerve-block anesthesia (block), obtained from the spectral data, are shown in Figure 1. The abscissa represents intensity levels in dB, and the ordinate represents the number of occurrences in percent. The total numbers of occurrences, that is, the total number of time samples for the

259

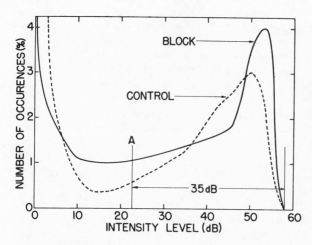

Figure 1. Distributions of intensity levels of normal (control) and anesthetized (block) speech. Percent number of occurrences is plotted as a function of intensity levels (dB). A threshold used for further analysis of data is indicated as A in the figure.

control and block conditions, were 8570 and 8329, respectively. The peaks at the lowest intensity levels represent pauses and low-energy portions of the utterances, since all time samples were involved in the analysis; that is, the distribution function is continuous from pause (no energy) to phonation (high energy). When the distribution pattern for the control speech is compared to that for the block condition, there are more very low-energy samples in the block condition, resulting in a less sharp distinction between pause and phonation segments. The distribution of intensity levels of background noise in the recordings was used to select a threshold of 35 dB below the maximum level for further analysis of speech. This threshold was selected to exclude pauses and very low-energy portions of the utterance from the analysis. Specifically, 38% of the total number of time segments was excluded from the block condition, and 49% of the segments from the control condition.

Vowel-to-Consonant Ratios. With the simultaneous display of plots of intensity levels and digital spectrograms, it was possible to determine vowel-to-consonant ratios for selected syllables in the two types of speech. The selection of syllables was governed mainly by the existence of clear spectral and intensive definitions of syllabic components in the digital spectrograms. Thus, for example, a number of glides, low-energy fricatives, and voiced stops and liquids, in which a steady state portion of the spectrum could not be easily identified, were excluded from the analysis. These sound classes were adequately represented, however, in the portions of the speech sample subjected to analysis. The ratios are summarized in Table 1, where the average vowel-to-consonant ratios (in dB) for various classes of sounds are shown for the control and block conditions. The measurements, of course, were made on the same syllables for both conditions. On the average, approximately 25 measurements were involved in calculating ratios for each class of sounds. Over-all average ratios were calculated from the individual ratio measurements. The average ratio of

260

TABLE 1. Vowel-to-consonant ratios in dB for various classes of consonants produced under the control and block conditions. The over-all averages are 10.2 dB and 13.1 dB for the control and block speech, respectively.

| | Consonantal Class | | | |
Speech Mode	Affricates and Stops	Fricatives	Nasals	Liquids
Control	14.1	10.0	9.4	6.3
Block	19.0	18.8	9.0	5.2

10.2 dB for the control condition is 3-5 dB smaller than that estimated from level measurements of vowels and consonants in Sacia and Beck's study (1926) or that given by Horii, House, and Hughes (1971). The vowel-to-consonant ratios for various classes of sounds in the control condition are comparable to those reported earlier (Fairbanks and Miron, 1957; House et al., 1965; Weiss, 1968) with, again, a tendency for the ratios in the present study to be smaller. This tendency probably is attributable to the absence of energy below approximately 250 Hz, and the consequent under-estimation of voiced sound levels.

Comparison of the control and block conditions reveals that, for fricatives and affricate-stops, the vowel-to-consonant ratios are significantly larger under the block condition. The ratios involving nasals and liquids, on the other hand, do not differ significantly in the two conditions. We recognize that our observations concerning the nasals are limited by the high-pass nature of the processing system.

Spectral Characteristics. The spectral characteristics of the utterances can be investigated in several ways. In Figure 2, for example, the amplitude distributions for different frequency regions are shown separately for speech in the control and block conditions. Pauses and low-energy samples have been ex-

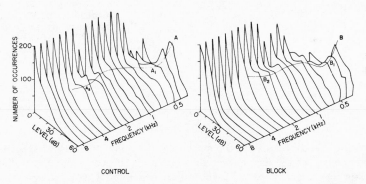

CONTROL   BLOCK

FIGURE 2. Amplitude distributions of normal (control) and anesthetized (block) speech for different frequency regions. Number of occurrences is plotted as a function of amplitude levels (dB) for each frequency region. Occurrences in excess of 200 are ignored for display purposes. The second peaks in the distribution are labeled as A and B (see discussion in the text).

261

cluded. In each case the vertical axis gives the number of occurrences and the horizontal axes give the amplitude levels and frequencies. The total number of occurrences, of course, is the same for all filters in a given portion of the figure. The displays for the control and block conditions have been normalized to make them directly comparable.

In general, distribution of amplitudes in the low-frequency regions is bimodal with one peak at the lowest intensity level and another at some higher level. As frequency increases, the second peak diminishes in size and the contour approaches a Poisson distribution. In the control condition, the second maximum (identified as. A in the figure) approaches the lower level as frequency increases, and then returns to a moderate level as frequency continues to increase. The maximum in the low-frequency region (A_1 in the figure) probably represents the average energy of the sonorants, and the maximum in the higher frequencies (A_2 in the figure) represents the average energy of the nonsonorant sounds. The block condition presents a similar distribution pattern, except there is much less high-frequency energy and the second maximum shifts to lower frequencies (see B_2 in the figure).

A long-time average spectrum of the speech is shown in Figure 3 where

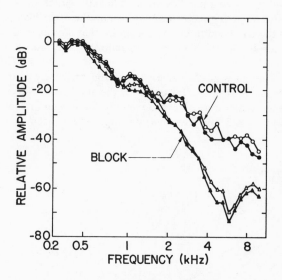

FIGURE 3. Long-time average spectra of normal (control) and anesthetized (block) speech for the first (open points) and second (closed points) halves of the passages exclusive of pauses and very low energy sounds. Amplitudes in dB relative to the maximum components are plotted as a function of frequency.

amplitude (in dB relative to the maximum component) is plotted as a function of frequency for the first and second halves of the passages. A threshold excluding pauses and very low-level sounds was used. These average long-time spectra for the control condition are similar to those reported by Dunn and White (1940). Clearly, speech produced while the subject is deprived of oral sensation has much less high-frequency energy (as already observed in the amplitude distribution for each filter), and there is not much difference between the first and second halves of the utterances. The latter finding also confirms the view that the long-time spectrum of a short utterance (about 30 seconds) is reasonably stable and not affected by the particular script used.

From a phonetic point of view, the average short-time spectrum is of great interest; those spectra studied were averaged over about 10 to 20 time samples (equivalent to 100 to 200 msec), much less than for the long-time spectrum, but much more than used in deriving an amplitude spectrum (that is, "section") with a standard sound spectrograph. Such spectra were obtained from the digital data for /s, ʃ, l, ɝ, ɑ, i/; the selection criterion was the existence of clearly defined phoneme segments in the digital spectrograms of both the control and block speech. Spectra were obtained for 20 occurrences of /s/, five occurrences of /ʃ/ and /l/, four occurrences of /ɑ/ and /i/, and seven occurrences of /ɝ/. For the vowels, only the relatively steady-state portions were analyzed.

The results of the short-time analyses are shown in Figure 4, where spectral

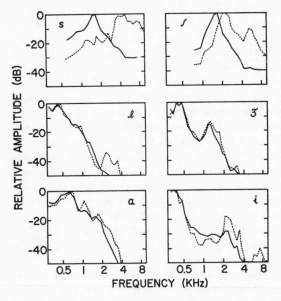

FIGURE 4. Short-time average spectra of /s, ʃ, l, ɝ, ɑ, i/. Dashed lines represent data for control condition, and solid lines for anesthetized condition. Amplitudes in dB relative to the maximum components are plotted as a function of frequency. The range of values displayed along the abscissa is from 0.25 to 9.5 k Hz.

envelopes for the control speech are represented by dashed lines and those for the block speech by solid lines. The measurements for the control condition are generally in agreement with those reported in the literature. For the fricative sounds, for example, the two prominent spectral maxima were near 4500 and 7800 Hz for /s/, and near 2100 and 5300 Hz for /ʃ/. Heinz and Stevens (1961) reported a lower maximum for /s/ between 3500 and 6400 Hz, and a second maximum between 8000 and 8400 Hz. For /ʃ/, they reported a lower maximum between 2200 and 2700 Hz, and a second maximum between 4300 and 5400 Hz.

263

Hughes and Halle (1956) reported a spectral maximum between 5000 and 7000 Hz for /s/, and between 2000 and 3000 Hz for /ʃ/. Strevens (1960) observed a maximum between 4000 and 5000 Hz for /s/ and between 1600 and 3500 Hz for /ʃ/, and also noted a sharp cut-off near 7000 Hz for /ʃ/ (also seen in this data). For /l/, Tarnoczy (1948) reported formants at 420, 1400, 2400, and 3200 Hz, in close agreement with the data in this study. The spectra for the vowels /ɑ/, /i/, and /ɝ/ show similar agreement with earlier reports (see, for example, Peterson and Barney, 1952; Lehiste and Peterson, 1961; Stevens and House, 1961; Holbrook and Fairbanks, 1962).

When the spectra of sounds produced in the control and block conditions are compared, significant changes in the fricatives are evident in the sensory-deprived productions. Spectral maxima were shifted down in frequency by as much as 3000 Hz in the case of /s/ and 1000 Hz for /ʃ/. Scott and Ringel (1971) and Prosek (1971) have described less close and more retracted places of constriction for /s/ and /ʃ/ in the speech of the same talker (and other talkers) when oral structures are anesthetized. The shifts of the spectral maxima for /s/ and /ʃ/ observed in our study are in the direction predicted by acoustic theory (see, for example, Fant, 1960; Flanagan, 1965) for such changes in articulation. When the oral structures of the talker were anesthetized, the major maximum in the spectrum of /s/ was centered at a frequency lower than that of /ʃ/, suggesting that perceptual confusions can occur between these sounds.

A different kind of change was observed in the spectra of the vowels /ɑ/ and /i/. The center frequencies of the formants did not change significantly, but the relative amplitudes of the formants, as well as the general contour of the spectral envelopes, were changed. (There were no obvious differences, however, between the /ɝ/ samples produced in the two conditions.) In the control speech, the levels of F2 for /ɑ/ and /i/ were 6 and 18 dB, respectively, below those of F1. In the block speech, the levels of F2 for /ɑ/ and /i/ were 12 and 28 dB, respectively, below the F1 levels. These changes in the relative amplitudes of formants may change the quality of the utterances since the difference limen for the amplitude of F2 is about 3 dB (Flanagan, 1957). Spectral changes under oral anesthesia may represent changes in the glottal spectrum brought about by the influence of oral anesthesia on laryngeal behavior; this matter requires further examination.

Fundamental Frequency. The fundamental-frequency characteristics of the speech materials were obtained with a simple version of a program based on cepstrum analysis (Noll, 1964). The speech was low-pass filtered at 4.8 k Hz and time-sampled at a 10-k Hz rate; the program calculated an F_0 value, whenever possible, for each 10 msec of speech. Specifically, the 512 data points in a time window of 51.2 msec were submitted to a fast Fourier analysis. The window had a Hamming weighting function where the nth value is given by $0.5 - 0.5 \cos (2 n/512)$. The returned coefficients were used to calculate logarithmic amplitude values which, in turn, were submitted to a fast Fourier analysis to provide the cepstrum. The program found the appropriate peak in the cepstrum and calculated its distance from the origin to determine the fundamental frequency. The time window was shifted by 10-msec intervals to yield one F_0 value every 10 msec. The accuracy of this method of calculating fundamental frequency for connected speech was tested informally by comparing the results to period-by-period manual measurements of high-quality oscillograms, and found to be satisfactory.

In the frequency analyses, only those portions of the utterances were used for which the program produced reasonable values for both control and block conditions. Distribution histograms based on approximately 2100 measurements for each talking mode are presented in Figure 5. These distributions show

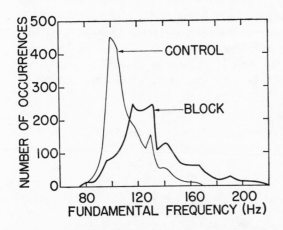

FIGURE 5. Distributions of fundamental frequencies for normal (control) and anesthetized (block) conditions. Approximately 2100 points are involved for each condition.

that, on the average, under nerve block the talker used a higher fundamental frequency (about 20 Hz (or 3 semitones) above his "normal" average of 108 Hz) and used larger frequency changes than those observed in the normal condition (manifesting a standard deviation of 24 Hz compared to 15 Hz). This finding agrees with the observation of Ringel and Steer (1963) that talkers with anesthetized oral structures used an average fundamental frequency higher than their normal performance. Since, at the time of the recording, "vocal effort" was not under experimental control, this rise in average fundamental frequency may be attributable to the greater vocal effort used by the talker trying to speak normally while deprived of oral sensation, rather than to some direct effect of the anesthetic.

Time Measurements. Since the effects of oral anesthesia on the temporal characteristics of speech have been reported before (Gammon, et al., 1971; Scott and Ringel, 1971), measures of speech rates and phonation-time ratios were made for comparison. The rate of utterance was calculated from the digital spectrograms by counting the number of words and dividing by the total time elapsed during the utterance, excluding pauses. Phonation-time ratios were a by-product of the program that calculated the fundamental frequencies of the utterances; the ratios were derived by dividing the total phonation time (that is, the voiced portions of the utterances) by the total utterance time, excluding pauses.

The time measures are summarized in Table 2. The rate of utterance de-

TABLE 2. Average rate (words per minute), phonation-time ratio (phonation time [seconds]/duration [seconds]), and duration of the speech sample.

Speech Mode	Rate	P-t Ratio	Duration
Control	198.5	0.63	85.9
Block	175.0	0.76	82.8

creased about 10% when anesthesia was introduced. The phonation-time ratio, however, was significantly larger in the block condition, suggesting that the block production was characterized by a prolongation of voiced segments or fewer pauses. Inspection of the digital spectrograms showed essentially that this was the case. A typical example is shown in Figure 6, where the digital

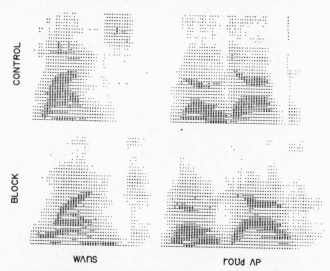

FIGURE 6. Digital spectrograms for the words *once* and *rode up* produced under block (lower spectrograms) and control (upper spectrograms) conditions. Note the prolonged voiced segments in general, the reduced high-frequency energy for /s/, and the less clear stop closure and burst for /d/ and /p/ for the block condition.

sound spectrogram of the block speech shows portions that, relative to the control speech, are noticeably prolonged.

DISCUSSION

The acoustic characteristics of connected speech produced by talkers de-

266

prived of oral sensation have been predicted previously by careful observers of articulation who used acoustic theory to extrapolate their descriptions. Our study serves to validate these predictions, as well as to demonstrate the utility of some simple methods of computer analysis in describing statistical properties of connected speech, both normal and abnormal. The statistics reported here should be characteristic, since 30 seconds or more of connected speech (without an a priori bias in the frequency of occurrence of particular phonemes) can be expected to have reasonably stable statistical characteristics (Li, Hughes, and House, 1969).

The results of the analyses of speech produced without oral sensation can be summarized as (1) a reduction in high-frequency spectral components, (2) some temporal disorganization (primarily manifested as decreased rate of utterance and prolongation of [voiced] syllabic nuclei), and (3) a higher and more variable fundamental frequency. In general, these results substantiate the conclusion of previous studies. Probably they are attributable primarily to a reduction in the accuracy with which the talker forms constrictions in the vocal tract. Both the location and degree of constriction seem to be changed by loss of tactile sensation. The temporal disorganization and the changes in fundamental frequency may be functions of the talker's increased effort to produce accurate speech without sensory feedback from the oral structures. The implications of these data for theories of articulatory control are obvious and are discussed in detail elsewhere (Scott and Ringel, 1971; Prosek, 1971; Mac-Neilage, 1970).

Changes in the spectral characteristics of some speech sounds are certainly correlated with changes in articulatory gestures. Whether such changes result in phonemic substitutions must be judged by perceptual experiments (but see Scott, 1970, and Prosek, 1971, for persuasive evidence to the contrary). Apparently the high intelligibility of speech produced by talkers deprived of oral sensation may be due, in part at least, to the condition's selective effect on classes of speech sounds, as well as to the adaptability of the human listener to systematic distortions of the speech signal.

The acoustic data presented here should supplement our understanding of the production and perception of speech. The computer programs used are applicable to analysis of speech in general, as well as to the analysis of diverse categories of disordered speech.

ACKNOWLEDGMENT

Cheryl M. Scott provided the speech materials on which this report is based and her contributions are acknowledged with gratitude. This investigation was sponsored in part by the Office of Aerospace Research, USAF, under the technical cognizance of Air Force Cambridge Research Laboratories, OAR, and by National Institute of Dental Research under award 1 R01 DE 02815-02. Arthur S. House is currently at the Institute for Defense Analysis, Princeton, New Jersey 08540.

REFERENCES

DUNN, H. K., and WHITE, S. D., Statistical measurements on conversational speech. *J. acoust. Soc. Amer.*, 11, 278-288 (1940).

FAIRBANKS, G., and MIRON, M. S., Effects of vocal effort upon the consonant-vowel ratio within the syllable. *J. acoust. Soc. Amer.*, 29, 621-626 (1957).

FANT, C. G. M., *Acoustic Theory of Speech Production*. The Hague: Gravenhage, Mouton (1960).

FLANAGAN, J. L., Difference limen for formant amplitude. *J. Speech Hearing Dis.*, 22, 205-212 (1957).

FLANAGAN, J. L., *Speech Analysis, Synthesis and Perception*. New York, Academic (1965).

GAMMON, S. A., SMITH, P. J., DANILOFF, R. G., and KIM, C. W., Articulation and stress/juncture production under oral anesthetization and masking. *J. Speech Hearing Res.*, 14, 271-282 (1971).

HEINZ, J. M., and STEVENS, K. N., On the properties of voiceless fricative consonants. *J. acoust. Soc. Amer.*, 33, 589-596 (1961).

HOLBROOK, A., and FAIRBANKS, G., Diphthong formants and their movements. *J. Speech Hearing Res.*, 5, 38-58 (1962).

HORII, Y., HOUSE, A. S., and HUGHES, G. W., A masking noise with speech-envelope characteristics for studying intelligibility. *J. acoust. Soc. Amer.*, 44, 1849-1856 (1971).

HOUSE, A. S., WILLIAMS, C. E., HECKER, M. H. L., and KRYTER, K. D., Articulation testing methods; Consonantal differentiation with a closed-response set. *J. acoust. Soc. Amer.*, 37, 158-166 (1965).

HUGHES, G. W., and HALLE, M., Spectral properties of fricative consonants. *J. acoust. Soc. Amer.*, 28, 303-310 (1956).

HUGHES, G. W., and HEMDAL, J. F., Speech Analysis. Purdue Research Foundation, Final Report, Contract AF 19(628)-305, Air Force Cambridge Research Laboratories, Bedford, Massachusetts, AFCRL-65-681 (July 1965).

LEHISTE, I., and PETERSON, G. E., Transitions, glides, and diphthongs. *J. acoust. Soc. Amer.*, 33, 268-277 (1961).

LI, K.-P., HUGHES, G. W., and HOUSE, A. S., Correlation characteristics and dimensionality of speech spectra. *J. acoust. Soc. Amer.*, 46, 1019-1025 (1969).

MACNEILAGE, P. F., Motor control of serial ordering of speech. *Psychol. Rev.*, 77, 182-196 (1970).

McCROSKEY, R., CORELY, N., and JACKSON, G., Some effects of disrupted tactile cues upon the production of consonants. *South. Speech J.*, 25, 55-60 (1959).

NOLL, M. A., Short-time spectrum and "cepstrum" techniques for vocal-pitch detection. *J. acoust. Soc. Amer.*, 36, 296-302 (1964).

PETERSON, G. E., and BARNEY, H. L., Control methods used in a study of vowels. *J. acoust. Soc. Amer.*, 24, 175-184 (1952).

PROSEK, R. A., An evaluation of the role of oral sensation in consonant production. Doctoral dissertation, Purdue Univ. (1971).

RINGEL, R. L., and STEER, M. D., Some effects of tactile and auditory alterations on speech output. *J. Speech Hearing Res.*, 6, 369-378 (1963).

SACIA, C. F., and BECK, C. J., Power of the fundamental speech sounds. *Bell Syst. tech. J.*, 5, 393-403 (1926).

SCOTT, C. M., A phonetic analysis of the effects of oral sensory deprivation. Doctoral dissertation, Purdue Univ. (1970).

SCOTT, C. M., and RINGEL, R. L., Articulation without oral sensory control. *J. Speech Hearing Res.*, 14, 804-818 (1971).

STEVENS, K. N., and HOUSE, A. S., An acoustical theory of vowel production and some of its implications. *J. Speech Hearing Res.*, 4, 303-320 (1961).

STREVENS, P., Spectra of fricative noise in human speech. *Lang. Speech*, 3, 32-49 (1960).

TARNOCZY, T., Resonance data concerning nasals, laterals and trills. *Word*, 4, 71-77 (1948).

THOMPSON, R. C., The effects of oral sensory disruption upon oral stereognosis and articulation. Paper presented at the 45th Annual Convention of the American Speech and Hearing Association, Chicago (November 1969).

WEISS, M. S., A study of the relation between consonant-vowel amplitude ratio and talker intelligibility. Master's thesis, Purdue Univ. (1968).

TACTILE PERCEPTION: FORM DISCRIMINATION IN THE MOUTH

ROBERT L. RINGEL, KENNETH W. BURK, CHERYL M. SCOTT

STEREOGNOSIS may be defined as the ability to recognize the form of objects through the sense of touch. This ability has been recognized as an important indicator of nervous system integrity and appropriate tests of this function are generally included in a neurological examination (Forster, 1962). It is generally accepted that impairments of stereognostic capacity (astereognosis) in the presence of otherwise intact sensory channels are indicative of a central nervous system pathology. Specifically, Wechsler (1947), McDonald and Chusid (1962), and Nielsen (1965) attributed astereognosis to lesions of the parietal lobe (post-Rolandic gyrus) and/or subcortical regions. In so far as stereognostic capacities may serve as a prototype of sensory discrimination, it may be hypothesized that information pertaining to the ability of persons to make judgements of object-shape upon the oral presentation of the stimuli may yield important insights into the nature of the oral sensory mechanisms which are believed to underly the speech monitoring system.

In clinical settings, stereognosis is tested by placing common objects such as keys, pens, and coins in the subject's hand. Obviously such practices are not applicable to the oral region. Modifications of stimulus materials and response modes were initiated by a number of investigators interested in this region. Some of these investigators have attempted to assess oral form perception abilities of persons with various forms of nervous system, oral structure, and communicative behaviour disturbances using two-dimensional geometric plastic forms in an oral-tactile to visual matching procedure. The findings of these investigators were reported in the first "Symposium on Oral Sensation and Perception" (Bosma, 1967) and additional findings are reported in the second Symposium (Bosma, 1968). The relation between the tasks modified for use in the oral region and traditional stereognostic testing has not been specified. In general, the results of studies of oral form functioning by different investigators are often inconsistent. Perhaps the variability of such results reflects the use of many different methodologies and stimulus materials. Consistent trends which do exist tend to support the view that persons with organic pathologies (nervous system and oral structure) and speech defects experience difficulty in oral form recognition tasks.

The conclusions reached in those studies and their implications in understanding the role of speech control systems must be viewed cautiously. The informants in such studies were usually allowed to use their visual systems in the process of matching the stimulus objects. As Weinberg (1968) noted, experiments have not measured oral sensory capacity by itself but rather some aspect of intersensory matching. The potential problems involved in tasks of intersensory matching would seem to place severe restrictions upon the information such oral form perception testing procedures might yield. For example, a patient who is "visually deficient" but "tactually normal" would exhibit poor oral sensory abilities if visual functioning were allowed to remain an integral part of the tactile matching task. This criticism becomes more pronounced if a traditional view of the speech servo-system is accepted. In such systems, visual process interaction with oral system

BRITISH JOURNAL OF DISORDERS OF COMMUNICATION, 1968, vol. 3, 150-155.

tactile monitoring is not implied. It appears therefore that a test which attempts to provide information about the tactile modality must be limited primarily to that modality and not lend itself to sources of contamination by involving other sensory channels such as vision.

The present test was constructed to eliminate the intersensory nature of the form matching tasks employed by previous investigators by using an oral referent for the discrimination. The experimenters also attempted to make the new test applicable to persons representing a wide range of ages, intellectual abilities, and physical states. To meet such requirements, the test used relatively few stimuli, and called for a simple discrimination type of response. Since the design of the test did not require form recognition per se, it may not be considered to measure stereognostic abilities in the traditional sense. Rather, the test was intended to serve as a measure of form discrimination.

METHOD

Subjects.—Sixteen females and four male university students served as the normal-speaking subjects in this investigation. Their age range was 19 to 25 years with a mean age of 22 years. All were judged free of speech defects, oral structure anomalies, and reported no past or present history of sensory and/or motor disturbances.

Nine female and 18 male students enrolled in the Purdue University Speech and Hearing Clinic for speech therapy served as articulatory-defective subjects. They ranged in age from 18 to 25 years with a mean age of 19 years. The articulatory-defective subjects reported no past or present history of sensory and/or motor defects, and gross abnormalities of the oral structures were not observed upon examination. Traditionally the articulation problems demonstrated by this group would be classified as "functional" in nature.

Articulatory-defective subjects were further subdivided into two groups, a mild articulation group (A_1), and a moderate articulation group (A_2). Twelve subjects were assigned to the first group and fifteen subjects were placed in the second group. Group assignments were made by an experienced clinical speech pathologist and were based on samples of spontaneous speech. The assignments took into consideration articulatory error features such as conspicuousness of error, frequency of occurrence of the misarticulated sound in conversational speech, consistency of error production, and the number of misarticulated sounds. By way of summary, at a clinical level, A_1 subjects represented mild articulation problems, while A_2 subjects represented moderate levels of articulation problems.

Stimuli.—The stimulus materials used in this investigation were drawn from the pool of 20 plastic geometric forms developed at the National Institute of Dental Research (NIDR 20's). Ten forms were drawn from this pool to represent a wide range of individual item difficulty and confusability, as reported by Moser et al. (1967). The ten forms shown in Figure 1 were subdivided into four geometric classes: triangular (1, 2), rectangular (3, 4, 5), oval (6, 7, 8), and biconcave (9, 10). The pairing of the forms made possible "within-class" (e.g., item 1-2, 7-8) and "between-class" (e.g., item 1-9, 3-8) stimulus pairs. Each stimulus pair was used only once, for example, pair 7-9 precluded the use of pair 9-7. The total 55 form-pairs thus generated were evaluated by each subject. Ten pairs, selected at random from the total group, were re-evaluated by each subject for purposes of reliability. In summary, each subject evaluated a total of 65 stimulus form-pairs.

270

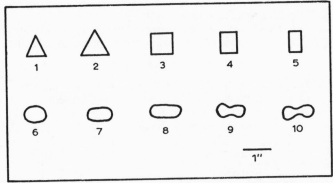

Fig. 1

Geometric forms employed in the oral sensory discrimination task.

Procedure.—The forms in each stimulus pair were presented successively to the subject. Each was placed by the investigator in the subject's mouth. The subject was allowed to retain the first form of a pair for a period of five seconds; a period of approximately five seconds intervened before the second form presentation. Once the form was in the subject's mouth, he was allowed to manipulate it in any fashion he desired. Upon removal of the second form of the stimulus pair, the subject was asked to indicate whether the two forms were the "same" or "different". This procedure was followed for each of the 55 pairs of forms. The stimulus pairs were randomized in presentation order. Following this testing the ten reliability items were presented using an identical procedure. To prevent visual and manual cues from influencing evaluations, subjects were blindfolded and not allowed to handle the stimulus materials.

RESULTS

The number of errors committed was determined for each subject. This was followed by computation of measures of central tendency and variability for subject groups and subgroups. These statistics, summarized in Table I, indicate that the articulatory-defective subjects as a total group made a larger average number of errors and were more variable in their performance than the normals. The exception was that the variability displayed by the articulation (A_1) sub-group was comparable

TABLE I

Average number and variability of errors for normal-speaking and articulatory-defective subjects*

Subject Group	N	Mean	Standard Deviation
Normal	20	4·00	1·71
Articulation (Total)	27	6·81	2·46
Articulation (A_1)	12	5·42	1·67
Articulation (A_2)	15	7·93	2·46

*A_1—mild articulation problem; A_2—moderate articulation problem.

to that of the normal speakers. It should be noted that the average number of errors increased with the severity of articulatory problem.

To assess the significance of the average difference in number of errors for subject groupings, t-tests for unrelated measures were applied to the data (Table 2).

TABLE II

Summary of t-tests for significance of difference in average numbers of errors for normal-speaking and articulatory-defective subjects

Group Comparison	t-value	Significance
Normal vs. Articulation (Total)	4·38	·01
Normal vs. Articulation (A₁)	2·82	·05
Normal vs. Articulation (A₂)	5·60	·01
Articulation (A₁) vs. Articulation (A₂)	3·03	·01

These findings, in conjunction with the results presented in Table 1, indicate that on the average the normal speakers produced significantly fewer errors than the total articulatory-defective group and its sub-groups. In addition, the two articulatory-defective sub-groups differed significantly in their average performance. Subjects in the articulation (A₂) group made a greater average number of mistakes.

A second analysis of the data compared errors made on within-class and between-class stimulus pairs. The results of this analysis, presented in Table 3,

TABLE III

Average numbers and variability of between-class and within-class errors for normal-speaking and articulatory defective subjects

Subject Group	N	Between-Class		Within-Class	
		Mean	Standard Deviation	Mean	Standard Deviation
Normal	20	·20	·41	3·80	1·76
Articulation (Total)	27	1·96	1·93	4·85	1·63

indicate that both the normal and articulatory-defective subjects made a greater average number of within-class than between-class errors. The variability associated with the group performances was similar with perhaps the exception of the normal group for between-class errors. Through application of a t-test for correlated data it was found that the difference in the average number of between-class and within-class errors was statistically significant for both groups (Table 4).

A further analysis of between-class and within-class errors suggested by the data evaluated the proportion of these two types of errors as they were represented in the performance of the normal speaking and total articulatory-defective groups. These proportions are shown in Table 5. It can be seen that the discrepancy in

TABLE IV

Summary of t-tests for significance of difference in mean number of between-class and within-class errors for normal-speaking articulatory-defective subjects

Subject Group	t-value	Significance
Normal	13·14	·01
Articulation (Total)	6·89	·01

TABLE V

Proportionate distribution of between-class and within-class errors for normal speaking and articulatory-defective subjects, and associated X^2 value

	Type of Error	
Subject Group	Between-Class	Within-Class
Articulation (Total)	·288	·712
Normal	·050	·950

$X^2 = 18·67$ (significant at ·01 level)

proportions is greatest for subjects with normal articulation. When the proportions for normals were treated as expected data and a X^2 test of significance applied, a value of 18·67 was obtained which is significant at the ·01 level of confidence. While this finding must be interpreted with caution since subjects may have disproportionately contributed to the error distributions, it does suggest that errors produced by the articulatory-defective subjects are distributed in a manner significantly different from that of the normals.

The reliability of subject responses was of considerable importance in the investigation. The extent of internal reliability is shown in Table 6. Seven normal speakers were completely consistent on retest and 13 showed only one disagreement. Twenty-one of the 27 articulatory-defective subjects had no more than one disagreement, with only one having as many as three. Considering the complexity of the task these data are interpreted as indicating a very satisfactory level of intra-subject reliability.

DISCUSSION AND CONCLUSIONS

Although the results of the present study cannot be directly compared to those of other investigations since different methodologies have been used, the present findings support the view that persons with defective articulation experience difficulty in tasks of oral form discrimination.

The ability to differentiate between normal-speaking and articulatory-defective young adults on the basis of their performance on a test of oral form discrimination is a significant finding. These results support the often hypothesized relation between oral sensory system functioning and articulation skill. Additional efforts at both experimental and theoretical levels are needed to specify the exact nature of the interactions of these and other factors which may serve to relate the oral sensory and speech production systems. At present, what appears to be most important

TABLE VI
Reliability: Extent of intra-subject response agreement during the second
presentation of 10 stimulus pairs

Subject Group	Number of Test-Retest Agreements	Number of Subjects
Normal (N=20)	10	7
	9	13
	⋮	⋮
	0	0
Articulation (Total) (N=27)	10	9
	9	12
	8	5
	7	1
	⋮	⋮
	0	0

is the fact that persons of college level intellectual ability who demonstrate what are
considered to be functional articulation errors make a greater number and proportionately different types of errors in tasks of oral form discrimination than are made
by a comparable group of normal speakers. Furthermore, performance on such
sensory tasks varies in accordance with the severity of the articulation defect.

These preliminary findings serve to question the appropriateness of the term
"functional" as it has been used traditionally to describe the basis of articulation
errors made by persons similar to those studied in this investigation. The orderliness
of the present findings in comparison to the inconsistencies reported by other
investigators using oral-tactile-visual matching procedures also calls into question
the rationale behind studies of oral form perception that require subjects to correlate
objects held in their mouth with similar objects displayed before them visually.
The need to explore a sensory basis for "functional" articulation problems is evident
and would strongly support the further use of the oral discrimination task described
in this study in subsequent investigations.

ACKNOWLEDGEMENTS
*This investigation was supported by a Public Health Service Research Career
Development Award (1KO3-DE 32614-01) from the National Institute of Dental
Research to R. L. Ringel.*

REFERENCES
Bosma, J. (Ed.). *Symposium on Oral Sensation and Perception.* Illinois: Thomas (1967).
Bosma, J. (Ed.). *Second Symposium on Oral Sensation and Perception.* In Press (1968).
Forster, F. *Synopsis of Neurology.* St. Louis: Mosby (1962).
McDonald, J. and Chusid, J. *Correlative Neuroanatomy and Functional Neurology.*
    California: Lange (1962).
Moser, H., LaGourge, J., Class, L. Studies of Oral Stereognosis in Normal, Blind and
    Deaf Subjects. In Bosma, J. (Ed.), *Symposium on Oral Sensation and Perception.* Illinois:
    Thomas (1967).
Nielsen, J. *Agnosia, Apraxia and Aphasia.* New York: Hafner (1965).
Wechsler, I. *Textbook of Clinical Neurology.* Philadelphia: Saunders (1947).
Wienberg, B., Lyons, M., Manchester, G. Studies of Oral Manual and Visual Form
    Identification Skills in Children and Adults. In Bosma, J. (Ed.), *Second Symposium on
    Oral Sensation and Perception.* In Press (1968).

INTRA-ORAL RECOGNITION OF GEOMETRIC FORMS BY NORMAL SUBJECTS[1]

WILLIAM N. WILLIAMS   AND   LEONARD L. LA POINTE

Summary.—Oral form recognition abilities were determined for 40 normal *S*s between the ages of 20 and 59 yr., using 12 different geometric forms in 8 sizes. The purposes were: (1) to explore such related variables as form complexity, form size, *S*s' age, sex and education level and *S*s' response time; and (2) to reduce the total number of test items to a more manageable level by selecting those shapes and sizes from the original test items which contribute most to the obtained oral stereognosis scores. There were no significant differences for sex or educational level, but significant relations were found among performance· levels and age groups. In addition, *S*s' performance tended to be inversely related to response time. Within the limits of several criteria, 10 forms were selected which can practically and effectively provide a measure of oral form recognition. And, these forms may permit assessment of oral sensory integrity.

Much information is available on sensation in various parts of the body, particularly in the extremities (3, 4); however, little is known about oral sensation and perception. Ringel and Ewanowski (9) have noted that ". . . lack of procedures for effectively evaluating the receptive capacities of this region is unfortunate inasmuch as it has been demonstrated that such information gathered from exploration of other regions of the body is extremely valuable at an applied level in the cl'nical assessment of various forms of neuro- and myopathologies."

In addition, the acquisition of information on oral sensation and perception is important to the speech scientist, and such investigators as McDonald (6) and McCall (5) have suggested that the role of kinesthesia and tactile sensation in the oral cavity may be more vital to the feedback processes in the perception of articulatory placement than audition, once speech patterns have been established.

The assessment of oral sensation and perception could be accomplished by testing such dimensions as two-point discrimination, light touch, and kinesthesia. Oral form recognition (oral stereognosis) no doubt utilizes all of these sensory parameters, therefore, varying levels of form recognition might indicate degrees of oral sensory integrity. Several studies of oral stereognosis have been completed and recently reported in a symposium (2), and many of the contributors

---

[1]The authors express their appreciation to Mr. Stanley Woodland, Dental Laboratory Technician, Veterans Administration Hospital, Gainesville, Florida, who aided in the construction of the different geometric forms, and to Dr. J. Thornby, University of Florida, for his assistance in the statistical analysis of the data. This study was supported in part by research funds from the VA Hospital, Gainesville, Florida, and by the College of Dentistry, University of Florida, Gainesville, Florida.

PERCEPTUAL AND MOTOR SKILLS, 1971, vol. 32, no. 2, 419-426.

to this symposium have indicated the need for additional research in this area. More specifically, Moser, LaGourgue, and Class (8) have called attention to research on the development of the assessment device. Such factors as form complexity, size, thickness, S's age, sex and education, and time required for identifying the form are significant variables in the assessment and understanding of oral stereognosis. One of the purposes of this study was to obtain and analyze data relative to these variables. The second purpose was to select the shapes and sizes which contributed most to the obtained stereognosis scores.

METHOD

Subjects

Forty normal Ss between the ages of 20 and 59 yr. were chosen for this study. Included were 5 males and 5 females in each of the following age groups: 20—29 yr., 30—39 yr., 40—49 yr., and 50—59 yr.

Form Construction

The forms were selected from the basic shapes used in the Southern California Kinesthesia and Tactile Perception Test developed by Ayres (1).[2] Fig. 1 shows the 12 geometric shapes used in the present study.

For intra-oral presentation these shapes were moulded from dental acrylic in four different two-dimensional sizes, with each size being moulded in two thicknesses. Table 1 lists the approximate dimensions of the eight sizes.

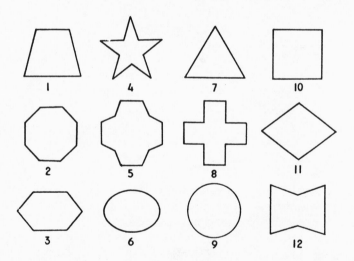

FIG. 1. The 12 geometric forms used in assessing stereognostic ability [Reproduced with permission of Dr. Jean Ayres from her Subtest M of the Southern California Kinesthesia and Tactile Perception Tests, published by Western Psychological Services, 1966.]

[2]Dr. Jean Ayres and Western Psychological Services, 12031 Wilshire Blvd., Los Angeles, Calif. 90025, graciously granted permission for our use of this material and reproduction of the geometric forms shown in Fig. 1.

TABLE 1
DIMENSIONS OF FORMS IN EIGHT DIFFERENT SIZES

Size	Width (in.)*	Thickness (in.)	Size	Width (in.)*	Thickness (in.)
1	1⅛	¼	5	½	¼
2	1⅛	⅛	6	½	⅛
3	¾	¼	7	⅜	¼
4	¾	⅛	8	⅜	⅛

*These values were obtained by measuring across the width of the square and represent the approximate width of the other forms.

As a precaution against accidental swallowing and in order to facilitate handling of the forms, a 6-in. piece of light monofilament line was embedded into the side of each form. This flexible line permitted more extensive oral manipulation of the form than if secured by a non-flexible shaft.

Administration

Each S was required to identify 96 forms (8 sizes, 12 shapes each). The 8 sizes and the 12 shapes within each size were randomly ordered for presentation to each S.

In order to lend evidence to the assumption that none of the Ss included in the study had a basic deficit in form discrimination, the Ayres Manual Stereognostic subtest was administered prior to presentation of the intra-oral forms. All Ss appeared to have adequate discrimination for these forms.

Standardized instructions were presented to each S. Ss were told to use free oral manipulation and then to indicate their selection by pointing to the picture of the form on a placard depicting all 12 shapes. Ss were instructed to close their eyes as each form was placed in their mouth and again after they made their selection when the form was being retrieved. Ss received no information as to whether their selections were correct or incorrect and were cautioned to make their selection of each form in reference to the "feel" it had for them and not in terms of any elimination process. Ss' responses were recorded in terms of accuracy and time. After testing each S, the forms were cleaned with an iodine based (Wescodyne) solution.

RESULTS

The mean number of correct responses for the 40 Ss for all 96 forms was 71.4. The 40 Ss presented a range of correct responses from 33 to 91, with a SD of 14.2. Following is a summary of the data regarding shape, size, thickness, age, sex, education and time.

Shape

Fig. 2 lists the hierarchy of difficulty for the 12 shapes and illustrates those shapes which were significantly harder than the others. For example, the star was identified on an average of 7.87 times out of a possible eight (eight dif-

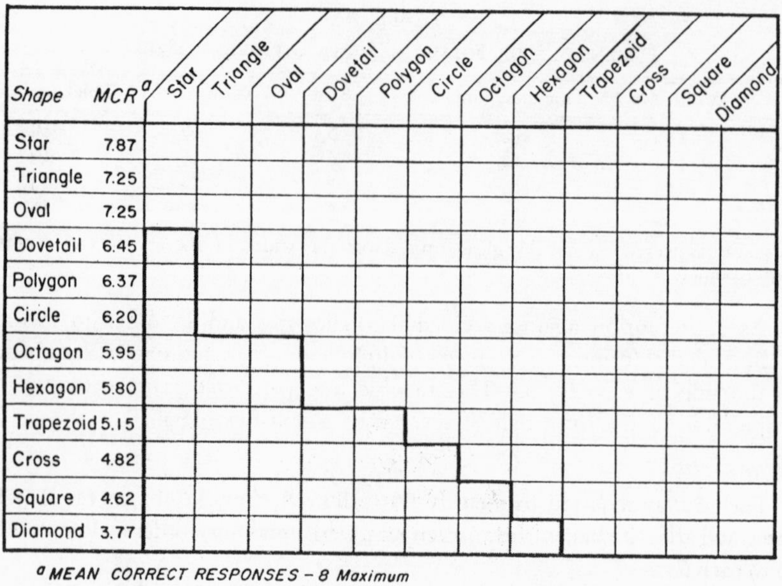

Shape	MCR[a]	Star	Triangle	Oval	Dovetail	Polygon	Circle	Octagon	Hexagon	Trapezoid	Cross	Square	Diamond
Star	7.87												
Triangle	7.25												
Oval	7.25												
Dovetail	6.45												
Polygon	6.37												
Circle	6.20												
Octagon	5.95												
Hexagon	5.80												
Trapezoid	5.15												
Cross	4.82												
Square	4.62												
Diamond	3.77												

[a] MEAN CORRECT RESPONSES – 8 Maximum

FIG. 2. Hierarchy of difficulty and significant differences of difficulty (shaded area) among the 12 geometric shapes

ferent sizes) by all 40 Ss. Those shapes included in the shaded area beneath any given shape listed across the top of the figure were significantly harder to identify ($P < .05$). For instance, the shaded area in the column below the circle indicates that the cross, square and diamond were significantly harder.

Size

Table 2 shows the hierarchy of difficulty for eight different sizes. Since there are 12 different geometric shapes within each size, the maximum number of correct responses for any given size is 12. From this table it can be seen that size 3 has the highest mean of correct responses (9.72 out of 12) while size 7 shows the most errors (7.62 out of 12). It is evident that there is no progressive relationship regarding size, i.e., the smallest size is not the hardest and the largest size the easiest although the two smallest sizes do appear to be the most difficult. A Tukey's multiple comparisons showed that performance on size 7 was significantly lower than for sizes 1 through 6 and performance on size 8 was significantly lower than on sizes 1, 3 and 5.

Sex and Age

An analysis of the responses for the 40 Ss yielded no statistically significant differences between the performances of males and females. When performance levels were examined by age groups, a *t* test indicated a significant difference ($P < .05$) for Age Group 1 and Age Group 4. The performance differences

278

TABLE 2

HIERARCHY OF DIFFICULTY FOR EIGHT SIZES (40 Ss)

Size*	Mean Correct Responses†	Size*	Mean Correct Responses†
3	9.72	4	9.08
1	9.50	2	8.95
5	9.32	8	8.22
6	9.20	7	7.62

*Size 1 = Largest Size; Size 8 = Smallest Size.
†12 Maximum.

among other age groups (cf. Table 3) were nonsignificant. The data suggest no stable performance plateau appears through the adult age range. Others, such as McDonald and Aungst (7), have noted that performance improves through adolescence, stabilizes through adulthood and then decreases in the geriatric population.

The data from this study suggest that age level, even within the adult population, might be important in oral stereognostic performance and therefore in the interpretation of oral stereognostic results.

Education

Ss ranged in years of education from 10 to 21, with a mean of 15.8, but educational level was not significantly related to stereognostic performance. In fact, when the 40 Ss were ranked according to years of education, those 20 Ss below the median in years of education had a higher mean stereognostic score (73.3) than the 20 Ss above the median (69.4).

Time

The time value for each S was determined by recording the number of seconds that elapsed from placement of the form in S's mouth until he made his selection. The total time value for all 96 forms for the 40 Ss ranged from 7 to 51 min., with a mean of 19 min. In order to determine the relationship between performance level and time, a correlation coefficient was computed.

TABLE 3

MEAN CORRECT RESPONSES OF FOUR AGE GROUPS

Age Groups*	Mean Correct Responses†
1 (20—29)	77.9
2 (30—39)	76.4
3 (40—49)	69.3
4 (50—59)	62.2‡

*10 Ss per group (5 males, 5 females).
†96 maximum.
‡Significantly different ($P < .05$) from the performance level of Age Group 1.

279

The value of —.33 suggests a slight inverse relationship between performance and time. That is, those who scored higher tended to take less time. A close look at the relationship between time and performance indicated that the top 10 performers had a mean time value of 11 min. while the 10 lowest performers had a mean of 21 min. A correlation coefficient of —.79 was obtained for these 20 Ss.

Learning-adaptation

The data were analyzed to determine if Ss' performance on the 96 forms varied systematically, which might be explained by either a learning or an adaptation effect. As discussed earlier, the eight sizes were randomly arranged so that the sequence of sizes presented was different for each S. It was found that scores in the early part of the sequence were significantly lower ($P < .01$) than scores obtained later in the sequence.

Fig. 3 is a graphic representation of performance change for the 40 Ss. The numbers along the abcissa refer to the temporal order of subtest presentation regardless of size. The values along the ordinate represent the mean correct responses for all 40 Ss for each subtest. A maximum score of 12 was possible since any given set was composed of 12 different shapes. It is evident from this figure that there is some learning throughout the task. This change can be explained by increased familiarity with the same 12 geometric shapes since the 12 shapes are presented eight different times (eight sizes). If the improved performance observed was due to learning the stereognostic task *per se*, one

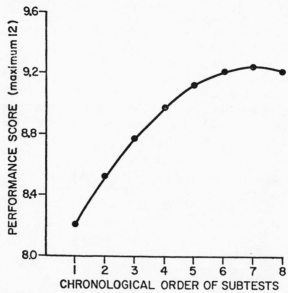

FIG. 3. Improvement in performance by 40 Ss on the eight different subtests

280

might expect to see improvement during the first set of 12 geometric shapes presented. However, when the score for the first six items within the first set of 12 shapes was compared with the score for the last six items of this set, no significant difference was found. It appears then, that with a short test of stereognosis, Ss perform just as well on early items as they do on items which appear later. In this sample there was no apparent adaptation or fatigue in Ss' performance.

Criteria for Final Form Selection

In order to be clinically practical, a test of oral stereognosis must not be excessively time consuming. One of the purposes of this study was to analyze the data in an attempt to select those forms which contribute most to the total test score, thereby creating an assessment device which would be more manageable in its administration. Several criteria were established to aid in selecting forms which were to be included in the final test. Consideration was given to the (1) correlation of scores on individual test items with total test scores. In order to determine which forms were efficient predictors of total test score, correlation coefficients were run for all 96 forms. Those forms with relatively low correlations were excluded. (2) Intelligibility value was examined. Intelligibility refers to the number of correct responses made to any given form. As can be seen from Table 2 and Fig. 2, a wide range of intelligibility existed for both the different geometric shapes and sizes. Forms of varying levels of intelligibility were selected in order to assure adequate variance. (3) Error spread was checked. Forms meeting the first two criteria were then analyzed and selected in terms of their error pattern. Error spread refers to the number of different forms that were chosen incorrectly when a particular form was presented. For example, 127 errors were made when the cross was presented, but these errors were distributed among only four other geometric shapes. However, 131 errors were made on the square, but these errors were distributed among nine different forms. Therefore, in this example the square has relatively large error spread and prediction of response pattern would probably be less accurate than for the cross. In order to lend a degree of predictability to response patterns, forms were selected that had relatively small error spread. (4) Variety of shape was examined. If other selection criteria were equal, form choice was then made to include shapes other than those already selected.

Using these criteria, nine different forms were selected. In addition, the star in size 6 was also selected because of its potential diagnostic significance in that it was never missed by any of the 40 normal Ss. Table 4 shows the final 10 forms which were selected, including approximate size and thickness of each form.

Reliability

Reliability of this 10-item test of oral stereognosis must still be established.

TABLE 4
FINAL 10 FORMS: GEOMETRIC SHAPE, WIDTH, AND THICKNESS

Form	Width (in.)	Thickness (in.)
Polygon	1	¼
Octagon	¾	¼
Octagon	¾	⅛
Hexagon	1	⅛
Dovetail	½	¼
Star	¾	⅛
Triangle	⅜	¼
Cross	⅜	¼
Trapezoid	⅜	⅛
Cross	⅜	⅛

However, preliminary test-retest results with these 10 forms suggest that reliability is adequate. Four Ss who were not included in the original sample were tested once and then again seven days later. A reliability coefficient of .92 was obtained.

The present data suggest that these 10 forms can be used to explore further the parameters of oral form recognition. Hopefully the development of a reliable and practical tool of oral stereognosis will prove valuable as a measure of the sensory integrity of the oral mechanism. This tool might then be applied to the study of the relationships among varying levels of oral sensation and perception and speech proficiency.

REFERENCES

1. AYRES, A. J. *Southern California kinesthesia and tactile perception tests.* Los Angeles, Calif.: Western Psychological Services, 1966.
2. BOSMA, J. F. (Ed.) *Symposium on oral sensation and perception.* Springfield, Ill.: Thomas, 1967.
3. DEJONG, R. N. *The neurologic examination.* (3rd ed.) New York: Harper & Row, 1967.
4. GELDARD, F. A. *The human senses.* New York: Wiley, 1953.
5. MCCALL, G. N. The assessment of lingual tactile sensation and perception. *J. speech hear. Dis.*, 1969, 34, 151-156.
6. MCDONALD, E. T. *Articulation testing and treatment: a sensory motor approach.* Pittsburgh: Stanwix House, Inc., 1964.
7. MCDONALD, E. T., & AUNGST, L. F. Studies in oral sensorimotor function. In J. F. Bosma (Ed.), *Symposium on oral sensation and perception.* Springfield, Ill.: Thomas, 1967. Pp. 202-220.
8. MOSER, H., LAGOURGUE, J. R., & CLASS, L. W. Studies of oral stereognosis in normal, blind and deaf subjects. In J. F. Bosma (Ed.), *Symposium on oral sensation and perception.* Springfield, Ill.: Thomas, 1967. Pp. 244-286.
9. RINGEL, R. L., & EWANOWSKI, S. J. Oral perception: I. Two-point discrimination. *J. speech hear. Res.*, 1965, 8, 389-398.

A COMPARATIVE STUDY OF TWO PROCEDURES FOR ASSESSMENT OF ORAL TACTILE PERCEPTION

Norman J. Lass, Mary E. Tekieli, and Marcia P. Eye

A contemporary discussion of speech production often includes the concept of a servosystem model.[1] This model likens the act of speaking to a servosystem in which sensory feedback provides essential information to the speaker and thus allows him to monitor his speech production. There appear to be at least three monitoring systems which provide information to the speaker to help him learn and subsequently to maintain adequate speech: (1) auditory feedback, (2) tactile feedback, and (3) kinesthetic feedback. Of the three feedback systems, the largest body of information is available on the auditory feedback system. However, the results of several investigations have led to increased interest in the tactile feedback system.[2,3,4] These

investigations have shown that elimination of tactile feedback from the tongue and certain other regions in the oral cavity by means of anesthetization produced adverse effects on the subjects' articulation and intelligibility. These findings have important implications in the field of speech pathology. It has been reasoned that since the subjects' articulatory precision was affected by experimental disruption of the tactile feedback system, the integrity of the tactile sensory system in individuals with articulatory defects should be questioned.

This increased interest in the role of the tactile feedback system in speech production has lead to the development of tests of oral stereognosis.[5,6,7,8] Stereognosis is the ability to recognize the form of objects by means of the sense of touch.

Norman J. Lass (Ph.D., Purdue University, 1968) is Assistant Professor of Speech Pathology-Audiology at West Virginia University; Mary E. Tekieli (B.S., West Virginia University) and Marcia P. Eye (B.S., West Virginia University) are research assistants in the Speech and Hearing Sciences Laboratory and graduate students in the Speech Pathology-Audiology program at West Virginia University. The authors wish to thank Dr. Edwin C. Townsend, Associate Professor of Statistics, West Virginia University, for his statistical consultation. Appreciation is also extended to Dr. Ralph L. Shelton, Professor of Speech Pathology, University of Kansas Medical Center, for providing the pictures used in the visual matching task in this study.

1 G. Fairbanks, "Systematic Research in Experimental Phonetics. I. A Theory of the Speech Mechanism as a Servosystem," Journal of Speech and Hearing Disorders, XIX (1954), 133-139.

2 R. L. McCroskey, "Relative Contribution of Auditory and Tactile Cues to Certain Aspects of Speech," Southern Speech Journal, XXIV (1958), 84-90.

3 R. L. McCroskey, N. W. Corley and G. Jackson, "Some Effects of Disrupted Tactile

Cues Upon the Production of Consonants," Southern Speech Journal, XXV (1959), 55-60.

4 R. L. Ringel and M. D. Steer, "Some Effects of Tactile and Auditory Alternations on Speech Output," Journal of Speech and Hearing Research, VI (1963), 369-377.

5 R. C. Grossman, "Methods for Evaluating Oral Surface Sensation," Journal of Dental Research, XLIII (1964), 301-307.

6 E. T. McDonald and L. F. Aungst, "Studies in Oral Sensorimotor Function," in J. F. Bosma (ed.), Symposium on Oral Sensation and Perception (Springfield, Illinois: Charles C Thomas, 1967), pp. 202-220.

7 H. Moser, J. R. LaGourge, and L. W. Class, "Studies of Oral Stereognosis in Normal, Blind, and Deaf Subjects," in J. F. Bosma (ed.), Symposium on Oral Sensation and Perception (Springfield, Illinois: Charles C Thomas, 1967), pp. 244-286.

8 R. L. Shelton, W. Arndt, and J. Hetherington, "Testing Oral Stereognosis," in J. F. Bosma (ed.), Symposium on Oral Sensation and Perception (Springfield, Illinois: Charles C Thomas, 1967), pp. 221-243.

CENTRAL STATES SPEECH JOURNAL, 1971, vol. 22, 21-26.

Tests of manual stereognosis are used routinely in clinical neurological examinations.[9] Since manual stereognosis provides useful information to the neurologist concerning the patient's overall sensorimotor functioning, oral stereognosis, the ability to recognize the form of objects placed in the mouth, may potentially be a very useful clinical tool to the speech pathologist in evaluating the functioning of the articulatory mechanism.

These tests of oral stereognosis usually involve the placement of objects of varying shapes in the oral cavity and the subject's visual identification of the shapes. However, the results of various studies employing these tests have been inconsistent and have led to a serious questioning of the value of standard methods of assessing oral stereognosis. Such tests have sometimes failed to differentiate between individuals with normal and those with abnormal patterns of articulation. Ringel, Burk, and Scott offer the following explanation for these inconsistencies:

The conclusions reached in those studies and their implications in understanding the role of speech control systems must be viewed cautiously. The informants in such studies were usually allowed to use their visual systems in the process of matching the stimulus objects. As Weinberg (1968) noted, experiments have not measured oral sensory capacity by itself but rather some aspect of intersensory matching. The potential problems involved in tasks of intersensory matching would seem to place severe restrictions upon the information such oral form perception testing procedures might yield. For example, a patient who is 'visually deficient' but 'tactually normal' would exhibit poor oral sensory abilities if visual functioning were allowed to remain an integral part of the tactile matching task. This criticism becomes more pronounced if a traditional view of the speech servosystem is accepted. In such systems, visual interaction with oral system tactile monitoring is not implied. It appears therefore that a test which attempts to provide information about

the tactile modality must be limited primarily to that modality and not lend itself to sources of contamination by involving other sensory channels such as vision.[10]

Ringel and his associates[11] developed a test procedure which eliminated the intersensory nature of the form matching tasks employed by previous investigators. This procedure involves the use of relatively few stimuli and requires a simple discrimination type of response from the subject. The discrimination ability of an individual is measured by his ability to tell the difference or sameness between two forms presented orally instead of matching an oral presentation with a visual duplicate. They found that their oral form discrimination procedure is capable of detecting deficiencies in oral sensory receptiveness which correlates well with defective articulation. Thus, they consider their procedure a more valid indicator of an individual's orosensory functioning than tests involving inter-sensory matching tasks.

The purpose of the present investigation was to compare the technique developed by Ringel, Burk, and Scott[12] with a procedure involving inter-sensory matching (Shelton, Arndt, and Hetherington[13]) in an attempt to determine if individuals exhibit differences in their performance between the two procedures.

METHOD

Three sessions were required of each subject: one screening and two experimental sessions. The screening session involved procedures for the selection of subjects. The two experimental sessions were used for administration of the two tests of oral tactile perception. A mini-

9 F. Forster, *Synopsis of Neurology* (St. Louis: Mosby, 1962).

10 R. L. Ringel, K. W. Burk, and C. M. Scott, "Tactile Perception: Form Discrimination in the Mouth," *British Journal of Disorders of Communication*, III (1968), 150-155.
11 *Ibid.*
12 *Ibid.*
13 Shelton, Arndt, and Hetherington.

mum of 24 hours was required between all sessions.

Subjects

Thirty females, all students at West Virginia University, served as subjects. All had normal articulation, hearing, neurological status, superficial tactile sensation, oral cavity structure, and vision. They ranged in age from 20 to 33 years, with a mean age of 22 years.

Screening Session

The following tasks were included in the screening session: (1) a hearing screening evaluation; (2) the reading of a standard prose passage; (3) an oral peripheral examination; (4) two tests of superficial tactile sensation; (5) a visual matching task; and (6) a questionnaire on neurological history and status.

The hearing screening evaluation was performed on a Beltone model 12 D portable audiometer from 250 through 8000 Hz at 20 dB. Individuals who failed any of the tested frequencies were excluded from the study.

The prose passage employed was Van Riper's 'My Grandfather'" passage.[14] The articulatory characteristics of each subject were determined from the reading of this passage by two graduate students in Speech Pathology-Audiology at West Virginia University. Those with articulation defects were not included as subjects in the study.

The oral peripheral examination was used to assess the structural integrity of the oral cavity. Individuals with structural abnormalities of the oro-facial region were eliminated from the study.

The "Test of Light Touch" and "Test of Tactile Agnosia"[15] were employed to

exclude individuals with defects in superficial tactile sensation. In the former test, the subject was instructed to close her eyes and to report by saying "yes" when she felt a wisp of cotton on her skin. Random presentations of a cotton wisp were made to the right and left hands, forearms, and face. A cotton-tipped applicator was used to assess sensation on the tongue. Individuals who reported no sensation on any single stimulus presentation were excluded from the study. In the latter test, the subject closed her eyes and was asked to identify by touch several common objects (e.g., spoon, watch, key,) which were placed in her right and left hands. Individuals who failed to identify any of the objects were excluded from the study.

The visual matching task involved matching graphic representations of the stereognosis forms.[16] Two sets of shapes were provided; one set was numbered and the other was not. The subject's task was to match each un-numbered shape with its numbered counterpart. This task was employed to assess visual acuity and visual form perception, necessary abilities for successful performance of tests involving visual matching tasks. Individuals who made more than two errors were excluded as subjects from the study.

The questionnaire on neurological history and status was employed to eliminate individuals with central nervous system disturbances.

Experimental Sessions

Two experimental sessions, one for each of the two techniques being investigated, was required of each subject. Each session, which lasted approximately 30 minutes, was held in the Speech and Hearing Sciences Laboratory at West

14 C. Van Riper, *Speech Correction: Principles and Methods* (Englewood Cliffs, New Jersey: Prentice-Hall, 1963), p. 484.
15 Mayo Clinic and Mayo Foundation, *Clinical Examinations in Neurology* (Philadelphia: Saunders, 1963).

16 R. Canetta, "Lingual Stereognosis: A Normative Study in Adults" (Ph.D. diss., University of Washington, 1967).

Virginia University. The techniques were administered in random order to each subject.

Test stimuli. The stimuli in both procedures were 11 forms drawn from a standard 20-item set developed at the Oral and Pharyngeal Section of the National Institute of Dental Research. The forms were selected to insure the multiple occurrence of items having the same gross geometric descriptions. The 11 forms used are shown in Figure 1. They can be subdivided into four geometric shapes: biconcave (1 and 2), oval (3, 4, and 5), triangular (6, 7, and 8) and rectangular (9, 10, and 11). All forms had handles attached to them.

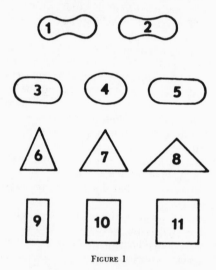

FIGURE 1

Inter-sensory matching task. In this procedure, a test booklet was placed before the subject and the following instructions were orally presented to her: "I have some small forms like these (show forms) and pictures like these (show pictures). The form will be put in your mouth for you to feel. You may move it around with the handle to help you feel it, but do not look at it. After feeling it with your tongue and mouth, circle the picture of the form which you think you have in your mouth. Take as much time as you like and guess if you are not sure. Are there any questions?"

The test booklet contained five pictures of similar shapes on each page. However, only one picture on each page represented the appropriate shape for each test form. The pictures used were obtained from the test of oral stereognosis developed by Shelton, Arndt, and Hetherington.[17] The order of presentation of the test forms was randomized for each subject. In addition, three of the 11 forms were repeated for subject reliability estimations. Thus, a total of 14 forms were presented to each subject.

Form discrimination task. In this procedure, the following instructions were presented orally to each subject: "I have some small forms like these (show forms) which I'm going to place in your mouth. I'll put one form in your mouth, take it out, and then put another form in your mouth. You may move the form around with the handle to help you feel it, but do not look at it. After feeling it with your tongue and mouth, I want you to tell me whether the two forms were the *same* or *different.* Take as much time as you like and guess if you are not sure. Are there any questions?"

A time interval of no more than five seconds was allowed between the presentation of the first and second forms of a given pair. The forms in each geometric shape subdivision were paired with each other (1-2; 3-4; 4-5; 3-5; 6-7; 7-8; 6-8; 9-10; 10-11; 9-11). In addition, one form in each of the four shape subdivisions was randomly selected and paired with itself (2-2; 3-3; 8-8; 11-11). Five pairs were randomly selected and repeated for subject reliability estimations. Thus, a total of 19 pairs were presented to each subject. The order of presentation of

17 Shelton, Arndt, and Hetherington.

286

pairs was randomized for each subject. In both experimental procedures, the forms were shielded from the subject's view by a piece of paper placed between the base of the subject's nose and her mouth. Moreover, she was never given information about the correctness of her responses during the experimental sessions. All test forms were sterilized. The sterilization procedure was performed on all forms prior to use with each subject.

RESULTS

Results of subjects' performances on the two tasks are presented in Table 1. The table indicates that subjects made a fewer percentage of errors on the visual matching task than they did on the form discrimination procedure. In fact, nine of the 30 subjects (30 per cent) made no

TABLE 1
NUMBER OF ERRORS MADE BY THE 30 SUBJECTS ON THE TWO PROCEDURES FOR ASSESSMENT OF ORAL TACTILE PERCEPTION

	Visual Matching Task	Form Discrimination Task
Number of Items	11	14
Total Errors	87	122
Mean	2.9	4.1
S.D.	1.2	1.8
Range	0-9	1-9
Percentage	26.4	29.3

errors in their performance of the visual matching task, while none of them received perfect scores on the form discrimination procedure. To determine if these differences were statistically significant, a chi square test was performed.[18] The obtained value, was significant beyond the .01 level.

Table 2 contains the number of errors made by the subjects for each of the four classes of geometric shapes. It shows that for both tasks, the largest number of errors made involved the triangular

[18] J. P. Guilford, *Fundamental Statistics in Psychology and Education* (New York: McGraw-Hill, 1965), pp. 227-251.

TABLE 2
NUMBER OF ERRORS OF THE 30 SUBJECTS FOR EACH OF THE FOUR CLASSES OF GEOMETRIC SHAPES REPRESENTED IN THE TWO TASKS

Shape	Visual Matching Task	Form Discrimination Task
Biconcave	17	33
Oval	15	27
Triangular	38	49
Rectangular	17	13

shapes (see Figure 1). A total of 44 per cent of the errors on the visual matching task and 40 per cent of the errors on the form discrimination task involved the three triangular shapes included in the tests.

In addition, subjects' performances appear to be more reliable on the visual matching task. Approximately 53 per cent of the subjects had perfect test-retest agreement on the visual matching task, while only seven per cent showed perfect agreement for the form discrimination procedure.

DISCUSSION

In view of the nature of the two tasks investigated, the findings in the present investigation are somewhat surprising. In terms of task difficulty, the form discrimination procedure appears to be an easier task for the subject to perform. Neither inter-sensory matching nor absolute identification of the objects is required. Rather, the task calls for a relatively simple discrimination type of response from the subject. The form discrimination test should yield higher scores than those obtained on the visual matching task. The probability of a subject giving the correct responses on the form discrimination test by chance alone is 0.5, while on the visual matching task the probability of such an occurrence is only 0.2. On the form discrimination test, there are only two possible choices available to the subject ("same" or "dif-

287

ferent"), while on the visual matching test there are five possible choices (any of the five pictures on each page of the test booklet). Yet, despite these facts, a larger percentage of errors was made by subjects on the form discrimination test.

A possible explanation for these findings pertains to the memory factor involved in the form discrimination procedure. Since there is a time lag of several seconds between the presentation of the first and second stimuli in each pair, the subject is required to rely on her memory for successful performance of the required task. Therefore, memory may be a confounding variable responsible for form discrimination procedure than on the visual matching task.

Another possible explanation was offered by the subjects in the study. Most of them thought that they were more successful in their performance of the visual matching task because they had had very little experience in the type of task required of them in the form discrimination test. Perhaps lack of experience and training in performing this type of discrimination task was responsible for the findings in the current investigation.

It should be noted here that the form discrimination task employed in this study is not identical to the procedure used by Ringel, Burk, and Scott.[19] A total of 11 different stimulus forms were employed in this investigation, while

Ringel and his associates used only 10 forms (all forms were identical with the exception of one additional triangular shape in our study). All of our forms had handles attached to them, while none of the forms used by Ringel and his associates had handles. Our task involved 14 pairs of forms (only within-class comparisons), while the procedure of Ringel and his associates involved 55 pairs (both between-class and within-class comparisons). The subjects in our study were allowed to keep the forms in their mouths for as long as they wished, while the subjects in the other study were allowed to retain the first form of a pair in their mouths for only five seconds. Ringel and his associates provided a pre-testing training session for each subject, while we provided no such training. Some of these differences may have accounted for the large discrepancy in percentage of errors made by the subjects in the present investigation (29 per cent) and those made by normal adult subjects in Ringel, Burk, and Scott's study (7 per cent).[20]

Because of the relatively large percentage of errors made by subjects on both tasks and the stringent requirements of normality met by all subjects, it is suggested that further investigation be made of tests of oral tactile perception and of variables pertinent to the performance of such tests.

[19] Ringel, Burk, and Scott.

[20] *Ibid.*

ASSESSMENT OF ORAL TACTILE PERCEPTION: SOME METHODOLOGICAL CONSIDERATIONS

Norman J. Lass, Richard R. Bell, Jeanne C. Simcoe,
Nancy J. McClung, and William E. Park

INTRODUCTION

The current increased interest in the role of the tactile feedback system in the speech production process, resulting from the findings of several investigations[1,2,3] has led to the development of a number of tests of oral tactile perception which exhibit a wide variety of procedural differences. (See footnotes 4-11.) However, the results of different studies employing these tests have been inconsistent and contradictory and have led to a serious questioning of the value of the current methods for assessment of oral tactile perception.[12]

The purpose of the present series of experiments was to investigate some methodological factors involved in assessing oral tactile skills to try to de-

1 R. L. McCroskey, "Relative Contribution of Auditory and Tactile Cues to Certain Aspects of Speech," *Southern Speech Journal*, XXIV (1958), 84-90.

2 R. L. McCroskey, N. W. Corley and G. Jackson, "Some Effects of Disrupted Tactile Cues Upon the Production of Consonants," *Southern Speech Journal*, XXV (1959), 55-60.

3 R. L. Ringel and M. D. Steer, "Some Effects of Tactile and Auditory Alterations on Speech Output," *Journal of Speech and Hearing Research*, VI (1963), 369-377.

4 E. T. McDonald and L. F. Aungst, "Studies in Oral Sensorimotor Function," in J. F. Bosma (ed.), *Symposium on Oral Sensation and Perception* (Springfield, Ill.: Charles C Thomas, 1967), pp. 202-220.

5 R. M. Mason, "Studies of Oral Perception Involving Subjects With Alterations in Anatomy and Physiology," in J. F. Bosma (ed.), *Symposium on Oral Sensation and Perception* (Springfield, Ill.: Charles C Thomas, 1967), pp. 294-301.

6 H. Moser, J. R. LaGourge and L. W. Class, "Studies of Oral Stereognosis in Normal, Blind, and Deaf Subjects," in J. F. Bosma (ed.), *Symposium on Oral Sensation and Perception* (Springfield, Ill.: Charles C Thomas, 1967), pp. 244-286.

7 R. L. Shelton, W. B. Arndt and J. J. Hetherington, "Testing Oral Stereognosis," in J. F.

Bosma (ed.), *Symposium on Oral Sensation and Perception* (Springfield, Ill.: Charles C Thomas, 1967), pp. 221-243.

8 R. L. Ringel, K. W. Burk, and C. M. Scott, "Tactile Perception: Form Discrimination in the Mouth," *British Journal of Disorders of Communication*, III (1968), 150-155.

9 W. B. Arndt, J. Gauer, R. L. Shelton, D. Crary, and L. Chisum, "Refinement of a Test of Oral Stereognosis," in J. F. Bosma (ed.), *Second Symposium on Oral Sensation and Perception* (Springfield, Ill.: Charles C Thomas, 1970), pp. 363-378.

10 E. T. McDonald and L. F. Aungst, "An Abbreviated Test of Oral Stereognosis," in J. F. Bosma (ed.), *Second Symposium on Oral Sensation and Perception* (Springfield, Ill.: Charles C Thomas, 1970), pp. 384-390.

11 H. M. Moser and R. E. Houck, "A Study of the Lingual Orientation of Normal and Articulatory Defective Speakers on a Test of Lingual Identification of Selected Arrangements of Haptic Forms," in J. F. Bosma (ed.), *Second Symposium on Oral Sensation and Perception* (Springfield, Ill.: Charles C Thomas, 1970), pp. 398-409.

12 E. T. McDonald and L. F. Aungst, "Apparent Independence of Oral Sensory Functions and Articulatory Proficiency," in J. F. Bosma (ed.), *Second Symposium on Oral Sensation and Perception* (Springfield, Ill.: Charles C. Thomas, 1970), pp. 391-397.

CENTRAL STATES SPEECH JOURNAL, 1972, vol. 23, 25-35.

termine those factors which are responsible for the inconsistent and conflicting findings. Four individual studies are presented, each representing the investigation of a single methodological factor. A different group of subjects was used in each of the four studies, with no subject participating in more than one study.

A test of oral form discrimination was used in each of the four experiments to investigate the methodological factors.[13] This test consists of 10 forms drawn from a standard 20-item set developed at the Oral and Pharyngeal Section of the National Institute of Dental Research, Bethesda, Maryland. The forms were selected to insure the multiple occurrence of items having the same gross geometric descriptions. The 10 forms are shown in Figure 1. They can be subdivided into four geometric

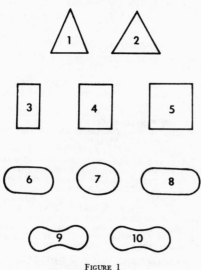

FIGURE 1

shapes: triangular (1, 2), rectangular (3, 4, 5), oval (6, 7, 8), and biconcave (9, 10). In this test, the subject's task was

[13] R. L. Ringel, K. W. Burk, and C. M. Scott, "Tactile Perception . . . "

to determine if two successively presented forms are the same or different. Each form was paired with every other form as well as with itself, for a total of 55 pairs. In addition, 10 pairs were randomly selected from the original 55 pairs and repeated for subject reliability estimations. Thus, a total of 65 pairs was presented to each subject. The order of presentation of the pairs, as well as the order of presentation of the forms in each pair, was randomized for each subject. No more than five seconds was allowed between the presentation of the first and second forms in each pair.

The following set of instructions was orally presented to each subject: "I have some small forms like these (show forms) which I'm going to place in your mouth. I'll put one form in your mouth, take it out, and then put another form in your mouth. You may move the form around, but do not make any attempt to look at it. After feeling it with your tongue and mouth, I want you to tell me whether the two forms were the *same* or *different*. Take as much time as you like and guess if you are not sure. Are there any questions?"

The subject was blindfolded throughout the entire experimental testing procedure. All forms were sterilized in an aqueous solution composed of one part of Zephiran Chloride to 750 parts of water prior to their use with each subject.

EXPERIMENT #1

Purpose

The purpose of this experiment was to determine if feedback information by the examiner concerning the correctness of the subject's responses significantly affected subject performance on a test of oral form discrimination.

Procedure

Three sessions were required of each

subject: one screening and two experimental sessions. The screening session included procedures for the selection of subjects. The two experimental sessions were used for administration of the two experimental conditions (feedback and no feedback) in the study. Subjects were not permitted to smoke, eat, or drink (except water) one-half hour prior to experimental testing.

Subjects. Thirty individuals, four males and 26 females, served as subjects. All were students at West Virginia University, and had normal articulation, hearing, neurological history and status, superficial tactile sensation, and oral cavity structure. They ranged in age from 18 to 23 years, and had a mean age of 20 years.

Screening session. The screening session consisted of: (1) a hearing screening evaluation; (2) the reading of a standard prose passage; (3) an oral peripheral examination; (4) two tests of superficial tactile sensation; and (5) a questionnaire on neurological history and status.

The hearing screening evaluation used a Beltone model 12D portable audiometer from 250 through 8000 Hz at 20 dB (re: ISO, 1964). Subjects who failed any of the tested frequencies were excluded from the study.

The prose passage employed was Van Riper's "My Grandfather" passage.[14] The articulation characteristics of each subject were determined from his reading of this passage. Those with articulation defects were excluded as subjects in the study.

The oral peripheral examination was used to assess the structural integrity of the oral cavity. Individuals with structural abnormalities of the orofacial region were eliminated from the study.

The "Test of Light Touch" and "Test of Tactile Agnosia"[15] were used to exclude individuals with defects in superficial tactile sensation. In the "Test of Light Touch" the subject closes his eyes and reports by saying "yes" when he feels a wisp of cotton on his skin. Random presentations of a cotton wisp are made to the right and left hands, forearms and face. A cotton-tipped applicator is used to assess sensation on the tongue. Individuals who felt no sensation on any single stimulus presentation were excluded from the study. In the "Test of Tactile Agnosia" the subject closes his eyes and identifies by touch several common objects (spoon, watch, key, fork, pencil, and cup) which are placed in his right and left hands. Those who failed to identify any of the objects were excluded.

A questionnaire on neurological history and status eliminated individuals with central nervous system disturbances.

Experimental sessions. Each of the two experimental sessions (one for each of the two experimental conditions of feedback and no feedback) lasted approximately 50 minutes and was held in the Speech and Hearing Sciences Laboratory at West Virginia University. The two conditions were administered in random order to each subject, so that 15 subjects received the feedback condition first and the no feedback condition second, while 15 subjects received the no feedback condition first and the feedback condition second. In the feedback condition, the subject was given information about the correctness of his responses for each of the 65 pairs presented to him. In the no feedback condition, no information was given concerning his responses. All forms had handles attached to them.

14 C. Van Riper, *Speech Correction: Principles and Methods* (Englewood Cliffs, N.J.: Prentice-Hall, 1963), p. 484.

15 Mayo Clinic and Mayo Foundation, *Clinical Examinations in Neurology* (Philadelphia: Saunders, 1963).

Results

Results of subjects' performance in the feedback and no feedback conditions appear in Table 1. The table indicates that subjects made a fewer number of

TABLE 1

NUMBER OF TOTAL, BETWEEN-CLASS, AND WITHIN-CLASS ERRORS MADE BY THE 30 SUBJECTS IN THE FEEDBACK AND NO FEEDBACK CONDITIONS

	Conditions	
	Feedback	No Feedback
Total Errors		
Mean	3.60	3.47
S. D.	1.92	2.01
Range	0-8	1-9
Percentage	6.55	6.30
Between-Class Errors		
Mean	0.57	0.57
S. D.	1.07	0.82
Range	0-4	0-4
Percentage	15.74	16.35
Within-Class Errors		
Mean	3.03	2.90
S. D.	1.57	1.49
Range	0-6	1-7
Percentage	84.26	83.65

errors when given no feedback information than when given information about the correctness of their responses. To determine if such differences were statistically significant, a chi square test was performed.[16] This test indicated no significant difference between the two experimental conditions (chi square = 0.08, df = 1).

Table 1 also contains the number of between-class and within-class errors made by the subjects in each of the two conditions. It shows that an identical number of between-class errors were made in both the feedback and no feedback conditions, with the feedback condition yielding a slightly larger number of within-class errors than the no feedback condition. In addition, the large majority of all errors were of the within-class type.

[16] J. P. Guilford, *Fundamental Statistics in Psychology and Education* (New York: McGraw-Hill, 1965), pp. 227-251.

Intra-subject reliability appears similar for both experimental conditions. Ninety per cent of the subjects showed 10 (perfect) or nine test-retest agreements in the feedback condition, while 93 per cent exhibited such test-retest agreements in the no feedback condition.

Discussion

The results of this experiment indicate that there are no significant differences in subject performance between the feedback and no feedback conditions. Twelve subjects (40 per cent) did better when feedback information was given about the correctness of their responses, 15 subjects (50 per cent) did better when no information was given to them, and three subjects (10 per cent) performed identically in both experimental conditions.

These findings are surprising; one would expect that giving a subject information about the correctness of his responses would improve his performance on the test. However, each form was paired with every other form as well as with itself only once (except for the 10 repeated pairs) in each experimental session. Therefore, the subject was never given another opportunity to respond to the exact pair on which he was given information. Nevertheless information about a given shape should help in recognition of that shape when it is paired with another form.

Another possible explanation pertains to the type of feedback information given to the subject. The subject was told simply whether his responses of "same" or "different" were correct or incorrect. He was never given information about the exact shape of the forms in his mouth. Perhaps such information is critical for improving performancce on the oral form discrimination test. Future research should explore this issue to determine the effect of more specific information about the shape and size of the forms on improving subject performance on the test.

EXPERIMENT #2

Purpose

The purpose of this experiment was to determine if a learning factor is operative in the assessment of oral form discrimination and, if the learning situation exists, to establish the nature of this learning factor.

Procedure

Each subject participated in five sessions: one screening and four experimental sessions. Subjects were not permitted to smoke, eat, or drink (except water) one-half hour prior to experimental testing.

Subjects. Subjects were 11 individuals, one male and 10 females. All were students at West Virginia University, and all had normal articulation, hearing, neurological history and status, superficial tactile sensation, and oral cavity structure. They ranged in age from 19 to 20 years, and had a mean age of 19.6 years.

Screening session. The tasks included in the screening session were identical to those described in experiment #1.

Experimental sessions. Each subject participated in four identical sessions, with one session occurring in each of four consecutive weeks. During each session, the examiner administered the test of oral form discrimination in the manner described earlier in the paper. The identical procedure was used in all four sessions. Each session, which lasted approximately 40 minutes, was held in a quiet room at the West Virginia University Medical Center. All forms had handles attached to them.

Results

Table 2 shows that more errors were made in the first experimental session than in the last session. However, the differences among sessions appear to be small. Results of a chi square test indicated that there were no significant differences in subject performance among the sessions (chi square = 1.72, df = 3).[17] Table 2 also contains the number of between-class and within-class errors made by the subjects in each of the four sessions. The majority of errors made were of the within-class type.

Intra-subject reliability improved steadily from session 1 to session 4. Seven

17 *Ibid.*

TABLE 2
NUMBER OF ERRORS MADE BY THE 11 SUBJECTS IN EACH OF THE FOUR TESTING SESSIONS

	Session 1	Session 2	Session 3	Session 4
Total Errors				
Mean	3.82	4.18	3.27	3.36
S. D.	1.78	1.42	1.55	1.43
Range	2-8	2-6	1-6	2-6
Percentage	6.94	7.77	5.95	6.11
Between-Class Errors				
Mean	0.45	0.09	0.09	0.18
S. D.	0.82	0.03	0.03	0.19
Range	0-2	0-1	0-1	0-2
Percentage	11.90	2.17	2.78	5.41
Within-Class Errors				
Mean	3.36	4.09	3.18	3.18
S. D.	1.96	1.32	1.34	1.33
Range	2-8	2-6	1-6	2-6
Percentage	88.10	97.83	97.22	94.59

293

of the 11 subjects showed 10 (perfect) or nine test-retest agreements in session 1, while eight showed such agreements in session 2, nine in session 3, and 10 in session 4.

Discussion

A trend is evident in the data of this study: subjects made fewer errors, and were more reliable in their performance in the last experimental session than in the first session. However, there is no clearcut progression from session 1 through session 4 and the differences in subject performance among all four sessions are not statistically significant. It would seem reasonable that no specific learning effect exists in oral form discrimination testing. It appears that the subjects' oral form discrimination skills do not improve with simply readministering the test. This finding provides useful information for future research on oral tactile skills. It allows for the readministration of the test of oral form discrimination without concern that improvement in subject performance resulted in part from previous exposure to the test. Therefore, improvement can be attributed to the variable under consideration, and not to a learning factor.

The findings also provide information on the consistency of subject performance. They indicate that subjects are consistent in their performance on the oral form discrimination test; they do not fluctuate sharply from one administration of the test to the next. We have further evidence of the reliability of the test of oral form discrimination, thus giving the experimenter more confidence in the results of subjects' performance on the test.

The above conclusions are based on four administrations of the oral form discrimination test; it is not possible to generalize to situations in which more than four administrations are provided.

In the present study, the tests were administered approximately one week apart. Therefore, it is not known if such conclusions would be reached if the tests were administered less frequently or more frequently than one week apart. For example, it is quite possible that administration of the tests one day apart would reveal a learning effect in the data. It is suggested that future research explore this issue further in an attempt to clarify the learning factor in oral form discrimination testing.

EXPERIMENT #3

Purpose

The purpose of this experiment was to determine if subject performance on a test of oral form discrimination is significantly affected by the handled-handleless condition of the sterognosis forms employed in the test.

Procedure

A total of three sessions, one screening and two experimental sessions, were required of each subject. Subjects were not permitted to smoke, eat, or drink (except water) one-half hour prior to experimental testing.

Subjects. Thirty persons, 15 males and 15 females, participated in the study. They ranged in age from 18 to 24 years, and had a mean age of 19 years. All subjects were students at West Virginia University and had normal articulation, hearing, neurological history and status, superficial tactile sensation, and oral cavity structure.

Screening session. The procedures included in the screening session in this study were the same as those described in experiment #1.

Experimental sessions. Two experimental sessions were used in this study, one for each of the two conditions (handled and handleless forms). The two conditions were administered in random order to each subject, with 15 subjects receiving the handled condition first and the handleless condition second, and 15 subjects receiving the handleless condition first and the handled condition second. In the handled condition, all 10 stereognosis forms had plastic handles attached to them. The subjects were allowed to use the handles to help them feel the forms in their mouth. In the handleless condition, no handles were available to the subjects, and manipulation of the forms was done entirely by the structures in the subjects' oral cavity. Each experimental session, which lasted approximately 45 minutes, was held in a quiet room at the West Virginia University Medical Center.

Results

Table 3 contains the results of subjects' performance in the two experimental conditions. It shows that the differences between the two conditions are very small. A chi square test[18] indicated

TABLE 3

Number of Total, Between-Class, and Within-Class Errors Made by the 30 Subjects in the Handled and Handleless Conditions

	Conditions	
---	Handles	No Handles
Total Errors		
Mean	4.43	4.10
S. D.	2.08	2.29
Range	1-8	1-10
Percentage	8.06	7.45
Between-Class Errors		
Mean	0.80	0.57
S. D.	1.19	1.48
Range	0-4	0-6
Percentage	18.05	13.82
Within-Class Errors		
Mean	3.63	3.53
S. D.	1.67	1.52
Range	1-8	1-9
Percentage	81.95	86.18

that these differences are not statistically significant (chi square = 0.42, df = 1).

18 *Ibid.*

Furthermore, the majority of errors were of the within-class type and the subjects exhibited a similar number of errors of both the within-class and between-class types for the handled and handleless conditions.

Intra-subject reliability was high and also very similar for both experimental conditions. A total of 19 of the 30 subjects in the experiment exhibited 10 (perfect) or nine test-retest agreements in both the handled and handleless conditions.

Discussion

The results of this study indicate that subject performance is not significantly affected by the handled-handleless condition of the stereognosis forms used in tht oral form discrimination test. Manipulation of the forms is not restricted by the handles, at least not enough to affect subject scores on the test. The handled-handleless condition of the forms does not appear to be an important factor in assessment of oral form discrimination abilities in subjects and should not be used to account for the differences in findings with different test procedures.

EXPERIMENT #4

Purpose

The purpose of this experiment was to determine if subject performance on a test of oral form discrimination is significantly affected by the location of placement of the stereognosis forms in the subject's oral cavity.

Procedure

Each subject participated in one screening and two experimental sessions. Subjects were not permitted to smoke, eat, or drink (except water) one-half hour prior to experimental testing.

Subjects. Subjects were 25 individuals, five males and 20 females. All were students at West Virginia University. The age range of the group was 18 to 22 years, and the mean age was 19 years. All subjects had normal articulation, hearing, neurological history and status, superficial tactile sensation, and oral cavity structure.

Screening session. The tasks included in the screening session were identical to those employed in experiment #1.

Experimental sessions. The two experimental conditions involved differences in the location of placement of the stereognosis forms in the subjects' oral cavity. In one condition, the forms were placed on the tongue tip of the subject, and in the other condition, they were placed on the subjects' tongue dorsum. "Tongue tip" was defined as that point which was 5.0 mm posterior to the leading margin of the tongue. "Tongue dorsum" was that point which was 25 mm posterior to the leading margin of the tongue. Testing at these two locations was done in the midline region, i.e., along the median sulcus of the tongue. To insure consistency of placement of the forms within as well as across all subjects, the two locations were marked with a dye (1 per cent Gentian Violet). The two conditions were administered in random order, so that 12 subjects received the tongue tip condition first and the tongue dorsum condition second, while 13 subjects received the tongue dorsum condition first and the tongue tip condition second. In both conditions, the examiner placed the stereognosis forms on the desired location and held the form in the subjects' mouth. Since an exact location was used for testing, the subjects were not allowed to move the form around in their mouth.

Results

Table 4 shows there are large differ-

TABLE 4

NUMBER OF TOTAL, BETWEEN-CLASS, AND WITHIN-CLASS ERRORS MADE BY THE 25 SUBJECTS IN THE TONGUE TIP AND TONGUE DORSUM CONDITIONS

	Conditions	
	Tongue Tip	Tongue Dorsum
Total Errors		
Mean	6.16	10.56
S. D.	3.70	4.92
Range	3-18	6-22
Percentage	11.20	19.20
Between-Class Errors		
Mean	2.64	6.12
S. D.	3.06	4.00
Range	0-14	0-15
Percentage	42.58	57.95
Within-Class Errors		
Mean	3.56	4.44
S. D.	1.15	1.73
Range	0-6	2-8
Percentage	57.42	42.05

ences in subject performance between the two experimental conditions. Subjects made much fewer errors when the forms were placed on the tongue tip than when they were placed on the tongue dorsum. Results of a chi square test[19] indicated that such differences between the two conditions were statistically significant (chi square = 34.13, df = 1).

The table also indicates that subjects made a larger number of both between-class and within-class errors when tested on the tongue dorsum than when tested on the tongue tip. More within-class errors were exhibited on the tongue tip than between-class errors; however, when tested on the tongue dorsum, subjects made more between-class errors.

Subjects appear to be more reliable when tested on the tongue tip than when tested on the tongue dorsum. Thirty-two per cent showed perfect test-retest agreements in the tongue tip condition, while only 16 per cent showed such agreements when tested on the tongue dorsum.

19 *Ibid.*

Discussion

The findings indicate that subjects' performance on the oral form discrimination test is affected by the location of placement of the stereognosis forms in the oral cavity. They made fewer errors when tested on the tongue tip than when tested on the tongue dorsum. This finding is in agreement with current knowledge on sensory innervation to the tongue.[20] It is also in agreement with previous findings on lingual two-point discrimination ability of normal individuals and general tactile sensitivity on the tongue.[21, 22, 23]

In comparing the results of the present study with those obtained in the previous three studies, it is evident that many more errors were made in the present experiment. One explanation for this finding is that only in this experiment were the subjects not permitted to manipulate freely the stereognosis forms in their mouths. The forms were held in the mouth by the examiner on the desired locations to prevent any variation in placement of the forms. This lack of freedom to explore the forms may have limited the amount of tactile information that could be obtained and thus resulted in more errors on the test.

In the case of the tongue dorsum, the number of subjects' between-class errors exceeded their within-class errors. This finding is unusual, since forms of grossly different geometric shape tend to be distinguished more easily than forms of the same geometric shape class.[24, 25] Perhaps the subjects' lack of freedom to manipulate the forms in their mouths may also be responsible for this surprising finding.

Conclusions

From the results of the four experiments described above, the following conclusions are offered:

(1) Feedback information to the subject concerning the correctness of his responses does not significantly affect his performance on a test of oral form discrimination.

(2) No specific learning effect appears to be operative in oral form discrimination testing; subject performance is consistent on the test from one administration to the next.

(3) Subject performance is not significantly affected by the handled-handleless condition of the stereognosis forms used in the test of oral form discrimination.

(4) The location of placement of the forms in the oral cavity is an important consideration and significantly affects subject performance on the test of oral form discrimination.

[20] R. C. Grossman and B. F. Hattis, "Oral Mucosal Sensory Innervation and Sensory Experience: A Review," in J. F. Bosma (ed.), *Symposium on Oral Sensation and Perception* (Springfield, Ill.: Charles C Thomas, 1967), pp. 5-62.

[21] R. C. Grossman, "Methods of Determining Oral Tactile Experience," in J. F. Bosma (ed.), *Symposium on Oral Sensation and Perception* (Springfield, Ill.: Charles C Thomas, 1967), pp. 161-181.

[22] N. J. Lass, C. L. Kotchek, and J. F. Deem, "Oral Two-Point Discrimination: Further Evidence of Asymmetry on Right and Left Sides of Selected Oral Structures," *Perceptual and Motor Skills*, XXXV (1972), 59-67.

[23] A. K. Pleasonton, "Sensitivity of the Tongue to Electrical Stimulation," *Journal of Speech and Hearing Research*, XIII (1970), 635-644.

[24] R. L. Ringel, K. W. Buck, and C. M. Scott, "Tactile Perception . . ."

[25] R. L. Ringel, A. S. House, K. W. Burk, J. P. Dolinsky, and C. M. Scott, "Some Relations Between Orosensory Discrimination and Articulatory Aspects of Speech Production," *Journal of Speech and Hearing Disorders*, XXXV (1970), 3-11.

The Effect of Memory on Subject Performance on a Test of Oral Form Discrimination

NORMAN J. LASS AND TERESA H. CLAY

THE CURRENT INTEREST in the role of the tactile feedback system in speech production has led to the development of various tests of oral stereognosis.[1] These tests usually involve the placement of objects of varying shapes in the oral cavity and the subject's visual identification of the shapes. However, the results of different studies employing these tests have been inconsistent and have led to a serious questioning of the value of standard methods of assessing oral stereognosis.

Ringel, Burk, and Scott offer the following as explanation for these inconsistencies:

> The informants in such studies were usually allowed to use their visual systems in the process of matching the stimulus objects ... The potential problems involved in tasks of intersensory matching would seem to place severe restrictions upon the information such oral form perception testing procedures might yield. For example, a patient who is "visually deficient" but "tactually normal" would exhibit poor oral sensory abilities if visual functioning were allowed to remain an integral part of the tactile matching task ... It appears therefore that a test which attempts to provide information about the tactile modality must be limited primarily to that modality and not lend itself to sources of contamination by involving other sensory channels such as vision.[2]

The authors wish to thank Sister George Marie Long and her staff at St. Francis Elementary School, Morgantown, West Virginia, for their cooperation in obtaining the children used as subjects in this study.

[1] Richard C. Grossman, "Methods for Evaluating Oral Surface Sensation," *Journal of Dental Research*, 43 (1964), 301; Eugene T. McDonald and Lester F. Aungst, "Studies in Oral Sensori-Motor Function," in *Symposium on Oral Sensation and Perception*, ed. J. F. Bosma (Springfield, Ill., 1967), pp. 202-20; Henry Moser, John R. LaGourge, and Lois W. Class, "Studies in Oral Stereognosis in Normal, Blind and Deaf Subjects," in Bosma, pp. 244-86; Ralph L. Shelton, William B. Arndt, Jr., and John J. Hetherington, "Testing Oral Stereognosis," in Bosma, pp. 221-43.

[2] Robert L. Ringel, Kenneth W. Burk, and Cheryl M. Scott, "Tactile Perception: Form Discrimination in the Mouth." *British Journal of Disorders of Communication*, 3 (1968), 150-51.

WESTERN SPEECH, 1973, vol. 37, no. 1, 27-33.

Therefore, Ringel and his associates developed a test procedure which eliminated the intersensory nature of the form matching tasks employed by previous investigators. This precedure involves the use of relatively few stimuli and requires a simple discrimination type of response from the subject. The discrimination ability of an individual is measured by his ability to tell the difference or sameness between two forms presented orally instead of matching an oral presentation with a visual duplicate. They found that this oral form discrimination task is capable of detecting deficiencies in oral sensory receptiveness which correlates well with defective articulation. Thus, they consider their procedure a more valid indicator of an individual's orosensory functioning than tests involving intersensory matching tasks.

However, in discussing this oral form discrimination task, Shelton asserts that although it removed the visual system from the subject's task, it "permitted a five second pause between stimuli. This should be eliminated to exclude memory as a confounding variable."[3]

In a recent study comparing the oral form discrimination task[4] with a visual matching task[5] for assessment of subjects' oral tactile functioning, Lass, Tekieli, and Eye found that 21 of their 30 subjects did better on the visual matching task than on the oral form discrimination procedure.[6] This finding was somewhat surprising in view of the nature of the two tasks investigated. In terms of both task difficulty and the laws of probability, the oral form discrimination procedure is an easier task and should yield higher scores than the visual matching procedure. One of the explanations for these findings offered by the authors pertained to memory:

> Since there is a time lag of several seconds between the presentation of the first and second stimuli in each pair [in the form discrimination procedure], the subject is required to rely on his memory for successful performance of the required task. Therefore, memory may be a confounding variable responsible for subjects' poorer performance on the form discrimination procedure than on the visual matching task.

The purpose of the present investigation was to determine if the memory factor has a significant effect on subject performance on the test of oral form discrimination.

METHOD

Three sessions were required of each subject, one screening and two

---

[3] Ralph L. Shelton, "Oral Sensory Function in Speech Production," Progress Report, National Institute of Dental Research, U.S. Public Health Service, Research Career Development Award #DE 31, 669-01, 1968.

[4] Ringel, Burk, and Scott.

[5] Shelton, Arndt, and Hetherington.

[6] Norman J. Lass, Mary E. Tekieli, and Marcia P. Eye, "A Comparative Study of Two Procedures for Assessment of Oral Tactile Perception," Central States Speech Journal, 22 (1971), 21-26.

experimental sessions. The screening session involved procedures for the selection of subjects. The two experimental sessions were used for administration of two experimental conditions, one at each of the two sessions. A minimum of twenty-four hours was required between all experimental sessions.

Subjects. The 30 adult subjects, 3 males and 27 females, were all students in the Speech Pathology-Audiology program at West Virginia University. They ranged in age from 19 to 22 years, with a mean age of 20 years. Of the 26 children in the study, 17 were females and 9 were males. All were students at St. Francis Elementary School, Morgantown, West Virginia. The age range for the children was 8 to 9 years, with a mean age of 8.4 years. All subjects had normal articulation, hearing, neurological status, superficial tactile sensation, and oral cavity structure.

Screening Session. The following tasks were included in the screening session: (1) a hearing screening evaluation; (2) evaluation of the articulatory characteristics of the subject; (3) an oral peripheral examination; (4) two tests of superficial tactile sensation; and (5) a questionnaire on neurological history and status.

The hearing screening evaluation was performed on a Beltone model 12 D portable audiometer bilaterally from 500 through 8000 Hz at 20 dB (re: ISO, 1964). Individuals who failed any of the tested frequencies were excluded from the study.

Assessment of the articulatory characteristics of subjects differed for children and adults. The adults read a standard prose passage, "My Grandfather."[7] The articulation of the children was assessed by means of the Arizona Articulation Proficiency Scale.[8] Those with articulation defects were not included as subjects in the study.

The oral peripheral examination was used to assess the structural integrity of the oral cavity. Individuals with structural abnormalities of the orofacial region were eliminated from the study.

The "Test of Light Touch" and "Test of Tactile Agnosia"[9] were employed to exclude individuals with defects in superficial tactile sensation.

The questionnaire on neurological history and status was designed to eliminate individuals with central nervous system disturbances.

Experimental Sessions. Two experimental sessions, one for each of the two conditions being investigated, were required of each subject. The two sessions, each of which lasted approximately 30 minutes, were held in the Speech and Hearing Sciences Laboratory at West Virginia University for

---

[7] Charles Van Riper, *Speech Correction: Principles and Methods*, 4th ed. (Englewood Cliffs, N. J., 1963), p. 484.
[8] J. Barker, *Arizona Articulation Proficiency Scale* (Beverly Hills, Calif., 1963).
[9] Mayo Clinic and Mayo Foundation, *Clinical Examinations in Neurology* (Philadelphia, 1963).

the adult subjects, and in a quiet room at St. Francis Elementary School for the children in the study. The conditions were administered in random order to each subject.

The stimuli in both experimental conditions were 11 forms drawn from a standard 20-item set developed at the Oral and Pharyngeal Section of the National Institute of Dental Research, Bethesda, Maryland (see Figure 1). The forms, selected to insure the multiple occurrence of items having the same gross geometric descriptions, can be subdivided into four geometric shapes: biconcave (1,2), oval (3,4,5), triangular (6,7,8), and rectangular (9,10,11). All forms had handles attached to them.

FIGURE 1

STEREOGNOSIS FORMS EMPLOYED IN ORAL FORM DISCRIMINATION TEST.

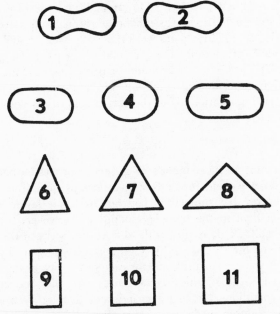

In the *no-delay* experimental condition, the following set of instructions was orally presented to each subject:

> I have some small forms like these [show forms] which I'm going to place in your mouth. I'll put two forms in your mouth at the same time. You may move them around with the handles to help you feel them, but do not make any attempt to look at them. After feeling them with your tongue and mouth, I want you to tell me whether the two forms are the *same* or *different*. Take as much time as you like and guess if you are not sure. Are there any questions?

In the *delay* condition, the following set of instructions was orally presented to each subject:

I have some small forms like these [show forms] which I'm going to place in your mouth. I'll put one form in your mouth, take it out, and then put another form in your mouth. You may move the form around with the handle to help you feel it, but do not make any attempt to look at it. After feeling it with your tongue and mouth, I want you to tell me whether the two forms are the *same* or *different*. Take as much time as you like and guess if you are not sure. Are there any questions?

A time interval of five seconds was allowed between the presentation of the first and second forms of a given pair in the delay condition. This time interval was determined by means of a stopwatch. However, the subject was allowed as much time as he wanted to explore each form.

In both the delay and no-delay experimental conditions, the forms in each geometric subdivision were paired with each other (1-2; 3-4; 4-5; 3-5; 6-7; 7-8; 6-8; 9-10; 10-11; 9-11). In addition, one form in each pair of the four shape subdivisions was randomly selected and paired with itself (2-2; 3-3; 8-8; 11-11). Five pairs were randomly selected and repeated for subject reliability estimations. Thus, a total of 19 pairs was presented to each subject. The order of presentation of pairs was randomized for each subject. In each experimental condition, the subject was blindfolded and was never given information about the correctness of his responses during the experimental sessions.

Results

Table I contains the mean number of correct responses for both conditions (delay and no-delay) and for both subject groups (children and adults). The table indicates that subjects in both groups made fewer errors in the delay condition than in the no-delay condition. However, the differences appear to be small. To determine if the differences between the two experimental conditions for the two subject groups were statistically significant, two sign tests[10] were performed, one for each of the two groups of subjects. These tests yielded no significant differences (p<.05) between the delay and no-delay conditions. Table I also indicates that for both experimental conditions, the children made more errors than did the adult group in the study. Results of two median tests[11] indicate that there is a significant difference between the performance of children and adults in the no-delay condition (p<.05) but no significant difference between them for the delay condition.

Table II contains the number of errors made by the subjects for each of the four classes of geometric shapes represented in the oral form discrimi-

---

[10] Sidney Siegel, *Nonparametric Statistics for the Behavioral Sciences* (New York, 1956), pp. 68-75, 111-16.
[11] *Ibid.*

TABLE I

NUMBER OF CORRECT RESPONSES OF THE CHILDREN AND ADULTS
IN THE DELAY AND NO-DELAY EXPERIMENTAL CONDITIONS.

	Children (N=26)		Adults (N=30)	
	No-delay	Delay	No-delay	Delay
Number of Correct Responses	222	234	293	302
Mean	8.54	9.00	9.77	10.07
S.D.	1.88	2.15	1.68	1.36
Range	5-13	4-12	6-12	7-14
Percentage	61.00	64.29	69.76	71.90

nation test. It shows that for both experimental conditions the largest number of errors made by both groups of subjects involved the triangular shapes (see Figure 1). For the group of children, a total of 34 per cent of the errors in the delay condition and 35 per cent in the no-delay condition involved the three triangular shapes included in the test. For the adult group, 36 per cent of the errors in the delay condition and 39 per cent in the no-delay condition involved these triangular shapes.

TABLE II

NUMBER OF ERRORS MADE BY THE TWO GROUPS OF SUBJECTS
FOR EACH OF THE FOUR CLASSES OF GEOMETRIC SHAPES IN THE STUDY.

	Children (N=26)		Adults (N=30)	
Shape	No-delay	Delay	No-delay	Delay
Biconcave	20	22	23	33
Oval	40	36	29	26
Triangular	50	48	50	46
Rectangular	32	24	25	13

Subject reliability appears to be higher for the adults in the no-delay condition but almost equal for both children and adult groups in the delay condition. Approximately 93 per cent of the subjects in the adult group had three or more test-retest agreements and 69 per cent had four or more test-retest agreements for the no-delay condition, while 86 per cent had three or more agreements and 55 per cent had four or more agreements for the delay condition. In the group of children, 65 per cent of the subjects had three or more test-retest agreements and 46 per cent had four or more agreements for the no-delay condition, while 88 per cent exhibited three or more agreements and 58 per cent had four or more agreements for the delay condition.

DISCUSSION

The findings of this investigation indicate that subjects did better in the delay than in the no-delay experimental conditions. One possible explanation for this finding pertains to the symmetry of oral cavity sensation and perception. When only one form is in the mouth at any one time, the form can be, and usually is, centered by the subject in the midline region of his tongue. When two forms are placed in the mouth simultaneously, however, it is impossible to center the forms in midline because of their size. As a result, one form usually lies on the tongue in a region lateral to the midline of the tongue, while the other form lies on the other lateral region. Since it has been shown that the midline regions of oral structures are more sensitive to tactile stimulation than the lateral borders of these structures,[12] the symmetry factor may partially explain why some subjects did poorer in the no-delay experimental condition.

The findings of this investigation indicate that the memory factor, as defined by a five-second delay between presentation of forms in a pair, did not have a significantly adverse effect on subject performance on the test of oral form discrimination. Therefore, memory cannot be validly considered as the factor responsible for the results of a previous study,[13] in which subjects performed better on a visual matching task than on a form discrimination test.

Future research in this area should pursue the issue of oral tactile memory in normal and articulatory defective individuals in an attempt to determine if delay times greater than five seconds will adversely affect subject performance on tests which assess tactile perception in the oral cavity.

---

[12] Robert L. Ringel and Stanley J. Ewanowski, "Oral Perception: 1. Two-Point Discrimination," *Journal of Speech and Hearing Research*, 8 (1965), 389-98; Gerald N. McCall, "The Assessment of Lingual Tactile Sensation and Perception," *Journal of Speech and Hearing Disorders*, 34 (1969), 151-56; Gerald N. McCall and Nancy R. Morgan, "Two-Point Discrimination: Two-Point Limens on the Tip and Lateral Margins of the Tongue," unpublished manuscript, Louisiana State University Medical Center, 1969.

[13] Lass, Tekieli, and Eye.

THE ASSESSMENT OF LINGUAL TACTILE
SENSATION AND PERCEPTION

Gerald N. McCall

Dental specialists and speech pathologists are becoming increasingly aware
of possible relationships between somesthetic sensory deprivation and abnormal oral motor behavior. In attempting
to understand these rᵉlationships, we
should be interested in the oral-facial
sensory system in general and in the
manner in which it provides an individual with the types of integrated information needed for learning movements
used in speaking, chewing, and swallowing.

The perception of motion of the
articulators probably is a synthesis of
different sensations, principally kinesthesis and touch. Researchers such as
Boyd (1940-41), Cooper (1953), and
Law (1954) have called attention to the
probable role of oral touch receptors in
subserving a proprioceptive function.
As Boyd theorized, it is possible that
the superficial sensations from the oral
area have come to play a particular role
in proprioceptive functioning, acting
vicariously for specilized muscular pro-
prioceptors.

Based on current knowledge of oral
physiology, we can postulate at least
four tactile sensory skills that appear to
have a priori relevance to the acts of
speaking, chewing, and swallowing: (1)
detection of the presence of tactile
stimuli and appreciation of minimal
changes in tactile stimulation; (2)
spatial discrimination and localization
of tactile stimuli; (3) temporal discrimination of tactile stimuli; and (4)
appreciation of simultaneous bilateral
tactile stimuli. A number of these

JOURNAL OF SPEECH AND HEARING DISORDERS, 1969, vol. 34, no. 2, 151-156.

sensory skills appear to be readily available for some degree of independent assessment through tests of tactile sensitivity, tactile acuity, two-point discrimination, tactile localization, and tactile extinction. Although adaptable for the assessment of sensation in the various parts of the oral-facial sensory system, I have employed the tests principally for the measurement of lingual sensation and perception.

METHODS FOR THE ASSESSMENT OF LINGUAL SENSATION AND PERCEPTION

Force variations associated with the presentation of stimuli during the assessment of lingual sensation and perception appear to require only gross control. The examiner should attempt to stimulate the tissues of the tongue in as consistent a manner as possible. McCall and Langhart (1966) have demonstrated that considerable variation in force can be tolerated without affecting the measurement of tactile sensation and perception on the tongue. Excessive drying of the lingual surface associated with prolonged tongue protrusion should be minimized by allowing a subject to draw his tongue into the mouth frequently. Ashby (1966) has shown that drying of the lingual surface affects measurement during the assessment of a number of tactile sensory skills.

TEST OF TACTILE SENSITIVITY. Tactile sensitivity refers to the detection of the presence of a tactile stimulus. Neurologists traditionally have assessed tactile sensitivity by noting a patient's ability to detect stimulation induced with a wisp of cotton. Although a wisp of cotton is gross, I have employed cotton as the instrument for assessing tactile sensitivity on the tongue. I employ a schedule of randomized stimulus presentations so that 10 stimuli are presented to a subject on each of three tongue areas: the tongue tip at midline and the lateral extremity of the tongue margin on each side of the body parallel to a point approximately 0.75 inch posterior to the tip along midline. A nontoxic coloring agent is used to insure reasonably exact points of stimulation. The subject's task is to indicate when he is aware of being touched. His performance on the test is scored by computing the percent of stimuli perceived on each of the three areas of the tongue.

My associates and I have used the Test of Tactile Sensitivity successfully with children as young as four years of age, junior high school students (Knight, 1966), and adults (Ashby, 1966; McCall and Langhart, 1966). The tongue is sufficiently sensitive to permit the normal subject to perceive 100% of stimuli produced with a wisp of cotton on the tip and lateral margins.

A second procedure traditionally used by neurologists is employed to detect unilateral tactile sensitivity impairment. A subject is stimulated alternately and repeatedly on the left and right margins of the tongue with a wisp of cotton and with an applicator stick. He is asked to make a judgment of the quality of sensations from the two sides of the tongue, i.e., do stimuli on the two sides of the tongue feel the same or different? A report of inequality of sen-

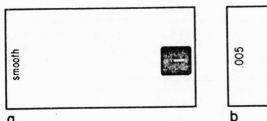

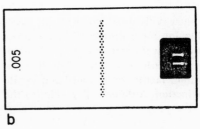

Figure 1. Examples of material employed in the Test of Tactile Acuity: (a) schematic drawing of ungrooved plate; (b) schematic drawing of plate with groove depth of 5 mils.

sations from the two sides of the body is interpreted as evidence of asymmetry in the tactile sensory system and suggests unilateral sensitivity impairment.

TEST OF TACTILE ACUITY. Tactile acuity denotes the ability to appreciate minimal changes in tactile stimulation. I use as a measure of tactile acuity a person's ability to detect a groove engraved on the otherwise smooth surface of a plastic plate. Eleven plates, each 1.5″ × 3″, are employed. All but one of the plates contain an engraved groove of uniform width and length but varied in depth. The grooves are approximately 1 in. long and 0.04 in. wide; the depth of the grooves ranges from 0.5 mil to 5 mils, in 10 steps of 0.5 mil each (Figure 1). The plates are passed in a vertical direction over the tongue tip and the subject reports his perception of the plate as smooth or grooved. Employing the method of minimal change, threshold is measured by averaging the groove depth required for perception on five ascending and five descending trials.

Data reported by Olroyd (1965), Ashby (1966), Knight (1966), and McCall and Langhart (1966) on nine- and eleven-year-old children, junior high school students, and adults demonstrate that the average groove depth required for perception by normal subjects on the Test of Tactile Acuity should be no more than 1.5 mils.

TEST OF TWO-POINT DISCRIMINATION. Two-point discrimination is measured using the modified caliper shown in Figure 2. Again, the method of minimal change is employed, threshold being measured by averaging the distance between two points required for two-point perception on each of five ascending and five descending runs. Increments of 0.025 in. are used for each run. Thresholds are established at points approximately 0.1 in. from the tongue tip at midline and approximately 0.1 in. from the lateral extremity of the tongue margins parallel to a point approximately 0.75 in. posterior to the tip along midline. The test areas are marked with a nontoxic coloring agent to facilitate intra- and intersubject threshold comparisons. Observations are made of the two point limens for each test area. Additionally, the degree of asymmetry in limen values for the tongue margins on each side of the body is noted.

When assessing two-point discrimination, the examiner should remember that the transition from one to two-point perception is not clear-cut (Jenkins, 1951; Ellender, 1968). Subjects

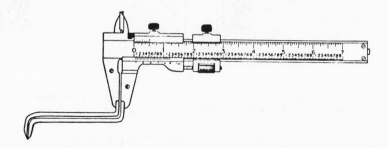

Figure 2. Schematic drawing of caliper adapted for sensory testing and employed in the Test of Two-Point Discrimination.

should be instructed to report "two points" only when they perceive two clearly distinct stimuli. They should be cautioned not to confuse a perceptual departure from singleness (i.e., line, circle, oval, or dumbbell) with clear duality.

Mean two-point limen values of 0.067 in. (1.7 mm),[1] 1.7 mm, 0.050 in. (1.3 mm), 0.047 in. (1.2 mm), and 0.038 in. (1.0 mm) have been reported for the tongue tip by McCall (1964), Ringel and Ewanowski (1965), Olroyd (1965), Ashby (1966), and Knight (1966), respectively. Olroyd (1965) and McCall and Morgan (1967) observed two-point limens on the lateral margins of the tongue to be significantly larger than limen values on the tongue tip. The latter investigators also noted evidence of asymmetry in two-point discriminatory capacity on the tongue margins of a high percentage of their "normal" subjects.

Present research evidence demonstrates that the normal two-point limen for the tongue tip is between 1 and 2

mm. Additional investigations are needed to establish norms for (1) other tongue areas and (2) differences in limen values that may be expected on the two sides of the tongue.

TEST OF TACTILE LOCALIZATION ABILITY. Tactile localization ability refers to the spatial localization of tactile stimuli. Tactile localization on the tongue is measured by stimulating each of six areas on the tongue 10 times in random order. In response to each stimulus the subject attempts to identify the area stimulated on a schematic drawing of the tongue (illustrated in Figure 3). The points of stimulation corresponding to those shown in Figure 3 are marked on the tongue with a nontoxic coloring agent as follows: (A) 0.1 in. from the tongue tip in midline; (B) 0.75 in. from the tongue tip in midline; (C-D) 0.1 in. from the lateral extremity of each tongue margin parallel to a point 0.75 in. posterior to the tip along midline; and (E-F) 0.1 in. from the lateral extremity of the tongue tip on each side of the body. A subject's performance is scored by noting the percent of stimuli localized correctly. Observations are also made of the direction and consistency of mislocalizations and

---

[1]Author's conversion from inches to millimeters.

the degree of asymmetry in localization ability indicated for the two sides of the tongue.

The Test of Tactile Localization Ability has been administered to more than 50 normal teenagers and young adults (Knight, 1966; McCall and Langhart, 1966). These subjects correctly localized 80% or more of the stimuli presented to the various tongue areas. The most common type of localization error involved a perceptual displacement anteriorly of stimuli presented posteriorly to the tongue.

TEST OF TACTILE EXTINCTION. Tactile extinction refers to an inability to appreciate simultaneous bilateral tactile stimuli. A subject is stimulated unilaterally on each of the tongue margins and simultaneously on both tongue margins at points approximately 0.1 in. from the lateral extremity of the tongue margins parallel to a point 0.75 in. posterior to the tip along midline. A randomized schedule is employed so that 10 stimuli are presented unilaterally to each tongue margin and 10 stimuli are presented bilaterally to both tongue margins. The subject's task is to indicate the side(s) of the tongue stimulated. His performance is evaluated by noting the percent of perceived simultaneous bilateral stimuli.

Data obtained by Knight (1966) and McCall and Langhart (1966) on teenagers and adults demonstrate that the normal subject should perceive 100% of simultaneous bilateral stimuli presented to the tongue.

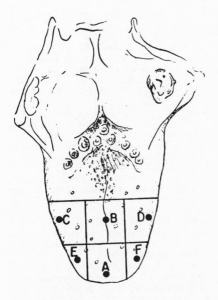

Figure 3. Schematic drawing of the tongue used by subjects to indicate perceived location of tactile stimuli on the Test of Tactile Localization Ability.

SUMMARY

Dental specialists and speech pathologists are becoming increasingly aware of the importance of studying the relationship between oral sensory functioning and motor behavior. In this article, a series of tactile sensory skills that appear to have a priori relevance to the acts of speaking, chewing, and swallowing are defined and test procedures appropriate for the assessment of a number of these sensory skills described, with guidelines to expected performance by normal persons on the tests.

ACKNOWLEDGMENT

The essentials of this paper were presented at the 1968 National Convention of the American Cleft Palate Association. The supportive and collaborating research by student investigators at the Louisiana State University Medical Center is gratefully acknowledged. David Rutherford, Northwestern University, designed the materials for the Test of Tactile Acuity.

REFERENCES

ASHBY, J. K., A study of the effects of drying of the lingual surfaces on certain measurements of lingual somesthetic sensibilities. Unpublished master's thesis, Louisiana State Univ. (1966).

BOYD, J. D., The sensory component of the hypoglossal nerve in the rabbit. *J. Anat.* (London), 75, 330-345 (1940-41).

COOPER, S., Muscle spindles in the intrinsic muscles of the human tongue. *J. Physiol.*, 122, 193-202 (1953).

ELLENDER, ELIZABETH Z., A methodological investigation of the transition from one to two-point perception. Unpublished master's thesis, Louisiana State Univ. (1968).

JENKINS, W., Somesthesis. In S. S. Stevens (Ed.), *Handbook of Experimental Psychology.* New York: Wiley (1951).

KNIGHT, D. P., JR., A study of the adequacy of certain methods for the assessment of lingual somesthetic sensibilities in a group of slow learners of junior high school age. Unpublished master's thesis, Louisiana State Univ. (1966).

LAW, MARY E., Lingual proprioception in the pig, dog and cat. *Nature*, 174, 1107-08 (1954).

MCCALL, G. N., Study of certain somesthetic sensibilities in a selected group of athetoid and spastic quadriplegic persons. Unpublished doctoral dissertation, Northwestern Univ. (1964).

MCCALL, G. N., and LANGHART, Marylen E., A study of the effect of variations in stimulus force on the measurement of lingual sensation and perception. Unpublished research, Louisiana State Univ. Medical Center (1966).

MCCALL, G. N., and MORGAN, NANCY R., Two-point discrimination: Two-point limens on the tip and lateral margins of the tongue. Unpublished research, Louisiana State Univ. Medical Center (1966).

OLROYD, MARIE H., Lingual somesthetic sensibilities of normal nine and eleven year old children. Unpublished master's thesis, Louisiana State Univ. (1965).

RINGEL, R. L., and EWANOWSKI, S. J., Oral perception: 1. Two-point discrimination. *J. Speech Hearing Res.*, 8, 389-398 (1965).

SOME RELATIONS BETWEEN OROSENSORY DISCRIMINATION AND ARTICULATORY ASPECTS OF SPEECH PRODUCTION

Robert L. Ringel

Arthur S. House

Kenneth W. Burk

John P. Dolinsky

Cheryl M. Scott

Man's ability to recognize the form of objects by means of his tactile sensory system provides the neurologist with diagnostic information that contributes to the overall assessment of sensori-motor functioning (Forster, 1962). Oral stereognosis, or the ability to recognize the form of objects placed in the mouth (presumably mediated by the oral tactile sensory system), therefore, can be a valuable tool to the speech pathologist in evaluating the functioning of the articulatory mechanism. The value of standard methods of assessing oral stereognosis has been open to question because of their failure to distinguish between persons with normal and persons with abnormal patterns of articulation, presumably because these methods depend on sensory systems other than those under test, and rely on absolute responses rather than on the subject's

JOURNAL OF SPEECH AND HEARING DISORDERS, 1970, vol. 35, no. 1, 3-11.

discrimination functions (Ringel, Burk, and Scott, 1968).

A further shortcoming of standard methods of testing oral stereognosis is their failure to distinguish between decisions made at different levels of discrimination activity, as exemplified by Ruch's (1951) discussion of the difference between the cone-vs.-pyramid (no edges vs. sharp edges) and pyramid-vs.-wedge (relation of geometrical planes) discrimination tasks. His example, and current theorizing about sensory processing—particularly the processing of speech and language—suggest strongly that useful tests of oral stereognosis should distinguish between failures to discriminate at different levels of sensory functioning. It is not enough to believe that the severity of an oral discrimination disability increases merely as the total error score increases; identification of the level of discrimination failure is crucial for understanding the sensory deficit in question and its potential effect on organized motor activities such as speech production.

Procedures for assessing oral stereognosis which attempt to incorporate this point of view have been described earlier, along with some preliminary results that differentiated between various degrees of articulatory proficiency—which prior tests of oral stereognosis failed to demonstrate (Ringel, Burk, and Scott, 1968). The subjects in the preliminary study were adults; the data they provided are highly reliable and have good face validity, at least when tested against the judgments of experienced speech pathologists.

The study reported here describes the application of the new test of oral form discrimination to children with a variety of articulatory abilities (and as such represents a portion of a standardization study in progress). In reporting these results, comparisons will be made to the earlier data provided by adult talkers.

METHOD

Stimuli

The 10 stimulus forms used in this investigation were drawn from a standard 20-item set used in many previous studies (Shelton, Arndt, and Hetherington, 1967). The items used are known to represent a wide range of absolute identifiability (Moser, La-Gourque, and Class, 1967) and were selected to insure the multiple occurrence of items characterized by the same gross geometric descriptions and differing essentially in some (undefined) size characteristic. Figure 1 shows the 10 selected forms used in this investigation.

Some items were triangular in shape (1, 2), some rectangular (3, 4, 5), some oval (6, 7, 8), and some were biconcave (9, 10).

Procedure

The task required a subject to decide whether two successively presented forms were the same or different. Each item in Figure 1 was paired with every other item in the figure and with itself, giving 55 pairs. To these pairs were added 10 additional pairs selected at random from the original 55 to serve as reliability check stimuli. The total

312

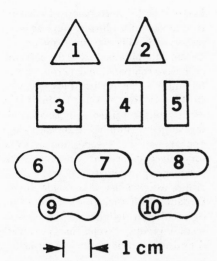

Figure 1. Forms used for the oral discrimination tasks. The material is a white, heat-resistant, inert plastic. The major dimensions of each item can be estimated from the scale in the figure; all thicknesses are approximately 3 mm.

experimental ensemble, therefore, consisted of 65 pairs of stimuli. The order of presentation was randomized for each subject, but the reliability check stimuli always were presented after the original test stimuli. The order in which the items of a given pair were "mouthed" was established a priori by chance.

Throughout the experimental session the subject was blindfolded and was not allowed to touch the stimulus materials with his hands. The experimenter put each item into the subject's mouth and allowed him to keep it there for five seconds. Once a form was in the subject's mouth he was encouraged to manipulate it there in any manner he desired. Upon removal of the first item of the pair, the second item was immediately placed in the subject's mouth; this maneuver usually required

about five seconds. Immediately after the second item was removed from his mouth, the subject indicated whether the two items of the pair were the same or different. During the pretesting training session the subjects were told that both same and different pairs of stimuli actually occurred in the test ensemble, but they were given no information about the proportion of occurrence of each class. An autoclave was used to sterilize each stimulus item before its use.

Subjects

Sixty children (30 boys and 30 girls) with so-called functional disorders of articulation constituted the experimental group of subjects. According to appropriate public school and/or clinic records these children had normal speech structures, sensory and motor capabilities and intellectual capacity, and were enrolled in grades one through five in local public schools. Their average age was eight years, one month. All were receiving speech therapy either in their schools or in the Purdue University Speech Clinic. The children were recruited so that three groups of 20 each, representing mild, moderate, and severe degrees of articulation problems, were formed. Assignment to a group was made by two or more experienced speech pathologists and was based upon such factors of articulation as the conspicuousness of errors, frequency of occurrence of misarticulated sounds in conversational speech, consistency of phoneme misproduction, and the number of misarticulated sounds. In general, subjects were judged to have a mild disorder of articulation if they produced one sound

313

incorrectly, a moderate disorder if they made two to four articulation errors, and a severe disorder if they consistently misarticulated more than four sounds. The mean ages in each of these groups was approximately the same as that of the total group, but no attempt was made to balance the number of boys and girls in the subgroups.

A control group of 60 elementary-school pupils was formed to parallel the experimental group in age and sex characteristics. According to public school records and the observations of two or more experienced speech pathologists, children in this group were free of speech defects, anomalies in oral structures, and history of sensory, motor, or intellectual impairments.

The data obtained from the 120 children were compared to data contributed by adults in an earlier study (Ringel, Burk, and Scott, 1968). In brief, the adult group consisted of normal-speaking subjects (number = 20, mean age approximately 22 years) and articulatory-defective persons (number = 27, mean age approximately 19 years). Subgroup assignments were made in accordance with the criteria used to assign children to the various experimental groups, except that no severe disorder group of adults was formed.

RESULTS AND DISCUSSION

The data of this study are the errors made on the task of oral form discrimination. The average performance of the various experimental groups is summarized in Table 1, along with the average performance of analogous adult subjects. In addition, the table contains an estimate of the response variability of the several groups. In general the tabulated data demonstrate that the subjects

TABLE 1. Average number of errors made on the 55-item test of oral form discrimination arranged according to subject's age and articulatory proficiency. The data for adults are taken from Ringel, Burk, and Scott (1968).

| | Children | | | Adults | | |
	N	Mn	SD	N	Mn	SD
Normal articulation	60	11.7	3.1	20	4.0	1.7
Mildly disordered articulation	20	12.4	4.2	12	5.4	1.7
Moderately disordered articulation	20	16.2	3.8	15	7.9	2.5
Severely disordered articulation.	20	20.1	7.4	—	—	—
Disordered articulation	60	16.6	6.5	27	6.8	2.5

with articulatory defects made more errors on the discrimination tasks than did the subjects with normal speech patterns, and that, furthermore, there was a clear tendency for errors to increase as a function of severity of articulation defect. The data also show, as might be expected, that children had more difficulty than adults with the discrimination task. In general, the magnitude of the variability data follows the trend established by the average scores.

To support the interpretation that discrimination errors increased as a function of the severity of the articulatory disorder, the differences between the various group averages in Table 1 were tested for significance. With two exceptions the differences were significant at the $p = 0.01$ level. The magnitude of the difference for one comparison that failed to reach this level (adults with normal speech vs. adults with mild articulatory defects) did exceed the 0.05 level of confidence, while the difference between the mean error scores of children with normal speech and children with mild articulation defects failed to reach even this level.

The number of times the subjects made the same decision when pairs were presented a second time (that is, the number of test-retest agreements) is a useful description of test reliability. The same decisions were made on 8 or more of the 10 reliability check items by 76% and 71% of the normal and articulatory defective children, respectively, and by 100% and 96% of the normal and articulatory defective adult subjects, respectively. This consistency of response supports the interpretation that the task was meaningful to the subjects and well within their performance capabilities. Furthermore, it is reasonable to conclude that the items generate a satisfactory level of response reliability, since consistency is varying only as a function of age. In other words, the children's responses were less reliable than those of the adults, but level of articulation proficiency did not appear to be a factor in test-retest performance.

The data presented thus far suggest strongly that a measurement of the ability to discriminate form in the mouth can differentiate between degrees of articulatory proficiency that have been established a priori by independent means. The assumption that tactile abilities in the mouth should function as a component of articulation is a general one, but has rarely been supported by experimental data. The agreement of the tabulated averages with this theoretical position is largely attributable to the experimental method, which minimized intersensory factors and utilized an actual discrimination task.

When a subject is exposed to a comparison pair, his task is to classify the general configuration of each item, to determine whether the items are in the same shape category, and to estimate the relative sizes of the two items. If two items are classified as having the same shape, the final judgment (same or different) reduces to a statement of relative size, but if the two shapes are judged to belong to different classes, the final judgment probably is a statement about their geometric shape. A judgment involving two items of similar shape and different size can be referred to as a within-class comparison, and a judgment involving items whose geometric shape differs categorically, as a between-class comparison.

In Table 2, the response errors have been arranged according to these classes, for the children and for the adults. The within-class errors—that is, errors involving the estimation of relative sizes of similarly shaped objects—failed to identify levels of speech proficiency. On the other hand, the tabulated data indicate that the performance of the various subject groups differs in number of between-class errors. When the error distribution of the normal talkers is used as the norm in a chi-square analysis, the difference in the proportion of between-class to within-class errors for both groups of articulatory defective subjects is significant. (All such comparisons exceeded the $p = 0.01$ level of confidence, except the comparison made for the children with mild articulation defects, which was significant at the $p = 0.05$ level.) It is interesting that the proportion of between-class errors for the children and the adults in-

creased monotonically as a function of severity of articulation defects. In summary, the ratio between within-class and between-class errors in the behavior of subjects with normal speech differed significantly from the between-class/within-class ratio obtained from subjects with disordered speech.

The within-class and between-class comparison tasks appear to be evaluating performance at different levels of discrimination activity. The between-class error scores are of particular interest to the speech pathologist since they appear to test discrimination processes whose integrity correlates positively with articulation proficiency. On the other hand, the within-class error scores do not distinguish between the experimental groups: the absolute values of these scores may be a function of the actual sizes of the items used in the test and, therefore, seem to reflect "acuity" measured at some level in the nervous

TABLE 2. Average number of between-class and within-class errors on the test of oral form discrimination arranged according to age and articulatory proficiency. Adult data derived from Ringel, Burk, and Scott (1968). The maximum averages are 37 and 18 for the between-class and within-class error categories, respectively.

| | Children | | Adults | |
	Between Class	Within Class	Between Class	Within Class
Normal articulation	1.7	10.0	0.2	3.8
Mildly disordered articulation	2.6	9.8	1.4	4.0
Moderately disordered articulation	5.0	11.2	2.4	5.5
Severely disordered articulation	8.6	11.5	–	–
Disordered articulation	5.2	11.1	2.0	4.9

system that is independent of speech function. These considerations suggest strongly, therefore, that a further refinement of testing methods for oral form discrimination should eliminate comparisons of the type we have called within-class.

This interpretation, of course, is limited by the fact that the test items used in the experiments do not allow for a precise division into within-class (size) and between-class (shape) categories. The triangles, for example, are not congruent, but vary between isosceles and equilateral types, while the rectangles include squares as well as parallelograms with equal angles and unequal sides. This failure to control "shape" rigorously makes it difficult to objectify the relative "size" of items, since the parameters underlying this judgment are not always easy to specify. Nevertheless, the analysis of data has assumed that only four gross shape categories—triangle, rectangle, oval, biconcave—were available to the subjects. In the further refinement of methods of testing the discrimination of form in the mouth this point should be clarified, of course, but the interpretation given here appears quite reasonable in the light of present data and theory.

The data reported here permit some further speculation about a hierarchy of form-discrimination ability across various levels of age and articulatory ability. That adults with defects of articulation performed with less errors than did children with normal articulation suggests strongly that age is a factor that facilitates performance in form discrimination (assuming merely that maturation correlates highly with chronological age). Maturational indices can be discussed as having at least

two major components—one related to physiological abilities as such, and another involving higher orders of organization of input to the organism. The adult may be more proficient in stimulus exploration than the child because of superior motor abilities that permit more appropriate manipulation of the stimulus forms. Similarly, the increased ratio of oral-cavity size to stimulus-form size in the adult as compared to that of the child may favor more adequate manipulation. McDonald and Aungst (1967), for example, have reported that the ability to identify forms in the oral cavity increases with age until the midteens and maintains a high level of accuracy during the middle years of life. They note that the leveling of the form-identification growth curve in the midteens parallels the completion of growth of oral and facial structures. Other factors which may favor the adult in discriminating form include his more developed motivational attitudes, and his attention and retention span. That is, the adult may have greater interest in participating, may attend more closely to the demands placed upon him, and may be more capable than the child of retaining sensory information for subsequent comparisons.

Retention, anatomical maturation, and motor development, factors that are said to be critical for the development of form discrimination abilities, are also said to underly the processes of speech. One can ask, therefore, whether sensory-discrimination abilities and speech development exist in a cause-effect relationship, or whether they both are related to more general factors such as neurological maturation and/or perceptual skill development. If the cause-effect hypothesis is accepted, oral sen-

317

sory disturbances can be considered as a new etiologic entity for defects of articulation, and ways of compensating for disturbed orosensory input channels should be sought. Such therapeutic approaches may take the form of prosthetic devices (Grossman and Bosma, 1963), drugs which either enhance or suppress the operation of an afferant channel (Ringel, 1968), and training aimed at developing the use of other input channels in lieu of the disturbed one (Chase, 1967).

The value of training speech-defective persons in oral-discrimination tasks must also be considered. If skills measured by the oral-form discrimination task do in fact underlie articulation, can articulatory proficiency be improved directly by training with appropriate orotactile discrimination tasks? If, on the other hand, sensory-discrimination abilities and speech development are merely related to more general factors, then a global approach to therapy seems indicated, such as that used with brain-injured or perceptually disturbed persons (Strauss and Kephart, 1955).

The ability to differentiate between normal-speaking and articulatory-defective persons on the basis of a task of sensory discrimination is of significance both from an applied and a theoretic point of view. Evidence supporting the view that normal articulation is reflected in orosensory functioning argues for the acceptance of a speech-production model that incorporate some servo-mechanical features, and for a variety of therapeutic practices that are compatible with such a model. Any theorizing about the processes of speech and language development and their maintenance must take into account the sensory mechanisms underlying articulatory activity.

ACKNOWLEDGMENT

This investigation was supported in part by Public Health Service Awards 1 KO3 DE 32614-03 and 1 RO1 DE 02815-01 from the National Institute of Dental Research, and by the Air Force Cambridge Research Laboratories under Contract AF 19 (628) -5051.

REFERENCES

CHASE, R. A., Abnormalities in motor control secondary to congenital sensory deficits. In J. F. Bosma (Ed.), *Symposium on Oral Sensation and Perception.* Springfield, Ill.: Thomas (1967), pp. 302-309.

FORSTER, F., *Synopsis of Neurology.* St. Louis: Mosby (1962).

GROSSMAN, R. C., and BOSMA, J. F., Experimental oral sensory prosthesis. *J. dent. Res.,* 42, 891 (1963).

MCDONALD, E. T., and AUNGST, L. F., Studies in oral sensorimotor function. In J. F. Bosma (Ed.) *Symposium on Oral Sensation and*

Perception. Springfield, Ill.: Thomas (1967), pp. 202-220.

MOSER, H., LAGOURQUE, J. R., and CLASS, LOIS W., Studies of oral stereognosis in normal, blind, and deaf subjects. In J. F. Bosma (Ed.), *Symposium on Oral Sensation and Perception*. Springfield, Ill.: Thomas (1967), pp. 244-286.

RINGEL, R. L., Tactile perception: Form discrimination in the mouth. Paper presented to the 44th Annual Convention of the American Speech and Hearing Association, Denver, Colorado (November 1968).

RINGEL, R. L., BURK, K. W., and SCOTT, CHERYL M., Tactile perception: Form discrimination in the mouth. *Brit. J. Disord. Commun.*, **3**, 150-155 (1968):

RUCH, T. C., Sensory mechanisms. In S. S. Stevens (Ed.), *Handbook of Experimental Psychology*. New York: Wiley (1951), pp. 121-153.

SHELTON, R. L., ARNDT, W. B., JR., and HETHERINGTON, J. J., Testing oral stereognosis. In J. F. Bosma (Ed.), *Symposium on Oral Sensation and Perception*. Springfield, Ill.: Thomas (1967), pp. 221-243.

STRAUSS, A. A., and KEPHART, N. C., *Psychopathology and Education of the Brain-Injured Child*, Vol. II. New York: Grune and Stratton (1955).

ARTICULATORY EFFECTIVENESS, STIMULABILITY, AND CHILDREN'S PERFORMANCES ON PERCEPTUAL AND MEMORY TASKS

RONALD K. SOMMERS

SHANNON COX

CYNTHIA WEST

The performances of 70 children, 35 from kindergarten and 35 from first grade, were studied on four auditory measures and one oral sensory discrimination task. Each group of 35 children included seven subjects with superior articulation, seven with deviant articulation and poor speech sound stimulability, seven with deviant articulation and good stimulability, seven with articulation defects and poor stimulability, and seven with articulation defects and good stimulability. Performances on a speech sound stimulability task were not found to be related to performances on any of the auditory measures and only slightly to the oral sensory task. Superior articulators had significantly better scores than the deviant and defectives on the oral sensory discrimination task, but scores on the auditory tasks were not significantly different. Comparison of the performances of /s/ and /r/ defectives revealed the latter group to be inferior on some auditory tasks compared with the superior articulators. Some relationships were found between subject performances on certain auditory tasks.

The ability of kindergarten and first and second grade children to correct misarticulations on a stimulability task has been linked to articulation change in a number of independent studies (Carter and Buck, 1958; Farquhar, 1961; Irwin, West, and Trombetta, 1966; Kisatsky, 1966; Sommers et al., 1961; Sommers et al., 1967; Stoia, 1961). The evidence is basically consistent to support this assertion, the only reported exception being a study of the effectiveness of articulation therapy for retarded children, in which stimulability performances were found not predictive of improvements (Sommers et al., 1970). The stimulability task can be described as the ability of the impaired subject to modify his defective phonemic productions toward normalcy as a function of simulation by the clinician. The present investigation attempted to identify factors which might relate to high and low achievement on stimu-

JOURNAL OF SPEECH AND HEARING RESEARCH, 1972, vol. 15, no. 3, 579-589.

lability tasks in children of the ages where such performances have been found to have clinical importance. Since some auditory perceptual and memory functions of articulatory defective children have been found to be inferior to normals (Mange, 1960; Sherman and Geith, 1967; Sommers, Meyer, and Furlong, 1969; Smith, 1967), we conjectured that children who are poor stimulators might be inferior to good stimulators on such tasks. In addition, we felt that the reported inferiority of articulatory defective children compared with normals on an oral sensory discrimination task (Ringel et al., 1970) might suggest that children having poor stimulability would be inferior in oral sensory discrimination to those having good stimulability scores.

A study of the performances of children having different degrees of articulatory proficiency (superior, deviant, or defective) on each of the four auditory and the oral sensory discrimination tasks also appeared important in view of the growing body of research suggesting that degree of articulatory effectiveness relates to performances on such tasks (Farquhar, 1961; Kronvall and Diehl, 1954; Sherman and Geith, 1967; Sommers, Meyer, and Furlong, 1967; Ringel et al., 1970). Ringel et al.'s (1970) study of oral sensory discrimination was repeated to determine whether the findings would obtain in younger subjects having less articulatory defectiveness.

METHOD

Subject Selection. From a sample of 122 kindergarten and first-grade children with misarticulations and a sample of 24 such children with superior articulation for their ages, 70 were selected as subjects. All subjects were drawn from schools in Haddonfield, New Jersey.

None of the subjects were receiving therapy or had received it in the past. All of the speech deviant and defective subjects were free of gross abnormalities of the oral/peripheral speech structure and had normal speed and accuracy of tongue movements (horizontally and vertically), reasonably normal dental occlusions, and normal velopharyngeal competency. All were free of hearing losses, based on a sweep-check audiometric test which examined 250, 500, 1000, 2000, and 4000 Hz at 25 dB (ISO) intensities. All subjects were considered by classroom teachers to be average or above average in academic performances and were drawn from three elementary schools located within a few miles of each other in neighborhoods having comparable socioeconomic levels. Two speech clinicians examined the 122 children having misarticulations on a revised version of McDonald's picture deep test of articulation and a modified version of the Carter-Buck Prognostic Speech Test (1958). Based on their performances on each of these tasks, 35 kindergarten and 35 first-grade subjects were selected according to the following scheme. Within each group of 35, seven subjects had superior articulation, seven had deviant articulation and poor stimulability scores (0-25%), seven had deviant articulation and good stimulability scores (36-100%), seven had articulation defects and poor stimulability scores, and seven had articulation defects and good stimulability. The complete design, therefore, consisted of 10 cells, each containing seven subjects.

Articulation Performances. Subjects termed superior articulated the following phonemes correctly in both three-word picture articulation tests and in spontaneous speech: /s/, /z/, /ʃ/, /tʃ/, /l/, /r/, /ɚ/, /ɝ/, /dʒ/, /θ/, /ð/, and /f/. Since misarticulation of these phonemes occurs frequently in the speech of five- and six-year-old children, their consistent and correct production was felt to denote superior performance. The articulatory deviant group was operationally defined as subjects having more than one but no more than two consistently misarticulated phonemic errors or no more than 60 phonetic contexts in error, as measured on a modified version of a picture deep test which measured each sound 15 times as a arrester and 15 times as an initiator of a syllable. A similar criterion was used to select those deemed to have articulation defects, except that such subjects were required to have three or four consistently misarticulated phonemes or the equivalent number of phonetic contexts in error as measured on the deep test. The means and standard deviations for the eight groups of articulatory deviant and mildly defective subjects, contained in Table 1, reflect their performances on both the deep test and stimulability task.

Dependent Variables. Four auditory perceptual tasks, two measuring short-term auditory memory, one thought to measure auditory synthesis of speech,

TABLE 1. Means and standard deviations of articulation and stimulability scores for eight experimental groups (Total $N = 56$ with seven per cell).

Group	Type	Articulation Errors Mean	SD	Stimulability Scores Mean	SD
A.	Kindergarten, deviant articulation, good stimulability	43.30	23.86	55.60	17.91
B.	Kindergarten, defective articulation, good stimulability	116.42	47.08	59.71	11.22
C.	Kindergarten, deviant articulation, poor stimulability	62.14	16.40	9.90	10.36
D.	Kindergarten, defective articulation, poor stimulability	138.14	36.31	10.90	7.01
E.	First grade, deviant articulation, good stimulability	36.00	15.31	70.71	24.71
F.	First grade, defective articulation, good stimulability	92.61	41.53	64.42	11.71
G.	First grade, deviant articulation, poor stimulability	55.30	17.21	13.43	9.94
H.	First grade, defective articulation, poor stimulability	98.92	27.72	16.00	6.15

and the other, speech sound discrimination, were administered to all 70 subjects. A fifth one, the oral sensory discrimination task devised by Ringel et al. (1970) was also given to all subjects. All of the auditory tests were given and scored according to directions provided in their respective manuals, and the oral sensory discrimination test was administered and scored exactly as Ringel and his associates described it.

All subjects were tested individually in reasonably quiet locations in schools. The testing order for each subject was the same. The Spencer Memory for Sentences Test (Spencer, 1958; McGrady, 1964) was administered first, followed by the Auditory Sequencing Sub-Scale from the ITPA (Kirk, Mc-Carthy, and Kirk, 1968). Both tasks appeared to assess to some extent short-term storage of auditory information, one meaningful speech (sentences), and the other less meaningful information (digits). The third auditory task was the Wepman Auditory Discrimination Test (1958), the fourth, the Auditory Closure Sub-Scale from the ITPA. The final dependent measurement, the oral sensory discrimination test, was then administered. Since repetition of Ringel et al.'s (1970) study was undertaken in the present investigation, the exact oral discrimination forms, testing procedures, scoring of responses, and reliability checks were performed. The only obvious difference was in the ages of the subjects, since subjects in the present study tended to be approximately two years younger, on the average, than those studied by Ringel and his colleagues.

Reliability. The mean percentage of agreement for the two examiners who completed the articulation testing was obtained by computing the number of correct responses each determined independently as the senior author examined seven subjects individually on the deep test. Each of the subjects was selected from a population of articulatory deviant or defective children not included in the study. Comparisons were based on a total of 660 phonetic contexts. The mean percentage of agreement between examiners was 91.6% for all phonemes studied and comparable to that reported in a number of investigations.

Reliability on the oral sensory discrimination test was determined and computed as Ringel et al. (1970) reported it. The procedure consisted of retesting 10 randomly selected pairs of forms for each subject and a comparison of the percentage of judgements in agreement. For all 70 subjects the mean percentage of agreement was 68.7%, the mean for 35 kindergarten subjects was 68.0, and the mean for the first-grade subjects was 69.4%. These reliability data are lower than those reported by Ringel et al. (1970) for older subjects. Apparently the task has a reasonable reliability index even at young age levels.

RESULTS

Articulatory Deviants and Defectives. A separate factorial analysis of variance was used to investigate the performances of the 28 subjects with articulatory deviant speech and the 28 with articulatory defects on each of

323

the five dependent variables. Each analysis examined the main effects of stimulability, articulation, and grade, and their interactions. The mean performances and standard deviations for the eight groups of subjects on each of the five dependent variables are presented in Table 2. First-grade subjects were superior to kindergarten subjects on the Wepman Auditory Discrimination Test ($F = 7.17$; $df = 1, 48$; $p < 0.01$). The means and standard deviations were 34.77 and 3.57, and 32.35 and 3.83 for first-grade and kindergarten subjects, respectively. First-grade subjects also were superior to kindergarten subjects on the Auditory Closure Sub-Scale of the ITPA ($F = 14.23$; $df = 1, 48$; $p < 0.001$). The means and standard deviations for first-grade and kindergarten subjects were 20.11 and 3.30, 17.42 and 3.18, respectively.

Superior and Inferior Groups: Auditory Measures. The mean performances of 14 superior speakers (seven kindergarten and seven first-grade subjects) were compared with the 28 articulatory deviant and 28 defective subjects on each of the four auditory measures. Comparisons were also made between the performances of the articulatory deviants and defectives. The first level of analysis consisted of independent t tests between groups using all subjects without regard to the types of phonemic errors made by ones from the articulatory inferior groups. A second analysis of mean differences was made by dichotomizing subjects so that 38 having a majority of their errors on /s/ and /z/, and 22 having the majority of their errors on /ɜ˞/, /ɝ/, and /r/ were compared with the superior speakers. None of the subjects having predominantly /s/ and /z/ errors were defective in /r/, /ɜ˞/, or /ɝ/, and the converse was also true.

For the first auditory measure, memory for sentences, none of the means of the articulatory deviant, defective, and superior articulators were significantly different. Also, mean differences between the /s/ and /z/ subjects were not significantly different (mean and standard deviations of the former group were 8.23 and 3.12, respectively, and 8.44 and 2.35 for the latter group). The results of the analyses of the means for the speech sound discrimination task indicated that the means for the deviant and defective groups were not significantly different, nor was there a significant difference between each of these means and that of the superior articulators. The mean of 22 subjects having errors on /r/, /ɜ˞/, or /ɝ/ was not significantly different from that of the superior articulators (mean and standard deviation for the former were 32.34 and 3.59, and for the superior group were 34.93 and 4.56). The mean score for 37 subjects defective in /s/ and /z/ was not significantly different from the superior articulators (mean and standard deviation of the former were 33.22 and 3.07, respectively).

None of the mean differences between the articulatory deviant, defective, and superior subjects were significant for the third articulatory measure, auditory sequencing. Neither were the differences between the mean scores of /r/, /ɜ˞/, or /ɝ/ and the superior articulators, and the /s/ and /z/ subjects and this group significantly different. Also differences between the mean scores on the auditory closure task were not significant between each of the

TABLE 2. Means and standard deviations based on the number of correct responses achieved by eight groups of subjects having inferior articulation on the five dependent variables ($N = 7$ per cell).

Group	Memory for Sentences		Speech Sound Discrimination		Auditory Sequencing		Auditory Closure		Oral Sensory Discrimination	
	Mean	SD	Mean	SD	Mean	SD	Mean	SD	Mean	SD
A. Kindergarten, deviant articulation, good stimulability	8.14	3.84	30.66	3.83	23.58	7.70	17.14	4.67	39.85	6.41
B. Kindergarten, defective articulation, good stimulability	8.13	1.30	32.12	4.48	28.58	6.67	16.42	2.44	38.85	5.27
C. Kindergarten, deviant articulation, good stimulability	8.28	2.19	33.00	3.40	29.28	9.01	17.28	3.30	37.85	7.40
D. Kindergarten, deviant articulation, poor stimulability	8.71	2.06	31.33	2.80	30.42	11.81	18.85	3.13	38.42	5.09
E. First grade, deviant articulation, poor stimulability	7.86	2.18	33.00	3.60	26.14	8.70	16.57	5.20	37.00	7.50
F. First grade, defective articulation, good stimulability	8.85	1.33	35.00	3.41	34.42	11.14	20.84	2.20	44.85	5.09
G. First grade, deviant articulation, poor stimulability	7.86	1.60	35.42	3.69	31.71	11.23	20.85	3.13	42.25	3.15
H. First grade, defective articulation, poor stimulability	8.86	1.35	35.00	2.79	27.71	6.77	22.14	2.27	37.71	7.44

three groups. A significant difference, however, was obtained when the performances of 22 subjects with errors on /r/, /ʒ/, or /ɝ/ were compared with the superior group ($t = 2.61$; $df = 34$; $p < 0.02$). The mean and standard deviation for the former were 18.09 and 3.35, respectively, and for the superior group, 21.36 and 3.86. No significant difference was found between the subjects who erred on /s/ and /z/ and the superior articulators.

Oral Sensory Discrimination. Table 3 contains the results of a series of

TABLE 3. Means and standard deviations for three groups of subjects on the oral form discrimination task.

Group	N	Mean	SD
Superior articulators	14	43.57	1.50
Articulatory deviant	28	39.25	1.61
Superior articulators	14	43.57	1.50
Articulatory defectives	28	40.10	1.14
Superior articulators	14	43.57	1.50
All /s/ defectives	38	38.84	0.98
Superior articulators	14	43.57	1.50
All /r/ defectives	22	39.54	1.21

t tests comparing the mean performances of subjects having different degrees of articulatory effectiveness and types of phonemic errors. The superior articulators were consistently better than the articulatory deviants and defectives on the task whether the phonemic errors were chiefly /s/ or /r/.

Types of Oral Sensory Discrimination Errors. According to Ringel et al. (1970), judgments involving two items of similar shape and different size can be referred to as within-class comparisons, while judgments involving items whose geometric shapes differ categorically are between-class comparisons. The between-class and within-class errors of subjects from each of the three articulatory groups were compared. The present results are compared with those of Ringel et al. (1970) in Table 4. With the exception of the superior articulators, all of the between-class mean errors are significantly greater than the within-class mean errors for the present results. This result is exactly the opposite of that determined by Ringel and his associates. In addition, for both the articulatory deviant and defective children, the between-class variance was significantly greater than the within-class variance ($F = 4.83$; $df = 1$, 26; $F = 7.16$; $df = 1$, 26, respectively). For the superior articulators, this variance ratio failed to reach significance.

DISCUSSION

The data failed to support the belief that some auditory perceptual and memory tasks would discriminate between groups of children having differ-

TABLE 4. A comparison of the average number of between-class and within-class errors on the test of oral-form discrimination arranged according to articulatory proficiency comparing the findings of Ringel et al. (1970) with those of the present investigation.

Category	Between Class Mean	SD	Within Class Mean	SD
Data from Ringel et al.				
Normal articulation	1.7	–	10.0	–
Mildly disordered articulation	2.6	–	9.8	–
Moderately disordered articulation	5.0	–	11.2	–
Data from our investigation				
Superior articulation	5.57	4.24	5.78	2.46
Articulatory deviant	9.18	5.74	6.32	2.61
Articulatory defective	8.82	5.48	6.53	2.05

ent degrees of speech sound stimulability. Although oral sensory discrimination scores were slightly related to the stimulability scores of the 56 subjects having inferior articulation, no significant differences were found between subjects having poor stimulability scores compared with those having good stimulability ones on the oral sensory discrimination task. In view of research evidence which tends to support the assertion that children having severe articulation disorders tend to be inferior on some auditory factors, it is possible that subjects in the present study were not defective enough to perform inferiorly. It is conceivable also that the present findings might not obtain if subjects eight years of age or older were studied.

The performances of 22 subjects predominantly defective in articulating /r/, /ɚ/, or /ɝ/ are of interest since a number of studies of auditory skills of /r/ defectives (McDonald and Aungst, 1967; Aungst and Frick, 1964; Mange, 1960) and two studies of their oral stereoagnostic skills found significant differences between their performances and those of normal-speaking children (Weinberg, Liss, and Holls, 1970; Aungst, 1965). Except for one study by Sommers, Meyer, and Fenton (1961), in which both /s/ and /r/ defectives were found significantly inferior to normals on a pitch discrimination task, comparable evidence to support the assertion that /s/ and /z/ defectives are less likely to perform poorly on auditory tasks does not appear to exist.

One suggestion from the results of the present study is that five- and six-year-old children having misarticulations of /r/, /ɚ/, or /ɝ/ may be inferior in speech sound discrimination and their abilities to recognize words with phonemes or syllables missing from them. Since both of these auditory tasks are linguistic, that is, both the discriminaton and the auditory closure tasks use words as stimulus material, it is also conceivable that the underlying inferiority tends to be a more general one involving language and special aspects of its processing. However, research to support the contention that /r/, /ɚ/, or /ɝ/ children tend to be inferior in other language skills does not appear to exist.

The moderate correlation (0.440) found between the scores of all 70 subjects on the speech sound discrimination and the auditory closure tasks tends to suggest that some underlying commonality exists. Perhaps more expected was the moderate relationship determined between the short-term memory tasks of auditory sequencing and memory for sentences.

Some findings from the present study tend to support those reported by Ringel et al. (1970). In the present study both the groups of subjects we termed articulatory deviant and articulatory defective were inferior on the oral sensory task to the superior articulators. In the Ringel et al. study, only their most severe group of subjects was inferior to normal articulating subjects on the same task. One explanation for these differences may rely on the developmental delay hypothesis of perceptual functioning frequently cited as causal in some speech and language disorders in children. It could be suggested that five- and six-year old children having superior articulatory skills may be neurologically more advanced than those who deviate from the normal for their age or are clearly delayed in their articulatory skills. Such a view might then suggest that as subjects reach age eight or older (the mean age of Ringel et al.'s subjects), many with fewer numbers of misarticulations catch up to normal children of the same age, but some with many articulation errors do not. Such a statement is consistent with reviews of the literature concerning speech sound discrimination presented by Winitz (1969) and Weiner (1967), and Weiner's conclusion that research findings generally support the statement that children below age nine with misarticulation have been found to be inferior to normal-speaking children on speech sound discrimination tasks. Additionally, Sommers, Meyer, and Furlong (1969) reported that both pitch discrimination and speech sound discrimination performances of children ages eight to 11 years were related to the degree of their articulatory defectiveness, and only the most severely defective were inferior to normals on each task. Evidence presented by Stitt and Huntington (1969) indicated that college students with misarticulations were inferior on a variety of auditory tasks, including pitch and speech sound discrimination. Further Weinberg, Liss, and Hollis (1970) found poor oral identification in teenage /r/ defectives. Again, this may tend to support the belief that some percentage of subjects with misarticulations continue to demonstrate inferior performances on some auditory perceptual, memory, and oral tasks.

Although poorer performances of children with misarticulations compared with superior speakers on an oral sensory discrimination task supports Ringel et al. (1970), the types of oral sensory errors were exactly opposite of those reported by them. The most apparent explanation for these findings stems from evidence summarized comprehensively by White (1963), which indicates that memory and perceptual functioning performances of children of the ages used in this study are qualitatively different from those of children of the ages used by Ringel and his associates. Children aged four, five, and six, according to White (1963), tend to begin having difficulties with the mechanism of inhibition which affects their learning and perceptual functioning.

Furthermore, research literature shows clearly that these ages tend to be transitional with an increased recognizable influence of language on learning. Studies concerned with response competition have demonstrated that first-learned responses, although suppressed, compete with second-learned responses (Spiker and Holton, 1958). This suggests a possible explanation for the large differences in the number of size and form errors compared to those reported by Ringel et al. (1970). The types of between- and within-class errors may reflect the language competency of the subjects. If so, our younger subjects made completely opposite error responses due to fewer abilities to cope with the competition in associate transfer. Thus, the first learned category or concept size (big/little) was successful in competing with the second learned category (shape), thus causing more errors of the latter. The expected superior language competency of the older subjects in the Ringel et al. (1970) investigation may, therefore, have been influential in reducing the competing effects of earlier learned responses through the mechanism of inhibition. Although other explanations appear to exist, this one seems most in keeping with the body of knowledge about the rather dramatic perceptual and learning performances for children aged four to six.

ACKNOWLEDGMENT

The authors are grateful for the assistance of Walter Moore and George McCandless who assisted in the statistical analyses.

REFERENCES

Aungst, L. F., and Frick, J. V., Auditory discrimination ability and and consistency of articulation of (r). *J. Speech Hearing Dis.*, 28, 76-85 (1964).

Aungst, L. F., The relationship between oral stereoagnosis and articulation proficiency. Doctoral dissertation, Pennsylvania State Univ. (1965).

Carter, E. T., and Buck, McK. W., Prognostic testing for functional articulation disorders among children in the first grade. *J. Speech Hearing Dis.*, 23, 124-133 (1958).

Farquhar, M. S., Prognostic value of imitative auditory discrimination tests. *J. Speech Hearing Dis.*, 26, 342-347 (1961).

Irwin, R. B., West, J. F., and Trombetta, M. A., Effectiveness of speech therapy for second grade children with misarticulations-predictive factors. *Except. Child.*, 32, 471-482 (1966).

Kirk, S., McCarthy, J., and Kirk, W., *Illinois Test of Psycholinguistic Abilities.* Chicago: Univ. of Illinois (1968).

Kisatsky, T. J., The prognostic value of Carter-Buck tests in measuring articulation skills of selected kindergarten children. *Penn. speech hearing Ass. Newslett.*, 7, 4-9 (1966).

Kronvall, E., and Diehl, C., The relationship of auditory discrimination to articulatory defects of children with no known organic impairment. *J. Speech Hearing Dis.*, 19, 335-339 (1954).

Mange, C. V., Relationships between selected auditory perceptual factors and articulation ability. *J. Speech Hearing Res.*, 3, 67-74 (1960).

McGrady, H., Verbal and nonverbal functions in school children with speech and language disorders. Doctoral dissertation, Northwestern Univ. (1964).

Ringel, R., House, A., Burk, K., Dolinsky, J., and Scott, C., Some relations between orosensory discrimination and articulatory aspects of speech production. *J. Speech Hearing Dis.*, 35, 3-12 (1970).

SHERMAN, D., and GEITH, A., Speech sound discrimination and articulation skill. *J. Speech Hearing Res.*, **10**, 277-281 (1967).

SMITH, C. R., Articulation problems and ability to store and process stimuli. *J. Speech Hearing Res.*, **10**, 343-353 (1967).

SOMMERS, R. K., COCKERVILLE, C. E., PAUL, C. D., BOWSER, D. C., FICHTER, G. R., FENTON, A. K., and COPETAS, F. G., Effects of speech therapy and speech improvement upon articulation and reading. *J. Speech and Hearing Dis.*, **26**, 27-38 (1961).

SOMMERS, R. K., LEISS, R. H., FUNDRELLA, D., MANNING, W., JOHNSON, R., OERTHER, P., SHOLLEY, R., and SIEGEL, M., Factors in the effectiveness of articulation therapy with educable retarded children. *J. Speech Hearing Res.*, **13**, 304-316 (1970).

SOMMERS, R. K., MEYER, W. J., and FENTON, A. K., Pitch discrimination and articulation. *J. Speech Hearing Res.*, **4**, 56-60 (1961).

SOMMERS, R. K., LEISS, R., DELP, M., GERBER, A., FUNDRELLA, D., SMITH, R., REVUCKY, M., ELLIS, D., and HALEY, V., Factors related to the effectiveness of articulation therapy for kindergarten, first, and second grade children. *J. Speech Hearing Res.*, **10**, 428-437 (1967).

SOMMERS, R. K., MEYER, W. J., and FURLONG, A. K., Pitch discrimination and speech sound discrimination in articulatory defective and normal speaking children. *J. aud. Res.*, **9**, 45-50 (1969).

SPENCER, E., An investigation of the maturation of various factors of auditory perception in pre-school children. Doctoral dissertation, Northwestern Univ. (1958).

SPIKER, C., and HOLTON, R., Associative transfer in motor paired associate learning as a function of amount of first task practice. *J. exp. Psychol.*, **56**, 123-132 (1958).

STITT, C., and HUNTINGTON, D., Some relationships among articulation, auditory ability, and certain other variables. *J. Speech Hearing Res.*, **12**, 576-594 (1969).

STOIA, L., An investigation of improvement in articulation in a therapy group and non-therapy group of first grade children having functional articulatory speech disorders. Doctoral dissertation, Columbia Univ. (1961).

WEINBERG, B., LISS, G., and HOLLIS, J., A comparative study of visual, manual, and oral form identification in speech impaired and normal speaking children. In J. F. Bosma (Ed.), *Second Symposium on Oral Sensation and Perception.* Springfield, Ill.: Charles C Thomas (1970).

WEINER, P., Auditory discrimination and articulation. *J. Speech Hearing Dis.*, **32**, 19-29 (1967).

WEPMAN, J., *Wepman Auditory Discrimination Test.* Chicago: Language Research Assoc. (1958).

WHITE, S., Evidence for a hierarchical arrangement of learning processes. In L. Lipsitt and C. Spiker (Eds.), *Advances in Child Development and Behavior,* Vol. II. New York: Academic, 187-219 (1963).

WINITZ, H., *Articulatory Acquisition and Behavior.* New York: Appleton-Century-Crofts (1969).

SPEECH-SOUND DISCRIMINATION AND TACTILE-KINESTHETIC DISCRIMINATION IN REFERENCE TO SPEECH PRODUCTION

CHARLES L. MADISON   AND   DONALD J. FUCCI

Summary.—The relationship between selected sensory discrimination variables and speech-sound production was investigated. Speech-sound discrimination, oral stereognostic discrimination, and articulation were measured in a group of 100 first-grade children. Ss had to have normal hearing; understand the concept of "same and different"; be less than 7 yr., 6 mo. of age; have no obvious neurological or physical impairment; and have a Columbia Mental Maturity Scale score of at least 85. A significant negative correlation between speech-sound discrimination in oral stereognostic discrimination was established. There was a significant difference in articulation scores between high and low speech-sound discrimination groups. The difference in articulation scores between high and low oral stereognostic groups was not significant. The possibility that the result of this and other studies could be explained by an age-linked dominant monitoring modality for articulation was discussed.

Articulation theorists have suggested that certain sensory modalities are of particular significance to speech production. In the Fairbanks' (1954) servosystem model, speech production is shown to be monitored by means of auditory and tactile-kinesthetic sensory feedback. In a recent discussion of articulation theory, Morley and Fox (1969) comment:

During the process of developing articulate speech the movements made by the child produce sounds, and he then experiences sensory feedback through what may be described as multiple internal loops. The receptor processes involved are (1) auditory, feedback through the auditory nervous system, and (2) the surface receptors, with tactile and proprioceptive feedback from the contacts and movements produced (p. 155).

McDonald (1964) views sensory discrimination as a vital element in the organism's ability to handle the continually more difficult differentiations of incoming stimuli necessary for articulatory refinement.

A number of researchers (Wepman, 1960; Kronvall & Diehl, 1954; Cohen & Diehl, 1963; Sherman & Geith, 1967) have shown speech-sound discrimination to be related to articulation. Others (Hall, 1938; Mase, 1946; Hansen, 1944) have not found such as relationship. Consequently, there has been conflict of opinion regarding the speech-sound discrimination-articulation relationship. Powers (1957) states,

... the great weight of evidence is against there being a systematic inferiority of functional articulatory defectives in ability to discriminate speech sounds (p. 742).

In a more recent review, Weiner (1967) points out that nearly every study involving children below the age of 9 yr. has shown a positive relationship between functional articulation and speech-sound discrimination, particularly where the articulatory difficulty was more severe.

PERCEPTUAL AND MOTOR SKILLS, 1971, vol. 33, 831-838.

Recently, oral stereognostic testing methods and materials have been developed to assess tactile-kinesthetic discrimination in the oral region (Hetherington, 1964; Woodford, 1964; McDonald & Aungst, 1967; Shelton, Arndt, & Hetherington, 1967). Research attempting to relate oral stereognostic discrimination to speech-sound production has been encouraging but not conclusive (Aungst, 1965; Thompson, 1969; Locke, 1969; Ringel, 1970).

Although much research has been conducted with respect to the auditory and tactile-kinesthetic senses as they affect articulation, studies attempting to relate the two areas are few. Consequently, the relative contribution of auditory and tactile-kinesthetic discrimination to articulation is not clear.

Research concerned with one or the other of sensory modalities in relation to functional disorders of articulation tends to ignore the possibility of multiple causation. Van Riper and Irwin (1958) suggest that the inconclusive results concerning speech-sound discrimination might have occurred because it is only one of several important etiological factors. Powers' (1957) contention that it makes good clinical sense to assume multiple causation for functional articulation cases is all too often ignored. The assumption of multiple causation reduces the likelihood that important etiological factors will be overlooked (Powers, 1957; Locke, 1968a, 1968b).

The present project examines the relationship between speech-sound discrimination and tactile-kinesthetic discrimination, and their etiological significance in functional articulation disorders. The study is designed to be sensitive to the possibility that non-organic deviant articulation may be a function of multiple influences. The following questions were investigated: (1) What is the relationship between speech-sound discrimination and tactile-kinesthetic discrimination in a group of first-grade children? (2) Is there a difference in articulation ability between groups of first-grade Ss who are high and who are low in speech-sound discrimination ability? (3) Is there a difference in ability to articulate between groups of first-grade Ss who are high and who are low in oral stereognostic discriminative ability?

METHOD

Subjects

From a pool of 118 first-grade children, 100 no older than 7 yr., 6 mo. were Ss. All Ss were public school children. There were 57 females and 43 males in the sample. The children ranged in age from 6 yr., 4 mo. to 7 yr., 6 mo., with a mean age of 6 yr., 10 mo.

First-grade children were chosen so that the discrimination variables under study might be operating to affect articulatory maturation. Work by Poole (1934) and Templin (1957) has suggested that for most children below the age of 7 yr., 6 mo. the maturation of articulation is not complete. Once adult-level articulation skill has been reached, it is, naturally, not then possible to measure the extent to which reaching this levels of skills was delayed by deficient discrimination skills. Possible functional relationships between articulation and discrimination skills are thus obscured.

In addition to age (10 children were eliminated on the basis of age), there were four other criteria for acceptance into the study. First Ss had to have hearing that was within normal limits. A pure-tone audiometric screening test was administered. The frequencies 500 Hz, 1,000 Hz, 2,000 Hz, and 4,000 Hz were tested bilaterally at a level of 25 dB (ISO). Any potential S not responding to more than one frequency in one ear or to the same frequency in both ears was excluded. Seven children failed to meet the hearing criteria. Second, the children had to show an understanding of the concept of "same and different." Ss were pretrained to the "same and different" concept using irrelevant visual stimuli to a criterion of three correct judgments out of three possible stimuli. If the criterion was not met, the concept was explained and S was checked again. A second failure would have resulted in dismissal from the study. However, all children were able to deal with the concept successfully. Third, 3 children having a known or observable neurological or physical impairment that could affect measures used in the study were excluded. Finally, in order to eliminate the effects of low intelligence on the measures being used, children with intelligence quotients of less than 85 on the Columbia Mental Maturity Scale were rejected (Sherman & Geith, 1967). Intelligence criteria accounted for the loss of 14 potential Ss.

Stimuli

The 100 Ss who met the selection criteria were given the following tests: Laradon Articulation Scale (Edmonston, 1963), Auditory Discrimination Test (Wepman, 1958), and an oral stereognostic discrimination task.

The oral stereognostic discrimination task was used to evaluate tactile-kinesthetic perception. The 20-item discrimination task required Ss to make "same or different" judgments about selected pairs of three-dimensional plastic forms from the National Institute of Dental Research (NIDR) Test of Oral Stereognosis (Bosma, 1967).

Ringel, Burk, and Scott (1968) used a 55-item "same or different" oral stereognostic discrimination task in a study of tactile-kinesthetic perception and articulation. To construct this task these researchers selected 10 of the NIDR forms and paired them in all possible combinations. The result was 45 "different" and 10 "same" pairs of forms. The oral stereognostic discrimination task used in the present study consisted of 20 pairs of forms randomly selected from the 55 pairs used by Ringel, Burk, and Scott. Ss were given two points per correct response on this task.

Procedure

The time needed to test each S was about 45 to 60 min. To avoid possible fatigue the testing was done in two sessions. In the first session, the Columbia and the Laradon were administered and scored according to recommended procedure. The discrimination testing was done in the second session. The discrimination tasks were alternated in order of presentation, with a 5-min. rest between them.

The Auditory Discrimination Test (i.e., Wepman) was administered according to the manual's specifications but not scored in the recommended manner. The Wepman can be invalidated by great numbers of errors (Wepman, 1958). For the purposes of this study, it was important that children with very poor speech-sound discrimination not be eliminated. Factors which can account for large numbers of errors on the Wepman—defective hearing, misunderstanding of the task, and low intelligence—were controlled.

To assure that presentation of the Wepman stimuli was consistent for all Ss, the test was audio tape recorded by an experienced speaker. Loudness, intonation, and inter-stimulus timing were held constant in preparing the tape. Ss were given one point for every correct response.

The procedure employed in the presentation of the oral stereognostic discrimination task was the same as that used by Ringel, Burk, and Scott (1968). Ss were instructed that two "little plastic forms" would be placed in their mouths and that they were to indicate whether they were the "same" or "different." The forms were placed in the children's mouths one at a time by the examiner. Ss were encouraged to feel them all over carefully and were allowed to retain them for approximately 5 sec. Three to 5 sec. elapsed between presentation of the first and second forms. Upon removal of the second form, Ss indicated whether the two forms were the "same" or "different."

RESULTS AND DISCUSSION

Table 1 provides the ranges, means, and standard deviations for the Laradon, Wepman, and oral stereognostic discrimination tasks.

A Pearson product-moment correlation (r) was used to determine the relationship between speech-sound discrimination and oral stereognostic discrimination scores for all 100 Ss. There was a statistically significant negative r of $-.52$ ($df = 98, p < .05$) between speech-sound discrimination and oral stereognostic discrimination. Children who scored high on a test of speech-sound dis-

TABLE 1

RANGE, MEAN, AND STANDARD DEVIATION OF LARADON ARTICULATION SCALE, AUDITORY DISCRIMINATION TEST AND ORAL STEREOGNOSTIC DISCRIMINATION TASK SCORES

Test	Range	M	SD
Laradon Articulation Scale	48-100	96.1	7.8
Auditory Discrimination Test	14- 38	32.8	3.6
Oral stereognostic discrimination task	16- 38	32.0	4.3

crimination tended to achieve low scores on a tactile-kinesthetic discrimination task. The correlations between articulation and scores on each of the discrimination tasks were also computed. The correlation between articulation and speech-sound discrimination was significant and positive ($r = .44, df = 98, p < .05$). Finally, the correlation between articulation and oral stereognostic discrimination indicated no significant relationship ($r = .03, df = 98, p > .05$).[1]

Sherman and Geith (1967) have demonstrated the advantage of selecting Ss on the basis of discrimination task performance prior to examining articulation proficiency. To determine the effect of high and of low performance on each of the sensory discrimination tasks on articulation the following procedure was used. First, from the sample of 100 Ss, the 25 Ss scoring highest on the Wepman were selected as a high speech-sound discrimination group. Second, the 25 Ss scoring lowest on the Wepman were selected as a low speech-sound discrimination group. Third, the high and low discrimination groups were matched for age (within 6 mo.) and sex. Finally, the mean articulation scores (Laradon) of the matched groups were analyzed.

When the matching procedure was carried out between the high and low speech-sound discrimination groups, two Ss were lost, leaving equal Ns of 23. Table 2 shows the ranges, means, and standard deviations of the Laradon scores for the high and low speech-sound discrimination groups.

TABLE 2

RANGE, MEAN, AND STANDARD DEVIATION ON LARADON ARTICULATION SCALE FOR HIGH AND LOW AUDITORY DISCRIMINTION TEST GROUPS

Auditory Discrimination Group	Range	M	SD
High	92-100	98.4	2.1
Low	48-100	92.2	12.3

Prior to testing the difference in articulation score means between the high and low speech-sound discrimination groups a test for homogeneity of variance was done. The variances for the two groups were not homogeneous. A Wilcoxon sign test showed that the high speech-sound discrimination group had achieved significantly ($p < .05$) higher articulation scores than the low speech-sound discrimination group.

A procedure similar to that used to analyze the articulation scores of the high and low speech-sound discrimination groups was applied to the high and

[1]Note that correlation between oral stereognostic discrimination and articulation with speech-sound discrimination partialled out was —.24; the correlation between oral stereognostic discrimination and speech-sound discrimination with articulation partialled out was —.57; and the correlation between speech-sound discrimination and articulation with oral stereognostic discrimination partialled out was .49.

TABLE 3
RANGE, MEAN, AND STANDARD DEVIATION OF LARADON ARTICULATION SCALE SCORES
FOR HIGH AND LOW ORAL STEREOGNOSTIC DISCRIMINATION GROUPS

Oral Stereognostic Group	Range	M	SD
High	70-100	96.1	8.4
Low	48-100	94.1	12.0

low oral stereognostic discrimination groups. The matching procedure resulted in a loss of 5 Ss, leaving equal Ns of 20. Table 3 shows the ranges, means, and standard deviations of the Laradon scores for the high and low oral stereognostic discrimination groups.

A test for homogeneity of variance between the high and low oral stereognostic groups showed them to be homogeneous. A standard t test for related means ($t = .530 < 2.101$, $df = 19$, $p > .05$) showed no significant statistical difference between the high and low oral stereognostic groups in articulation proficiency. Oral stereognostic discrimination as measured in the present study does not appear related to articulation proficiency in first grade Ss.

The case for speech-sound discrimination being an important factor related to articulation ability in first-grade children is strengthened. In the present study both the simple correlation and detailed examination of high and low speech-sound discrimination groups confirm the importance of the relationship. These results are consistent with those of several other investigators (Kronvall & Diehl, 1954; Wepman, 1960; Cohen & Diehl, 1963; Sherman & Geith, 1967).

The present study showed no significant difference between the high and low oral stereognostic groups in articulatory proficiency. Those children who performed well on an oral stereognostic discrimination task did not demonstrate better articulation ability than children who scored low on such a task. The correlation between articulatory ability and tactile-kinesthetic ability confirmed the point.

A predominating modality concept in articulation control has been implied by Van Riper and Irwin (1958). They hypothesize that,

. . . younger children are monitoring their articulation mainly by means of the auditory feedback. As their new articulation skills became stabilized, they turn over the monitoring to the kinesthetic and tactual feedback systems with less interference to the thought processes (p. 158).

The above hypothesis is definitely strengthened when the growing research information in speech-sound discrimination and tactile-kinesthetic discrimination is considered. Research projects using older Ss (adults or older elementary children) have not shown speech-sound discrimination to be related to articulation. Studies involving younger children (under 8 or 9 yr. of age) have shown speech-sound discrimination to be related to articulation proficiency (Weiner, 1967).

In the area of oral stereognostics the situation regarding age has generally been the reverse. Several studies (Robertson, Fucci, & Fokes, 1969; Ringel, Burk, & Scott, 1968) using adult Ss have found oral stereognostic discrimination to be related to articulation ability. Other studies (Aungst, 1965; Locke, 1969), as well as the present study which used children, have not shown tactile-kinesthetic discrimination to be related to sound learning and articulation skill. The only possible exception is the recent results reported by Ringel, House, Burk, Dolinsky, and Scott (1970). It may be important to note, however, that although the Ringel group used children as Ss, they were older elementary school pupils.

One of the more plausible explanations for a shift in monitoring of articulation from the auditory to the tactile-kinesthetic systems may be related to the internalization of articulation as an automatic motor act. The servo-system application to speech production (Fairbanks, 1954) and the extension of this concept by McDonald (1964) in the form of a sensory motor approach to articulation testing and treatment support the internalization-automatic process.

Available literature seems to indicate that 7 to 9 yr. of age may be a critical time related to phonological development and related skills. During this age-time span we can expect both articulation development and speech-sound discrimination ability reach a point of maturational stability (Poole, 1934; Templin, 1957; Weiner, 1967). Age, however, may not be the only important variable related to feedback monitoring of articulation. Perkell (1969) discusses the possibility of a different monitoring basis for vowel production than for consonant production.

The determination of whether or not the negative correlation between speech-sound discrimination and oral stereognostic discrimination found in the present study may be related to the predominating modality hypothesis of Van Riper and Irwin must await further research. The results of this study strongly indicate the need for examination of the articulation-monitoring process across age levels. A longitudinal research paradigm could do much to help determine whether there is a shift from the auditory to the tactile-kinesthetic systems with articulatory maturation.

REFERENCES

AUNGST, L. F. The relationship between oral stereognosis and articulation proficiency. Unpublished Ph.D. dissertation, Pennsylvania State Univer., 1965.

BOSMA, J. (Ed.) Symposium on oral sensation and perception. Springfield, Ill.: Thomas, 1967.

COHEN, J. H., & DIEHL, C. F. Relation of speech-sound discrimination ability to articulation-type speech defects. J. Speech hear. Disord., 1963, 28, 187-190.

EDMONSTON, W. Laradon Articulation Scale. Beverly Hills: Western Psychological Services, 1963.

FAIRBANKS, G. Systematic research in experimental phonetics: 1. A theory of the speech mechanism as a servosystem. J. Speech hear. Disord., 1954, 19, 133-139.

HALL, M. E. Auditory factors in functional articulatory speech defects. J. except. Educ., 1938, 7, 110-132.

HANSEN, B. F. The application of sound discrimination tests to functional articulatory defectives with normal hearing. J. Speech hear. Disord., 1944, 9, 347-355.

HETHERINGTON, J. J. Testing oral stereognosis in first grade, third grade and college students. Unpublished M.A. thesis, Univer. of Missouri at Kansas City, 1964.

KRONVALL, E. L., & DIEHL, C. F. The relationship of auditory discrimination to articulatory defects of children with no known organic impairment. *J. Speech hear. Disord.*, 1954, 19, 335-338.

LOCKE, J. L. Questionable assumptions underlying articulation research. *J. Speech hear. Disord.*, 1968, 33, 112-116. (a)

LOCKE, J. L. A study of oral stereognosis, auditory memory span, articulation, and production of non-English phones in a natural group of kindergarten and first grade children. Unpublished Ph.D. dissertation, Ohio Univer., 1968. (b)

LOCKE, J. L. Short-term auditory memory, oral perception, and experimental sound learning. *J. Speech hear. Res.*, 1969, 12, 185-192.

MASE, D. J. *Etiology of articulatory speech defects.* New York: Teachers Coll., Columbia Univer., Bur. Publ., 1946. (Contr. to Educ., No. 921)

McDONALD, E. T. *Articulation testing and treatment: a sensory-motor approach.* Pittsburgh: Stanwix House, 1964.

McDONALD, E. T., & AUNGST, L. F. Studies in oral sensorimotor function. In J. Bosma (Ed.), *Symposium on oral sensation and perception.* Springfield: Thomas, 1967. Pp. 202-220.

MORLEY, M. E., & FOX, J. Disorders of articulation: theory and therapy. *Brit. J. Dis. Communication*, 1969, 4, 151-165.

PERKELL, J. *The physiology of speech production: results and implications of a quantitative cineradiographic study.* Cambridge, Mass.: M.I.T. Press, 1969. (Res. Monogr. 53)

POOLE, I. Genetic development in articulation of consonant sounds in speech. *Elem. English*, 1934, 11, 159-161.

POWERS, M. H. Functional disorders of articulation-symptomatology and etiology. In L. E. Travis (Ed.), *Handbook of speech pathology.* New York: Appleton-Century-Crofts, 1957. Pp. 707-768.

RINGEL, R. L. Oral sensation and perception: a selective review. Paper presented at the Conference on Speech and the Dento-Facial Complex, New Orleans, 1970.

RINGEL, R. L., BURK, K. W., & SCOTT, C. M. Tactile perception: form discrimination in the mouth. *Brit. J. Dis. Communication*, 1968, 3, 150-155.

RINGEL, R. L., HOUSE, A. S., BURK, K. W., DOLINSKY, J. P., & SCOTT, C. M. Some relations between oral sensory discrimination and articulatory aspects of speech production. *J. Speech hear. Disord.*, 1970, 35, 3-11.

ROBERTSON, J. H., FUCCI, D. J., & FOKES, J. B. "Functional" defective articulation: an oral sensory disturbance. Paper presented at the 45th Annual Convention of the American Speech and Hearing Association, Chicago, 1969.

SHELTON, R. L., ARNDT, W. B., & HETHERINGTON, J. J. Testing oral stereognosis. In J. Bosma (Ed.), *Symposium on oral sensation and perception.* Springfield, Ill.: Thomas, 1967. Pp. 222-243.

SHERMAN, D., & GEITH, A. Speech sound discrimination and articulation skill. *J. Speech hear. Res.*, 1967, 10, 227-280.

TEMPLIN, M. C. *Certain language skills in children.* Minneapolis: Univer. of Minnesota Press, 1957.

THOMPSON, R. C. The effects of oral sensory disruption upon oral stereognosis and articulations. Paper presented at the 45th Annual Convention of the American Speech and Hearing Association, Chicago, 1969.

VAN RIPER, C., & IRWIN, J. V. *Voice and articulation.* Englewood Cliffs: Prentice-Hall, 1958.

WEBER, B. A. Effects of high level masking anesthetization of oral structures upon articulatory proficiency and voice characteristics of normal speakers. Unpublished M.S. thesis, Pennsylvania State Univer., 1961.

WEINER, P. S. Auditory discrimination and articulation. *J. Speech hear. Disord.*, 1967, 32, 19-28.

WEPMAN, J. *Auditory Discrimination Test.* Chicago: Language Research Assoc., 1958.

WEPMAN, J. Auditory discrimination, speech, and reading. *Element. Sch. J.*, 1960, 60, 325-333.

WOODFORD, L. D. Oral stereognosis. Unpublished M.A. thesis, Univer. of Illinois, 1964.

"FUNCTIONAL" DEFECTIVE ARTICULATION: AN ORAL SENSORY DISTURBANCE

DONALD J. FUCCI AND JOHN H. ROBERTSON

Summary.—Some sources of disordered articulation may be related to oral sensory disabilities alone. One method of evaluating oral sensory functioning is to test for lingual stereognostic capability. Two groups, aged 12 to 16, of 10 children considered to be normal speakers (Group A) and 10 children considered to have "functional" articulation (Group B) as judged by a speech pathologist were free of sensory and motor defects. 20 geometric plastic forms, developed by the National Institute of Dental Research (NIDRs 20) were used to assess perceptual discrimination: eye, finger tip, tongue tip, and tongue blade. In general, larger mean differences were found between the normal and "functional" articulation groups than within them. The groups differed consistently in the general performance levels on the oral stereognostic tasks and in the oral-tactile performance not only within groups but between groups. *S*s with "functional" articulation disorders (Group B) made more and different types of errors than normal speakers. Articulation disorders considered "functional" might be studied in relation to classical therapeutic procedures.

Literature on articulatory disorders suggests that normal development and maintenance of articulation presupposes, to some degree, the adequacy of gross and specific motor and sensory functioning within the oral region (Powers, 1957). Some sources of disordered articulation may reflect a basic oral-sensory disability. As a child learns to speak, he auditorily compares his speech-sound productions with those of his adult model. On a learning theory basis, when the child perceives his own utterances as similar to those of his adult model, tactile and kinesthetic cues from the articulators used to produce those utterances are said to be reinforced. With continued practice, this tactile and kinesthetic feedback is sufficiently stabilized to serve as the dominant automatic control for speech. Methods have been proposed for measuring oral-sensory functioning, e.g., test of lingual stereognostic capability (Grossman, Hattis, & Ringel, 1965).

Oral stereognosis may be defined as the ability to recognize the form of objects through the sense of touch within the oral region. This ability has been cited by Forster (1962) as indicative of the integrity of the nervous system, whereas, astereognosis in the presence of intact sensory channels is indicative of a nervous system pathology. Astereognosis is attributed to lesions of the parietal lobe (Post-Rolandic Gyris) or subcortical regions (Wechsler, 1947). Therefore, it may be contended that information about the quality of oral sensory functioning may lead to important insight into the nature of oral-motor proficiency. In other words, it may be hypothesized that there is a relationship between oral stereognosis and oral articulation. Although Bosma (1967) points out that such a relationship must remain purely speculative, studies of oral

PERCEPTUAL AND MOTOR SKILLS, 1971, vol. 33, 711-714.

stereognosis capability have indicated that a significant relationship between oral stereognosis and disordered articulation exists (Class, 1956). A significantly high incidence of lingual agnosia has been observed in speech defective samples (Palmer, Wurth, & Kincheloe, 1963). In addition, it appears that alterations of normal speech-related oral-tactile perception results in disturbances of speech output. Therefore, the speech production considered to be "functional" as defined by Van Riper (1962) may show an etiological oral-sensory disturbance which could be studied through the use of oral stereognostic forms. Further study of this possible relationship seems feasible.

Thus, we may ask (1) Do normal speakers and individuals with functional speech disorders vary consistently in their general performance levels on the oral stereognostic task, (2) Is there a consistent difference in oral-tactile performance at various loci in the oral region (tongue tip, tongue blade) within and between such groups, (3) Is there a difference in the number of correct responses in the oral stereognostic performance for structures outside the oral regions (eye, finger tips) and those in the oral regions (tongue tip, tongue blade) within and between such groups, and (4) Do the types of correct responses made by these two groups vary within and between the sets of shapes (pointed versus curved)?

METHOD

Twenty children were selected from a junior high school to compose two groups ranging in age from 12 to 16. They were screened by a competent speech therapist who used the Templin-Darley Screening Test of Articulation. The children in Group A were considered normal speakers, while the children in Group B were considered to have "functional" articulation disorders characterized by two or more defective and incorrect sounds. The mean age for Group A was 13.7 yr. The mean age for Group B was 14.2 yr. The articulatory-defective and normal speaking subjects reported no past or present history of sensory or motor defect; no gross abnormality of oral structures was noted.

The stimulus materials were 20 plastic geometric forms. Each form was attached to a 2-in. wand. These forms were developed by the National Institute of Dental Research (NIDRs 20). For the purposes of this study, the forms were divided into two geometric classes: points and curves. This division of the forms made possible the "within class" and "between class" stimulus groupings.

Four stereognostic tasks were administered to all Ss. The 20 stereognostic forms were randomized prior to presentation. Since each task was primarily one of intersensory matching, i.e., eye to picture, finger tip to picture, tongue tip to picture, and tongue blade to picture, it was anticipated that an individual who was "visually deficient" would exhibit poor oral sensory abilities (Ringel, Burk, & Scott, 1968). Therefore, the visual proficiency of each S was examined first. In Phase I, each S was presented the entire set of 20 forms and asked to match each form with the picture of his choice. Then in Phase II, each form was placed in the fingers of the preferred hand. S was asked to point to the picture of the form of his choice while the form was held in his fingers. He was not able to see the form. During Phase III, the forms were placed on the tongue tip. During Phase IV, sterilized forms were placed on the tongue blade. Each form was shielded from S's view with E's cupped hand. During each task, S was asked to point to the picture of the form thought to be in his mouth. He was allowed to retain and manipulate it in any fashion he so desired for 15 sec. The instructions approximated those suggested by Shelton, Arndt, and Netherington (1967).

340

The number of correct responses and the errors within classes and between classes of forms were recorded for all 20 Ss for the 20 forms. For each loci of form presentation, the total number of responses possible was 20.

Homogeneity of variance was checked using the Cochran test (Winer, 1962). For a .01 level test the critical value of $C_{.99}$ $(7,9)$ $= .3751$. The observed value of .13 does not exceed the critical value, showing asumptions of homogeneity of variance are tenable. The data were then submitted to a 3-factor repeated measures (case I) analysis of variance.

Fig. 1 (object, finger tip, tongue tip, tongue blade) represents graphically the mean distributions for Groups A and B of correct responses. The mean scores for Group A were 19, 16, 13.5, and 10.5 respectively. The mean scores for Group B were 18, 13.5, 8, and 5.7. The analysis of variance showed a significant difference between groups ($F = 23.93, p < .01$) and between places (object, finger tip, tongue tip, tongue blade) ($F = 76.48, p < .01$). Thus the groups differed consistently in the over-all performance of the oral stereognosis tasks. The oral-tactile performance of the parts of the oral regions were consistently different not only within each group but between them. Both groups made consistently more errors within the oral region (tongue blade); however, Group B's errors increased more than Group A's. Although Group A did make incorrect responses at all loci tested, Group B made markedly increased errors at oral loci.

Fig. 2 (object, finger tip, tongue tip, tongue blade) represents graphically

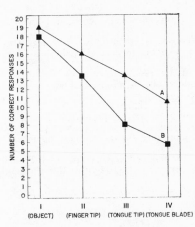

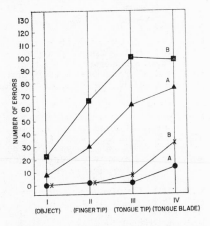

FIG. 1. Comparison of the mean distributions of Groups A and B and the levels of performance at each locus of the stereognostic task

FIG. 2. The total number of errors made by each group on each specific task. Group A is designated by a triangle for in-class errors and a circle for between-class errors. Group B is designated by a rectangle for within class errors and an (X) for between-class errors.

the mean distributions of within-class and between-class errors of Groups A and B. Group A's within-class errors were: 9, 63, 63, and 76 respectively. Comparative scores for Group B were 23, 66, 110, and 109 respectively. The analysis of variance gave no statistically significant difference between the classes (points and curves; $F = .59, p > .01$).

What appeared to be most important is that Ss considered to have "functional" articulation disorders made fewer and proportionately different types of correct responses in tasks of oral form discrimination than were made by a comparable group of 10 normal speakers. These findings suggest that the term "functional" may not be appropriate for people having articulation disorders such as those found in Group B of this experiment. These results also indicate that the therapeutic procedures for articulation disorders which are considered to be "functional" in nature might be further studied as to the appropriateness of such procedures. Utilization of an oral-tactile approach may be more suitable as a rehabilitative method. The data for both groups agree with recent research which indicates that the tongue tip appears to be more sensitive than other oral structures in identifying forms (Grossman, Hattis, & Ringel, 1965). Both groups showed consistently more correct responses made for the tongue tip than they did for the tongue blade. In this preliminary study of the appropriateness of the term "functional" for people having articulation disorders as in Group B, only a "trend" has been indicated. Research is needed.

The following conclusions were drawn: (1) normal speakers and individuals with "functional" speech disorders vary consistently in the general performance levels on the oral stereognostic tasks; (2) there are consistent differences in oral-tactile performance both within and between groups; (3) these differences in oral stereognostic performance are larger for structures not in oral regions (eyes, finger tips) than structures in oral regions (tongue tip, tongue blade) as expected, and (4) the within-class and between-class responses vary within and between groups of Ss.

REFERENCES

BOSMA, J. *Second symposium on oral sensation and perception.* Springfield, Ill.: Thomas, 1967.

CLASS, L. A comparative study of normal speakers and speech defectives with regard to the tactual-kinesthetic perception of form with the tongue. Unpublished M.A. thesis, Ohio State Univer., 1956.

FORSTER, F. *Synopsis of neurology.* St. Louis: Mosby, 1962.

GROSSMAN, R., HATTIS, B., & RINGEL, R. Methods of determining oral-tactile experience. *Arch. oral Biol.,* 1965, 10, 691-705.

NIELSEN, J. *Agnosia, apraxia, and aphasia.* New York: Hafner, 1965.

PALMER, M., WURTH, C., & KINCHELOE, J. The incidence of apraxia and agnosia in functional disorders in articulation. *ASHA,* 1963, 5, 10.

RINGEL, R., BURK, K., & SCOTT, C. Tactile perception: form discrimination in the mouth. *Brit. J. Disord. Communication,* 1968, 3, 150-155.

SHELTON, R., ARNDT, W., & NETHERINGTON, J. Testing oral stereognosis. In J. Bosma (Ed.), *Symposium on oral sensation and perception.* Springfield, Ill.: Thomas, 1967. Pp. 221-243.

VAN RIPER, C. *Speech correction: principles and methods.* Englewood Cliffs, N. J.: Prentice-Hall, 1962.

VAN RIPER, C., & IRWIN, J. *Voice and articulation.* Englewood Cliffs, N. J.: Prentice-Hall, 1962.

WECHSLER, I. *Textbook of clinical neurology.* Philadelphia: Saunders, 1947.

WINER, B. J. *Statistical principles in experimental design.* New York: McGraw-Hill, 1962.

ORAL FORM RECOGNITION TRAINING
AND ARTICULATION CHANGE[1]

RALPH L. SHELTON, VALERIE WILLIS, ANITA F. JOHNSON

AND WILLIAM B. ARNDT

Summary.—10 children with articulation disorders were given training in recognition of forms through oral exploration of those forms. Training materials were divided into sets. Fewer trials were required to reach performance criteria from one set to another, and fewer errors were made as Ss progressed from set to set. The control procedure used indicated that information gained through oral study of the forms contributed to performance but was not necessary to performance improvement. No gains were observed in any of four articulation measures.

Persons with articulation defects have been found to be inferior to normal speakers in performance on oral form recognition (stereognosis) tasks (Ringel, *et al.*, 1970).[2] Also, persons low in oral form recognition performance have proved to be inferior in learning to articulate phones foreign to their language (Locke, 1968).

Wilhelm (1970) converted a test of oral form recognition (Arndt, *et al.*, 1970) into an instrument for use in oral training. The 35 forms used in the test were divided into six sets—one for orientation and five for training. Six series of multiple-choice drawings were prepared for each form. Wilhelm then presented the items in each training set to his 4½-yr.-old Ss until they performed to a preset criterion. A single-subject, repeated-measures design was used. The first 3 Ss were required to match forms studied orally with drawings presented visually. Later 5 Ss were studied under other conditions such as (1) manual form recognition training and (2) articulation testing only. Ss were tested for correctness of articulation of several classes of articulation items. Wilhelm concluded that oral form recognition training when combined with repeated articulation testing resulted in improved articulation.

The purpose of the current study is similar to Wilhelm's, i.e., to determine whether oral form recognition training influences articulation in young children who have articulation problems. In the current study, however, all Ss received the treatment Wilhelm provided his first 3 Ss.

[1]This study was supported by Public Health Service Research Grant No. DEO3350 from the National Institute of Dental Research. The authors wish to thank Dr. Leija McReynolds, Miss Joyce Lim, Miss Marcie O'Brien, Miss Sue Kagen, and Mrs. Jennifer Noel for their assistance. Special acknowledgement is due Dr. Charles Wilhelm whose research motivated this study. We also wish to thank for their cooperation the children and staff members from the Catalina United Methodist Church, Campus Center Nursery School, Candy Cane Nursery School, and the Amphitheater Nursery School.
[2]The terms oral form recognition and oral stereognosis are used synonymously here.

The first question in the current study concerned whether performance in oral form recognition improved with training. This question was studied in three ways. As described below, forms used in training were divided into several sets of six objects each. Each training set was accompanied by six series of multiple-choice drawings. If oral form recognition performance improved, Ss should need to use fewer of the series of drawings to meet criterion as they progressed from one training set to another. Consequently, number of drawings used to reach criterion for each set was used as a performance measure. Ss who used the same number of drawing series in reaching criterion for a set could still differ in number of errors they made during that set. Therefore, number of errors per set was used as a second index to performance on the oral form recognition training task. Arndt's oral stereognosis test was administered to Ss during the first and last study sessions. The difference between the two scores was used as a third index to change in oral form recognition performance.

The second question asked was whether articulation change during a period of oral stereognosis training differed in magnitude from change measured during a baseline period. Four articulation test categories were analyzed. The first was total score on the revised Templin-Darley Diagnostic Articulation Test. The second was total score on a 34-item syllable test. The third and fourth categories involved the 31 /r/ and 17 /s/ items from the Templin-Darley test. Data from each articulation test were processed for the subject-group and for each individual S. These analyses involved consideration of score patterns during baseline, training, and post-training periods. Consideration of performance by individual Ss enabled the authors to determine whether the performance of any individuals differed from any group trend that was identified.

PROCEDURE

Subjects

Ss were solicited from nursery schools in Tucson. When children were referred by the schools' staff members, the study was explained to the parents in writing. Ss were the first 10 children who met criteria and whose parents gave permission for participation. Criteria for inclusion in the study were as follows: (1) fall one standard deviation or more below the mean on the revised Templin-Darley diagnostic articulation test; (2) pass an audiometric screening test at 25 dB ISO for the frequencies 500, 1K, 2K, and 4K Hz; and (3) make 10 or more errors on Arndt's oral stereognosis test. Children referred were engaged in conversation to determine if they made a sufficient number of articulation errors to warrant further testing. The sounds /s/, /r/, and /l/ were each sampled at least five times. Children who misarticulated phones from two phonemes—including one of the three just mentioned—one or more times were then administered the Templin-Darley test which was scored live by the examiner.

A total of 86 children were referred by teachers. Sixty-three were dismissed

344

because they were not observed to misarticulate phones from any two phonemes. Twenty-three of the children were tested further. Eight of these were dismissed because they did not score 1 or more standard deviations below the Templin-Darley mean score for their age. Four children were dropped because of bilingualism which would confound the study. One child refused to cooperate in preliminary testing and was not studied further. The remaining 10 children constituted the sample.

These 7 boys and 3 girls ranged in age from 4-1 through 6-4 ($M = 5$-2). Prior to the first baseline session, Ss were administered several tests that measure variables that may be related to articulation improvement with training. Four subtests of the Illinois Test of Psycholinguistic Abilities were administered. They were Auditory Association ($M = 35.1, SD = 7.0$),[3] Grammatic Closure ($M = 36.3, SD = 9.1$), Auditory Closure ($M = 37.3, SD = 6.1$), and Sound Blending ($M = 31.0, SD = 5.3$). Ss' standard scores on these four subtests were compared with the corresponding mean standard scores of the test standardization group which are reported in the test manual. This was done by use of t test procedure (Walker & Lev, 1953, p. 145, formula 7.2). Only one difference was significant at the .05 level. The current Ss were below the standardization group in sound blending. The Peabody Picture Vocabulary Test was also administered to Ss ($M = 99.7, SD = 3.2$).

Two additional children were studied for control purposes. These girls were 5-4 and 4-9 yr. of age. Their standard scores on the Peabody Picture Vocabulary Test were 114 and 108. They met the same articulation and hearing criteria as did the other Ss. They were also recruited from nursery schools; however, they were not identified and studied until data from the first 10 Ss were gathered and analyzed.

Training and Testing

The study plan called for baseline, training, and post-training periods. As shown in Fig. 1, the three periods were of approximately equal duration. The total procedure was administered over a 3-wk. period and involved 14 sessions, each of which lasted approximately 30 min. The first 3 sessions were baseline sessions; the next 7 were training or probe sessions, and the last 3 were post-training. Baseline and post-training sessions involved articulation testing only. Training time was ample for influencing articulation scores.

The training materials were based on the objects and drawings from the Arndt stereognosis test and were the same as those prepared and illustrated by Wilhelm (1971). Each S was to study an object in his mouth with his tongue tip and to choose the one of five drawings that matched the object. Six sets of drawings were used for each object in order to increase Ss' dependence on information gained by oral study of the objects. The 35 forms from the Arndt test,

---

[3]Means and standard deviations reported in this paragraph are for standard scores.

SESSION AND TYPE	1		2		3			4	5	6	7	8	9	10	11		12		13		14			
	B 1		B 2		B 3			T 1	P 1	T 2	T 3	P 2	T 4	T 5	P 3		E 1		E 2		E 3			
DAY	1	2	3	4	5	6	7	8	9	10	11	12	13	14	15	16	17	18	19	20	21
WEEK			1						2								3				

FIG. 1. Calendar reflecting duration of the study and the days during which baseline, training, probe, or post-training activities were conducted. B = baseline, T = training, P = probe, E = post-training.

each of which was attached to a handle, were divided into a practice set of five objects and five training sets of six objects each (Fig. 2). Six series of drawings were prepared for the practice set and for each training set. Each drawing series contained a card for each object, and each card presented five drawings. Four of the drawings were similar in form to the training object, and one matched the object.

Each training session began with the practice items which were studied manually rather than orally. S, without seeing the object, felt it with his hands. At the same time, S was shown an answer sheet with five drawings on it from

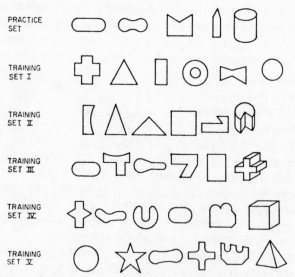

FIG. 2. Groups of forms used in oral form recognition training (after Wilhelm, 1971)

346

which he was to select the one which most closely resembled the object he had in his hand. For each incorrect response, he was shown the nylon object and the correct choice. This procedure was repeated until three practice items were correctly identified consecutively.

Upon completion of the practice items, the first training set was introduced. S was first presented with object 1 from training set 1. He was also presented with the card from the first drawing series that corresponded with the object presented. S was told to point to the one of five drawings which most closely resembled the object which had been in his mouth. No oral training object was shown to S, and when he made a mistake he was not shown which drawing was the correct choice.

The examiner presented the six objects in the training set sequentially regardless of whether S selected the proper drawing out of the five included on the card. When S selected a correct drawing, E placed a marble in a jar in S's view. If S made correct responses to all objects in a training set when the first card series was used, the session was terminated. If, however, one or more errors were made in response to card series A, the examiner presented the second card series from the same training set. Training was continued on training set 1 until S made no errors on the six forms within a given card series. If S made an error when the sixth card series was used, E returned to the first series. When a training set was completed, S was given a piece of candy or a star sticker.

During a probe session, S was again presented with the practice items manually and required to achieve the original criterion of successfully identifying three objects in a row. He was then presented orally all training sets that he had previously passed. Again, he had to succeed on all objects during the presentation of a card series. After the above review, articulation was tested. At the beginning of each training session, S also reviewed the practice set and all training sets previously passed. Original criteria were again met. No prizes or information about response correctness were given during probe sessions or the review portion of the training sessions.

The two control Ss were not given repeated articulation testing, i.e., they did not undergo the baseline and post-training articulation testing. However, they received the same training as the other Ss with the exception that they did not study the objects orally. Rather, they were asked to look at the cards in each drawing series and to guess which picture the examiner had in mind. Following correct guesses, the examiner placed a marble in a jar. Use of the control Ss permitted the authors to determine whether the study procedure could influence performance even in the absence of oral sensory information.

The revised Templin-Darley Diagnostic Articulation test and a syllable articulation test were administered imitatively during baseline, probe, and post-training sessions. Twenty-three of the items in the syllable test consisted of single consonants followed by the vowel /a/. The remaining items consisted of /r/ or

347

/s/ clusters followed by /a/. Responses were scored by the examiner and were also tape-recorded for later evaluation by three additional judges. Neither dates nor Ss' names were recorded on the tapes. Rather code numbers were used. Articulation responses were recorded on a Uher 4400 tape recorder. After all tapes were gathered, they were played back in a random order to three judges through an Ampex AG 350-2 tape recorder, a Grayson Stadler Model 162K amplifier, and a Calrad 12-in. CR-12A loudspeaker. Only one judge listened to the tapes at a time. The judges marked each response as either correct or incorrect. The incorrect category was to be used unless the judge was certain the response was correctly articulated. Judges were permitted to listen to a given response no more than twice. Scorings from the three judges were compared and consensus scores (agreement of two judges) were obtained.

The three judges were university students majoring in speech pathology. For orientation to the judging task, each judge was required to score five tape-recorded /s/ sound production tasks which had been obtained from grade school children who were inconsistent in their correctness of /s/ phone articulation. Consensus scores from the sound production tasks had been obtained from three other judges whose reliability had been established in a previous study. Each judge scored each item as either correct or incorrect and then compared his decision with the previously obtained consensus score. Percentages of agreement between the judges' scores and the consensus scores averaged 70%.

RESULTS AND DISCUSSION

Means and standard deviations for the number of series of drawings the experimental Ss used to reach criterion for each training set and for the number of errors they made throughout each set are reported in Table 1. Corresponding data for the two control Ss are also reported. Both the control and experimental Ss reduced the number of drawing series required to reach criterion as they progressed through the training sets. Also, they tended to make fewer errors from set to set. Scores for series IV were poorer than scores from series III for both

TABLE 1

MEANS AND STANDARD DEVIATIONS FOR NUMBER OF DRAWING SERIES
EXPERIMENTAL Ss USED IN ACHIEVING CRITERION FOR EACH TRAINING SET
AND FOR NUMBER OF ERRORS MADE

Training Set	Number of Series Used				Number of Errors Made			
	Experimental Ss		Control Ss		Experimental Ss		Control Ss	
	M	SD	S_1	S_2	M	SD	S_1	S_2
I	7.4	2.3	14	20	15.7	7.3	34	44
II	5.9	2.6	10	9	10.1	6.4	14	25
III	4.4	3.3	8	11	6.0	6.3	16	16
IV	5.0	1.7	10	11	7.9	4.6	26	25
V	2.3	0.9	7	5	2.1	1.4	10	9

Note.—Corresponding scores for control Ss are also reported.

control and experimental Ss. The control Ss required more drawing series and made more errors within each training set than the experimental Ss. The experimental Ss made more correct responses on the 35-item Arndt oral stereognosis test after training ($M = 28.4$, $SD = 1.3$) than before ($M = 9.0$, $SD = 4.0$).

The baseline, probe, and post-training scores from the four articulation measures used were averaged across Ss, and standard deviations were computed. These results are illustrated in Figs. 3 and 4. From inspection, it is evident that no articulation improvement was shown by any of the measures.

All scores for each S were plotted and inspected to determine whether any S might have improved his articulation during the treatment regimen. Both consensus scores and scores assigned by the examiner at the time of administration were studied. Subject 6 appeared to have improved his articulation of /r/ phones. However, since that S did not improve his articulation of /s/ phones and since

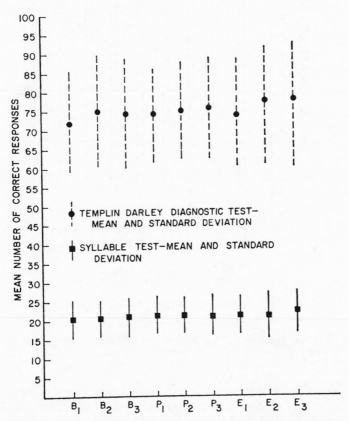

FIG. 3. Means and standard deviations for the Templin-Darley Diagnostic Articulation Test (rev.) and for the 34-item syllable test. Entries are included for baseline, probe, and post-training (E) test administrations. ● Templin-Darley $M \pm 1$ SD; ■ Syllable test $M \pm 1$ SD.

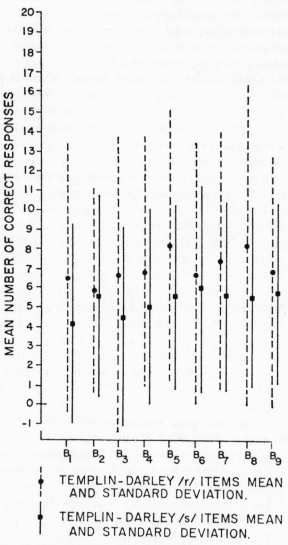

FIG. 4. Means and standard deviations for the /s/ and /r/ items from the Templin-Darley Diagnostic Articulation Test. Maximum possible scores were 31 for /r/ items and 17 for /s/ items.

none of the other Ss appear to have made improvement on any of the articulation measures, we must conclude that the treatment used did not influence articulation.

Throughout training, the experimental Ss required fewer drawing sets and made fewer errors than the control Ss. This indicates that oral study of the forms did contribute to performance within each training set. However, since both experimental and control Ss improved their performance as they progressed from set to set, it seems unlikely that improvement in performance involved use of oral form recognition. It is also unlikely that oral form recognition skill increased. As the training procedure progressed, Ss gradually learned and remembered which drawings constituted the correct choices. By the time the experimental Ss began the second or third training set, most were able to point to appropriate drawings from previously passed training sets without having the forms placed in the mouth. By probe 3, two Ss were able to point to every review drawing correctly without taking the forms into the mouth. Perhaps the information provided when a correct response was made was all that was needed to assure improved performance across training sets. However, Ss may also have improved their test taking ability through the course of the study.

The findings did not show improvement in articulation in the children who underwent the oral task and repeated articulation testing. Wilhelm concluded that his study, which used the same training procedure, did show such improvement. Since different articulation tests were used in the two studies, it is possible that Wilhelm's Ss may have had more serious articulation problems and consequently had greater opportunity for improvement. However, Ss in the current study were far from ceiling performance on any articulation measure used. In the current study, the 141-item Templin-Darley test and the 34-item syllable test were administered nine times whereas Wilhelm administered his 296-item test 11 times. Also, his test included isolated phones whereas the current testing did not. Consequently, Wilhelm's procedures provided a greater amount of articulation practice and stimulation with more kinds of items than were used in the current study. The two studies also used different procedures for scoring articulation test results. Rather than using consensus scores, Wilhelm assigned a point for each of the three judges who marked a given response correct. Thus, for Wilhelm's 296-item test, the maximum score possible was 888. The authors plan to compare these two scoring procedures in research in progress.

The current results indicate that the oral form recognition training used by Wilhelm and duplicated here is not a suitable treatment for disordered articulation. Research cited earlier indicates that articulation and oral sensation are related. Such a relationship, however, does not indicate that manipulation of one variable is an effective means for influencing the other.

REFERENCES

ARNDT, W. B., ELBERT, M., & SHELTON, R. L. Standardization of a test of oral stereognosis. In J. F. Bosma (Ed.), *Second symposium on oral sensation and perception.* Springfield, Ill.: Thomas, 1970. Pp. 379-383.

LOCKE, J. L. Oral perception and articulation learning. *Perceptual and Motor Skills*, 1968, 26, 1259-1264.

RINGEL, R. L., HOUSE, A. S., BURK, K. W., BOLINSKY, J. P., & SCOTT, C. M. Some relations between orosensory discrimination and articulatory aspects of speech production. *Journal of Speech and Hearing Disorders*, 1970, 35, 3-11.

WILHELM, C. L. The effects of oral form recognition training on articulation in children. Unpublished Ph.D. dissertation, Univer. of Kansas, 1971.

OROSENSORY PERCEPTION, SPEECH PRODUCTION, AND DEAFNESS

MILO E. BISHOP *and* ROBERT L. RINGEL

ARTHUR S. HOUSE

The oral form-discrimination abilities of 18 orally edu ated and oriented deaf high school subjects were determined and compared to those of manually educated and oriented deaf subjects and normal-hearing subjects. The similarities and differences among the responses of the three groups were discussed and then compared to responses elicited from subjects with functional disorders of articulation. In general, the discrimination scores separated the manual deaf from the other two groups, particularly when differences in form shapes were involved in the test. The implications of the results for theories relating orosensory-discrimination abilities are discussed. It is postulated that, while a failure in oroperceptual functioning may lead to disorders of articulation, a failure to use the oral mechanism for speech activities, even in persons with normal orosensory capabilities, may result in poor performance on oroperceptual tasks.

The positive relationship between speech skills and the ability to recognize and compare the form of small plastic objects by means of oral exploration is well established. Five independent investigations (Moser, LaGourgue, and Class, 1967; Ringel et al., 1968; Rossman, 1970; Edwards, 1970; Weinberg, Liss, and Hillis, 1970) have shown that articulatory-defective speakers with no known organic or structural pathologies have less success than their normal-speaking counterparts in recognizing forms placed in the mouth. Furthermore, Ringel et al. (1970) have shown that measurements of oral form discrimination differentiate between degrees of articulatory proficiency established a priori by independent means. The nature of the relationship between speech skills and oral form recognition, however, is not clear. Assuming that retention, anatomical maturation, and motor development are underlying processes for both speech and oral form recognition, the question of whether sensory-discrimination abilities and speech development exist in a cause-effect relationship, or whether they are both related to more general factors, such as neurological maturation or perceptual skill development, is an open one.

The nature of this relationship is clarified, in part at least, by Edwards' (1970) results, showing that articulatory defective talkers who had performed worse than their normal-speaking peers on a test of oral form discrimination

JOURNAL OF SPEECH AND HEARING RESEARCH, 1973, vol. 16, no. 2, 257-266.

did not perform inferiorly when the forms were explored in the hand. This finding indicates that differential performance on oral form discrimination is not attributable to differences in the development of general perceptual skill or general neurological maturation, but rather to deficits related to the ability to process, store, recall, and compare sensory/motor information received from the oral periphery.

MacNeilage (1970) hypothesizes that a talker develops a spatial concept of his oral cavity for use when he integrates tactile and kinesthetic feedback from an articulator with its projected motor activity to effect an accurate movement of that articulator toward a particular target position within the oral spatial field. Consequently, the inability of a talker to accomplish this will result in deviant speech patterns. Since many of the same skills are involved in tasks of oral form recognition, it is reasonable to postulate that performance on a test of oral form discrimination is a reflection of the ability to use these skills in speaking.

The relationship between orosensory discrimination and speech development is of particular importance to the speech development of deaf children. When auditory function is lost, the talker must rely on the orosensory mechanism for tactile, kinesthetic, and proprioceptive information to acquire and stabilize the motor gestures of speech. A deaf child's ability to use orosensory information may determine his ability to acquire intelligible speech. Nevertheless, relatively little is known about the characteristics of the orosensory processes in the deaf population. Bishop, Ringel, and House (1972) tested the orosensory acuity and form discrimination of congenitally deaf high school students who routinely use manual communication. Compared to a similar group of hearing students, the deaf group possessed essentially normal sensory acuity as indicated by measures of two-point discrimination, but performed poorly on the oral form-discrimination task. Subsequent testing revealed that when the forms were explored in the hand, the deaf and normal students made essentially the same number of errors, suggesting that the differential performance of the manual deaf on oral form discrimination was not due to some general cognitive deficit, but rather to deficits related to the oral channel of sensory input. The present report summarizes an investigation of the oroperceptual abilities of deaf individuals who use speech as their primary means of communication and compares its results to those obtained earlier.

PROCEDURES

The stimulus ensemble was a restricted version of one developed by Rossman (1970) to investigate the relative importance of size and shape difference to oral form discrimination. The Rossman ensemble consisted of 12 forms representing four geometric categories, with each category occurring in three sizes. The index of size was taken arbitrarily to be area. Nine forms from this earlier ensemble were selected for use and are identified in Figure 1. The test forms, therefore, represent three geometric categories (triangle, square, and

353

parallelogram) each in three sizes. They consist of a clear, heat-resistant inert plastic, approximately ⅛ inch thick. This ensemble provided a total of 45 comparisons when each form was paired with every other form and itself; nine comparisons were of the same tokens (that is, identical forms presented consecutively), and 36 comparisons were of different tokens (that is, the forms in each pair differed in shape or area).

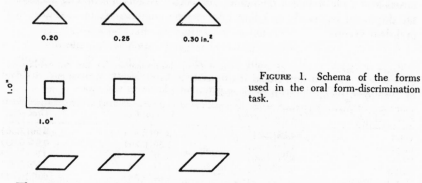

FIGURE 1. Schema of the forms used in the oral form-discrimination task.

The testing procedures were similar to those described earlier by Bishop et al. (1972). In essence, a test form was placed in the mouth of a blindfolded subject who was allowed to manipulate it within the oral cavity. The form was then removed and in its place a comparison form was immediately introduced. The subject's task was to specify whether the second form was the *same* as the first form, or *different*. Instructions to the subjects were given orally or manually, and responses were made orally or manually. Before data collection, informal testing was done to ensure that the task was understood. The order of presentation of pairs was randomized for each subject, and the order of presentation of the two items of a given pair was established by chance a priori. In the testing, response bias in favor of *different* was minimized by allowing the identical or *same* pairs to be presented an additional time. Before data analysis, these additional *same* items were removed so as not to confound the data by mixing responses to pairs compared twice with those compared only once.

A group of 18 deaf high school students, orally trained at the Clarke School for the Deaf, served as subjects. According to school records, each student had, since birth, a better-ear hearing loss in the speech-frequency range of more than 90 dB ISO. The ages of the students ranged from 15 to 18 years; all subjects were of normal intelligence. This group of subjects was selected to be comparable to the two groups of subjects tested previously by Bishop et al. (1972). The earlier groups each contained 18 subjects matched approximately for age, sex, and intelligence. One group had normal hearing and attended public high schools, while the other group was made up of deaf subjects enrolled at the Indiana School for the Deaf where their training was primarily in the manual mode.

The data of this study are the errors made on the oral form-discrimination task. Errors result when the subject asserts that two forms are different which are of the same size and shape (identical error), and when the subject asserts that two forms are the same which are of different size (size error), different shape (shape error), or both (size and shape error). The mean number of errors and their standard deviations for each category (including the total) are displayed separately in Table 1 for the normal-hearing, manual-deaf, and oral-deaf groups.

TABLE 1. Mean number of errors in oral form discrimination for the normal-hearing, manual-deaf, and oral-deaf groups. Each mean is based on 18 observations. Standard deviation associated with each mean is in parentheses following that mean.

Error Category	Normal Hearing	Manual Deaf	Oral Deaf
Total	4.83(2.24)	9.39(2.87)	5.56(2.36)
Identical	1.72(1.09)	1.50(0.96)	0.94(0.85)
Size	2.11(1.66)	4.11(1.37)	3.50(2.22)
Shape	0.61(0.59)	1.72(1.04)	0.50(0.69)
Size and shape	0.39(0.75)	2.06(1.58)	0.67(0.82)

To facilitate interpretation of the data, a separate analysis of variance was conducted for each of the four error categories (Winer, 1971, p. 149). These analyses revealed there was a significant difference among the groups in total errors ($F = 16.23$; $df = 2,53$; $p < 0.001$), size errors ($F = 5.60$; $df = 2,53$; $p < 0.01$), shape errors ($F = 12.19$; $df = 2,53$; $p < 0.001$), and size and shape errors ($F = 10.89$; $df = 2,53$; $p < 0.005$). There were no differences among the groups in the identical error category ($F = 2.89$; $df = 2,53$). In the categories where differences were found, a Newman-Keuls probing technique (Winer, 1971, p. 195) was used to determine which of the groups differed significantly. In the shape error category, size and shape error category, and total errors, differences among groups were the result of differences between the manual-deaf group and the other two groups; in these categories, the oral deaf and the normal hearing were not different from each other but both differed from the manual deaf. In the size error category, the manual deaf and the normal hearing were different from each other, but were not different from the oral deaf.

These results show that the oral-deaf group and normal-hearing group made essentially the same number of errors in each category. This is not the case for the oral-deaf and manual-deaf groups. The oral-deaf scores resembled the manual-deaf scores only in the identical and size error categories; the oral deaf made significantly fewer errors than the manual deaf in the shape and the size and shape error categories.

The comparisons made here are always within one of the error categories. To compare performances in the various error categories it is necessary to convert mean errors into error percentages, since the opportunity for error was not the same in each category. Error percentages for the three groups were computed separately for each of the error categories by dividing the number of errors made in a given category by the number of opportunities for error in that category. The resulting percentages reflect the rate at which errors occurred; these error rates are displayed in Table 2. As shown in the first line

TABLE 2. Oral form-discrimination error rates (%) for the normal-hearing, manual-deaf, and oral-deaf groups.

Error Category	Normal Hearing	Manual Deaf	Oral Deaf
Total	11	21	12
Identical	20	17	10
Size	23	44	39
Shape	7	19	6
Size and shape	2	12	4

of the table, the oral-deaf group made essentially the same percentage of total errors as the normal-hearing group, while the manual-deaf group made nearly twice that many. Essentially the same relationship existed in the two error categories where shape was a critical parameter. In each of these categories the error rates for the normal-hearing and the oral-deaf groups were very similar, while the error rates for the manual-deaf group were nearly three times greater.

In the size and identical error categories the relationship between the groups changes. The oral deaf failed to detect size differences at a rate 16% higher than the normal-hearing group, but 5% lower than the manual-deaf group. In the identical error category the relationship between the oral-deaf and normal-hearing groups is reversed, with the oral-deaf group making half as many errors (10% fewer) as the normal-hearing group. In this category, the manual-deaf and the normal-hearing groups performed essentially the same. Examination of the confusions for the shape error categories shows that the normal-hearing and oral-deaf groups behaved approximately the same.

TABLE 3. Oral form-discrimination error rates (%) associated with each shape combination.

Shape Combination	Normal Hearing	Oral Deaf	Manual Deaf
Triangle vs square	0	1	5
Triangle vs parallelogram	11	12	34
Square vs parallelogram	0	0	3

This similarity is reflected further in Table 3, which displays the percentage of errors made by the three groups for each of three possible shape combinations. In this table, shape errors and size and shape errors have been pooled so that the numbers in the table represent all errors incident to a particular shape combination. Clearly the normal-hearing and oral-deaf groups had no difficulty distinguishing triangles and parallelograms from squares, as evidenced by the fact that the oral-deaf subjects made only one such error (0.3%), and the normal group made no errors of that type. The manual-deaf group, however, experienced some difficulties in making this discrimination, as reflected in an average error rate of 5% for triangles vs squares and 3% for squares vs parallelograms. The fact that the majority of the errors occurred when triangles and parallelograms were paired suggests that angle, rather than the number of sides, was the principal parameter upon which decisions involving shape were based. Considering the overall similarity in the behavior of the oral-deaf and normal-hearing groups, it is perplexing that the oral-deaf made 10% fewer identical errors and 16% more size errors than the normal-hearing group. If the errors made in these two categories are pooled, however, the resulting error rates are once again very similar, being 22 and 25% for the normal-hearing and oral-deaf groups, respectively. It is possible, therefore, that errors made in these categories are not independent.

Recall that a size error is a failure to detect a difference between the sizes of identically shaped forms; on the other hand, an identical error is the "detection" of a nonexistent difference between identical stimuli. In performing the form-discrimination task the observer must establish internal criteria upon which to base his decision of *same* or *different*. These criteria can be set, for example, to avoid identical errors by permitting a judgment of *different* to be made only when differences are absolutely identifiable. Such a strategy, while eliminating identical errors, increases the number of size or shape errors. In the present study the effect of such a strategy would be greater on size than on shape errors, since differences in size were more difficult to detect than differences in shape. Of course, when the observer selects criteria designed to eliminate errors when tokens differ, the effect would be reversed.

In our investigation the oral-deaf group "detected" nonexistent differences only 10% of the time they had the opportunity to do so, and failed to detect actual differences in size 39% of the time. Their performance is consistent with a strategy that seeks to reduce identical errors at the cost of size errors by responding *same* when they are uncertain. However, when shape was the critical parameter, the oral deaf had essentially the same error rate as the hearing group.

Comparison of the oral-deaf and manual-deaf groups shows the manual deaf made approximately 8% more errors in each category, indicating that although they used a similar response strategy, they were unable to perceive differences in the forms with the same efficiency as either the normal-hearing or oral-deaf groups. This is particularly evident for the shape errors, where the manual deaf made three to six times more errors than the oral-deaf and normal-hearing subjects. It is this category of error which has consistently differentiated between normal and defective talkers in previous studies (Ringel et al., 1968, 1970; Rossman, 1970; Edwards, 1970).

357

DISCUSSION

These results can be compared directly to responses collected from a group of normal talkers and a group of talkers with functional defects of articulation (Rossman, 1970); the latter made errors on 17% of their total trials, while the former made errors 11% of the time. To facilitate the comparison of Rossman's findings with those of this experiment, the results of both investigations are shown in Table 4.

TABLE 4. Oral form-discrimination error rates (%) from Table 3 along with results for normal and articulatory defective subjects from Rossman (1970).

Error Category	Normal Hearing	Oral Deaf	Manual Deaf	Articulatory Defective	Normal Speaking
Total	11	12	21	17	11
Identical	20	10	17	45	24
Size	23	39	44	27	24
Shape	7	6	19	9	2
Size and shape	2	4	12	3	1

There are a number of similarities in the results of these experiments; in both, the normal subjects performed at an overall error rate of 11% and generated similar percentages of errors for identical and size categories, suggesting that the two groups employed equivalent response strategies. In the remaining error categories, however, where shape is a critical parameter, Rossman's normal subjects made fewer errors than the normal subjects in the Bishop et al. (1972) experiment.

When the manual-deaf and articulatory-defective groups are compared, similarities as well as differences can be observed. Both groups made substantially more errors (total) than their normal controls. The distributions of errors, however, suggest the two groups employed different response strategies. The relatively high level of identical errors for the articulation-defective group suggests they used very relaxed criteria for responding *different*, while the manual-deaf group, with its low level of identical errors, required gross differences before responding *different*. This interpretation is compatible with the fact that these two groups generated grossly different error rates in categories where shape is a critical parameter. If, for example, the articulatory-defective group actually used, as suggested, a response strategy which called for responding *different* whenever differences were suspected, the number of errors resulting from a failure to detect a difference would be reduced. Consequently, shape errors would occur less frequently, since they result from a failure to detect a difference in shape.

In spite of apparent difference in response strategy, the fact remains that the manual-deaf and the articulatory-defective groups made substantially more errors than their normal-hearing and speaking controls. Furthermore, when the effect of response strategy is partially neutralized by pooling the identical and size errors, the behavior of these two groups becomes more alike. It is tempting to speculate, therefore, that deficiencies in oral form discrimination may be a sign of deficit in some underlying mechanism central to the development and refinement of speech articulation.

If we can assume, as Ladefoged (1967) has suggested, that speech is a skilled body action like typing, piano playing, or golfing, then the facility with which the motor patterns of speech are acquired and refined is related to the efficiency with which sensory information is stored and processed and finally integrated with motor activity. Presumably this delicate sensory/motor interaction plays a major role in restructuring and refining executed articulatory patterns so as to make them consistent with patterns appropriate to the talker's phonological competence. The differential abilities of athletes to coordinate, refine, and stabilize motor patterns is well known. It seems reasonable that analogous differences also characterize the abilities of talkers to develop, refine, execute, and synergize the actions required for speech. If individuals are differentially endowed with these abilities as previously suggested, their distributions over the human population can be expected to approximate a gaussian function. Individuals whose poor orosensory faculties place them far to the left of the means of these putative distributions, all other factors being equal, would be likely candidates to exhibit delayed articulation or so-called functional disorders of articulation. Conversely, individuals far to the right of the means of such distributions would learn to execute articulatory gestures with better than normal success.

Experimental support for this hypothesis has been reported by Ringel et al. (1970) and Locke (1968). Ringel et al. demonstrated, for example, that measurements of oral discrimination similar to those used in our experiment could differentiate between degrees of articulatory proficiency established independently a priori. In other words, their results showed that subjects who had been judged previously to have severe disorders of articulation performed more poorly than subjects judged to have moderate disorders. Locke (1968) tested the ability of subjects having widely different orosensory abilities to learn speech sounds strange to their native language. He found that subjects who had done well on tasks of oral form discrimination learned the strange sounds more readily than those who had done poorly on the discrimination tasks.

The ideas that articulatory proficiency is a function of the talker's ability to coordinate sensory information and motor activity, and that this ability differs in various talkers, are compatible with the finding that the oral-deaf and the manual-deaf groups demonstrated real differences in discriminating oral forms. These ideas are not sufficient to explain these differences, however, since it seems incorrect to assume that the manual students (attending the Indiana School for the Deaf) are all poorly endowed with the potential abilities that allow articulatory skills to develop adequately. In fact, these students were not classified (that is, determined to be) manual on the basis of their failure to develop speech skills, but rather on the basis of the manual mode of communication and instruction emphasized at the school they attended.

If both groups of deaf subjects were, in fact, equally prepared to develop speech skills, how can the better performance on oral form discrimination of the oral deaf be explained? An answer might be sought in the method used to form the groups, which in this study was done according to the mode of communication and instruction used at the schools the subjects attended (without regard for their actual speech skills). The manual-deaf group routinely used manual methods in school; the oral-deaf group routinely used oral methods and received daily assistance in developing speech skills. Conceivably their performance differences are a function of their practice in using speech skills. Such an interpretation suggests that the normal development of the ability to integrate orosensory and oromotor activity in tasks such as those used in these studies is retarded when speech activities are reduced! An alternative argument might be that the admission practices at Clarke School for the Deaf are selective enough to guarantee that the oral-deaf group differs significantly from the manual-deaf group on some intellectual or cognitive dimension that is reflected in the oral form-discrimination scores. Such a point of view should predict that the manual-deaf group also will perform poorly when form discrimination is tested in the hand—and this, of course, is not the case. We are led, therefore, to the conclusion that the different abilities of these deaf groups in discriminating forms in the month is indicative of their abilities to effectively integrate orosensorimotor functions underlying speech articulation. Furthermore, the reduced ability of the manual deaf to integrate such activity is not attributable to some deficit or difference in innate capacity, but rather the result of not having used speech enough to adequately develop this integrative behavior.

These observations should not be interpreted as an argument against the idea that a failure in oroperceptual functioning may lead to disorders of articulation. Even in persons with normal orosensory capabilities, a failure to use the oral mechanism for speech activities may result in depressed functioning on tasks involving oroperception, and there may be an interactive relationship between speech functions and orosensorimotor control mechanisms. While the ability to refine speech performance is contingent upon the ability to integrate orosensory and oromotor activity, the development of this integrative ability, in part at least, depends on articulatory practice.

ACKNOWLEDGMENT

Appreciation is expressed to the faculty and students of the Indiana State and Clarke schools for the deaf for their cooperation and assistance in this investigation. This investigation was supported in part by Public Health Service Awards 2 RO1 DE 02815-04 from the National Institute for Dental Research, and the Air Force Cambridge Research Laboratories.

REFERENCES

BISHOP, M. E., RINGEL, R. L., and HOUSE, A. S., Orosensory perception in the deaf. *Volta Rev.*, 74, 289-298 (1972).

EDWARDS, E. R., A comparative study of form perception, kinesthetic and spatial orientation abilities in articulatory defective and normal-speaking children. Master's thesis, Purdue Univ. (1970).

LADEFOGED, P., *Three Areas of Experimental Phonetics*. London: Oxford Univ. Press (1967).

LOCKE, J. L., Oral perception and articulation learning. *Percept. mot. Skills*, 26, 1259-1264 (1968).

MACNEILAGE, D. F., Motor control of serial ordering of speech. *Psychol. Rev.*, 77, 182-196 (1970).

MOSER, H., LAGOURGUE, J. R., and CLASS, L., Studies of oral stereognosis in normal, blind and deaf subjects. In J. F. Bosma (Ed.), *Symposium on Oral Sensation and Perception*. Springfield, Ill.: Charles C Thomas (1967).

RINGEL, R. L., BURK, K. W., and SCOTT, C. M., Tactile perception: Form discrimination in the mouth. *Brit. J. dis. Commun.*, 3, 150-155 (1968).

RINGEL, R. L., HOUSE, A. S., BURK, K. W., DOLINSKY, J. P., and SCOTT, C. M., Some relations between oral sensory discrimination and articulatory aspects of speech production. *J. Speech Hearing Dis.*, 35, 3-11 (1970).

ROSSMAN, A., The effects of controlling stimulus size and shape upon oral form discrimination in articulatory defective and normal speakers. Master's thesis, Purdue Univ. (1970).

WEINBERG, B., LISS, G. M., and HILLIS, J., A comparative study of visual, manual and oral form identification in speech impaired and normal speaking children. In J. F. Bosma (Ed.), *Second Symposium on Oral Sensation and Perception*. Springfield, Ill.: Charles C Thomas (1970).

WINER, B. J., *Statistical Principles in Experimental Design*. (2nd ed.) New York: McGraw Hill (1971).

ORAL PERCEPTION: 1. TWO-POINT DISCRIMINATION

ROBERT L. RINGEL *and* STANLEY J. EWANOWSKI

Various oral structures were evaluated in 25 normal subjects, in order to gather normative data for selected parameters of tactile perception. Results revealed a significant progression of maximal to minimal discriminatory capacity and a tendency toward increased discriminatory ability at the midline aspect of the structures.

The importance of auditory, kinesthetic, and tactile sensory feedback in the total speech servo-mechanism has been hypothesized by Fairbanks (1954), Van Riper and Irwin (1958), and Mysak (1959). These authors have stated that a disruption in the proper functioning of such input channels may result in disordered speech output.

To date the principal source of information related to the speech monitoring mechanism has centered about the auditory system. This system has been explored extensively and data (i.e., acuity, retention, discrimination) are available which have proved useful in understanding the neuro- and psycho-physiological mechanisms which underlie the auditory system and which facilitate the evaluation of responses from persons who do not develop normal speech due to suspected auditory disturbances.

Although much normative information is available for assessing the functioning of the auditory mechanism, relatively little data that would allow similar understanding and evaluation of the tactile system have been presented.

For the most part, the only information regarding the contribution of tactile monitoring during speech production, by itself or in interaction with other sensory feedback channels, has been inferential in nature and has resulted from studies dealing with experimentally induced states of oral region tactile deprivation (McCroskey, 1958; Ringel and Steer, 1963) and from observations of the speech performance of persons with neuro-sensory diseases which produce somato-sensory disturbances (McDonald and Chusid, 1962). In general, it appears that alterations of normal speech related oral-tactile perceptions result in speech output disturbances. In addition, it has been observed that a significantly high incidence of lingual agnosia occurs among speech defective populations (Palmer, Wurth, and Kincheloe, 1963) and that perceptual difficulties, involving the various sensory modalities, may serve as a causative factor in speech and language agenesis (Lorenze, Sokoloff, and Cruz, 1962; Berry and Eisenson, 1956). While these observations are of clinical importance, they are related to

JOURNAL OF SPEECH AND HEARING RESEARCH, 1965, vol. 8, 389-398.

experimental or clinical observations of relatively severe conditions of sensory deprivation and provide limited insight into the more subtle states of sensory dysfunctioning that may contribute to rendering speech "disordered."

The lack of normative data on "oral-region tactile system" functioning and the associated lack of procedures for effectively evaluating the receptive capacities of this region is unfortunate inasmuch as it has been demonstrated that such information gathered from exploration of other regions of the body is extremely valuable at an applied level in the clinical assessment of various forms of neuro- and myopathologies. Specifically, it is a recognized fact that characteristic modes of perceptual response to tactile stimulation are associated with such disease entities as tabes dorsalis, Brown-Sequard syndrome, neuritis, multiple sclerosis, and muscular dystrophy (McDonald and Chusid, 1962; Forster, 1962). It has also been reported that patients suffering with "motor disorders" showed significantly poor performances on tests of tactile acuity and discrimination (Wienstien, 1954, 1955).

At a more basic level, information regarding the oral region's discriminatory capacity may provide, in part, the foundation for the further elaboration of theories of cutaneous sensitivity. It is apparent that the classical Pressure, Gradient, and Tension theories of skin sensitivity are based upon the nature of responses subjects gave to various forms of stimulation (Geldard, 1953). More recently, Nafe and Kenshalo (1960), in rejecting these earlier theories in favor of one claiming "movement of non-specific nerve terminations" as the effective common stimulus for cutaneous sensation, state that detailed sensory testing procedures are an essential element of the most direct approach for gaining insights into the mechanism of cutaneous sensation.

The application of techniques and instrumentation developed for the study of tactile receptivity in many regions of the body is often inappropriate for the study of oral region mechanisms due to the relative inaccessibility of many of the oral structures and to the obvious disadvantages of interfering with normal structure functioning. In addition, the histologically and functionally unique characteristics of the oral region severely limit generalizations to oral structures from data obtained from "non-speech" involved regions (Gairns, 1955; Silverman, 1961).

Within this framework a series of investigations was undertaken. The purpose of these studies was to develop a battery of procedures for use in tactile assessments of the oral region and to provide a store of normative data against which information obtained from subsequent investigations with speech deviant persons might be compared, and upon which theoretical constructs might be built. Separate reports, of which this is the first, will discuss each of the various aspects of the total research program.

TWO-POINT DISCRIMINATION

It has been reported that measures of two-point discrimination, the minimum separation of two punctiform stimuli that can be discriminated as two, provide an index to a basic discriminatory process; one that may be considered the prototype of sensory discrimination in all sense modalities (Ruch, 1951).

Early theorists hypothesized that the relationship between the size of the skin area served by a single neuron (a sensory circle) and the presence of interposed unexcited fibers between two such "circles" provide the neurophysiological basis of "two-point" perceptions. Present evidence, however, does not confirm this static concept but rather supports a more dynamic view of such perceptions. This latter approach involves a process, executed within the nervous system, in which a spatial discrimination involves the interaction of such factors as the size and density of innervation of the receptive field, the intensity and location of the stimulus, and the effects of afferent inhibition of areas surrounding the site of stimulation. A detailed description of these interactions is presented by Mountcastle and Powell (1959).

Tests of two-point discrimination are generally included in neurological evaluations. Standard texts of clinical neurology, which provide the examiner with procedural instructions and normative data for selected regions of the body, state that valuable diagnostic and therapeutic insights into a patient's level of perceptual functioning may be gained through this test (Forster, 1962; McDonald and Chusid, 1962). As noted earlier, however, the available techniques are generally not appropriate for use in the oral region. The purpose of the present investigation was to establish such procedures and normative data as are applicable in evaluating the two-point discriminatory capacities of selected oral structures.

METHOD

Subjects. Twenty female and five male university students served as subjects in this investigation. The age range of this group was 18-29 years, with a mean age of 20.6 years. All of the subjects were judged free of speech defects, reported no present or past history of neuro-sensory and/or neuro-motor disturbances, and indicated a right-hand preference. Each subject had refrained from eating or smoking for at least 30 minutes prior to the test session.

Instrumentation. The oral esthesiometer developed for use in this study is shown in Figure 1. This instrument facilitated the investigation of two-point

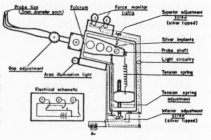

FIGURE 1. The oral esthesiometer. This instrument permits investigations of two-point discrimination capacity at both extra-oral and relatively inaccessible intra-oral sites under regulated conditions of contactor-skin (mucosa) force and stimulus point separation.

discrimination capacity at extra-oral and relatively inaccessible intra-oral sites. The esthesiometer also provided a means for calibrating and controlling the distance between the two stimulus points and the contactor—skin (mucosa) force. This latter factor was deemed important since it has been shown that tactile sensitivity varies with the force the transducer exerts against the skin surface (Bartley, 1958). Specifically, a pair of lights mounted on the instrument allows the experimenter to monitor, and thereby control, the amount of force exerted upon the skin surface by the stimulus points.

When the instrument is "unloaded," that is, when less than one gram of force is exerted in a downward direction on the probe points, the force of the tension spring is great enough to pull the shaft downward and cause it to contact the tip of the inferior adjustment screw. This contact results in a "closed circuit" and a subsequent illumination of the posterior bulb. When a force greater than one gram is exerted upon the probe points, as might occur when the points are displaced through contact with the skin surface, the shaft is lifted from its rest position and is balanced about a fulcrum between the two screws until the force exceeds three grams. At this point (> 3 grams) the shaft is lifted to the extent that it contacts the superiorly inserted screw and thereby closes the circuit associated with the anteriorly situated light bulb. Both the probe shaft and the adjustment screw tips were "silvered" to facilitate circuit closure. Hence the investigator was able to maintain a force $> 1 < 3$ grams on the probe points by keeping both lights off (both circuits open). Measurements of two-point limen were taken only during such periods. The distance between the stimulus probe points (the gap) is adjusted by means of a calibration knob which is mounted on the horizontal aspect of the probe arms; this knob is calibrated in .5mm increments and allows for a range of probe tip separation from 0-10mm.

The force and gap measures are calibrated by weight suspension and micrometer procedures respectively. The force range of 1-3 grams was found satisfactory for this study in pilot investigations; other ranges can be set, however, via the adjustment of screw insertion depth and spring tension. That is, the greater the distance between the superior screw tip and the shaft, the greater is the force necessary to bring them into contact, and the greater the tension of the spring, the greater is the force necessary to overcome its downward pull and thereby lift the shaft from its contact with the inferior screw tip.

Procedure. Each subject was blindfolded and seated in a dental chair with his head cradled in the head rest at a 45° angle. The specific anatomical areas under investigation were marked with a dye to insure consistency of location in successive stimuli presentations. The subjects were instructed to indicate whether they felt one or two stimulus points by depressing a signal button in a previously instructed manner. A period devoted to subject orientation and familiarization with the experimental task was conducted prior to collecting data.

The stimuli were presented to the selected regions at contactor—skin (mucosa) force levels within the predetermined range in both ascending and descending patterns (successive increments or decrements in distance between probe points respectively) in discrete steps of 0.5mm. The probe tips were left in contact with the skin surface for approximately a two sec period. The procedure followed was a modification of the technique of "limits" described by Stevens (1951).

Both ascending and descending procedures were followed three times in accordance with a random order; the median value of each of the two series was determined; subsequently these median values were converted into a mean score which was used to represent a subject's two-point limen score. Hence, the values presented in this study represent those obtained from three ascending and three descending trials.

The subjects were cautioned to report "two-points," in the ascending series, as soon as clear duality was noted and not when a hint of departure from singleness was experienced. This caution was in accordance with the philosophy that the former (clear duality) is the true two-point limen, and in recognition that the transition from one to two points is not perceptually clean-cut but rather passes through a series of intermediate stages (i.e., point, line, circle, oval, etc.) before it becomes two clearly distinct points (Jenkins, 1951). Response to different aspects of this transition may result in variable limen measures.

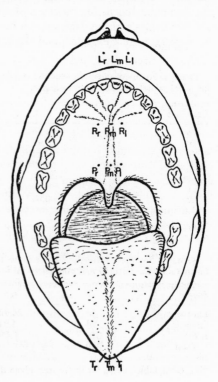

FIGURE 2. Selected oral region sites of two-point stimulation. Key: T—tonguetip, L—upper lip, P—soft palate, R—alveolar ridge, l—left side, m—midline, and r—right side.

Cautions bearing upon the effects of the reverse of this phenomenon during the descending trials were also given to the subjects.

The above procedures were used to test each subject's two-point discrimination ability at the upper lip, tongue tip, alveolar ridge, and soft palate at three positions; right side, midline, and left side as indicated in Figure 2. In addition, two extra-oral sites were stimulated, the thenar eminence of the right hand and the finger tip of the right middle finger. These 14 regions were stimulated in a random order.

RESULTS AND DISCUSSION

The mean and standard deviation two-point limen values, as determined for the selected anatomical regions, are shown in Table 1. These values indicate that differential discriminatory capacities exist among the structures evaluated and that, in general, the progression from maximal to minimal awareness of two-point stimulation involves the tongue tip, finger tip, lip, soft palate, alveolar ridge, and thenar structures in that order, respectively. To determine the possible significance of these variations, the data were subjected to an analysis of variance procedure. The results of this analysis, summarized in Table 2, indicate the presence of significant differences ($p = .05$) among the values representing the two-point limens for various oral and/or extra-oral anatomical structures. Further analysis of the data through the application of critical difference tests (at $p = .05$) were conducted, and the results are summarized in Table 3. It is

TABLE 1. Summary table of mean and standard deviation two-point limen values (in mm) for selected oral and extra-oral locations.

Locations	Mean	S.D.	Locations	Mean	S.D.
Tm[*]	1.70	0.46	Pm	2.64	1.10
Tr	1.72	0.47	Rm	2.66	1.09
Tl	1.82	0.41	Pl	2.95	1.17
F	2.09	0.57	Pr	3.06	1.26
Lm	2.31	0.72	Rr	3.20	1.29
Ll	2.47	0.84	Rl	3.21	1.39
Lr	2.49	0.69	TH	5.60	1.45

[*]Key: T—tonguetip, F—fingertip, L—upper lip, P—soft palate, R—alveolar ridge, TH—thenar region, l—left side, m—midline, and r—right side.

TABLE 2. Summary of analysis of variance to test differences among the mean two-point limen values for selected oral and extra-oral locations.

Source	df	ms	F	F.₀₅[*]
Locations	13	24.02	34.81	1.75
Subjects	24	4.04	5.85	1.52
L & S	312	0.69		
Total	349			

[*]F.₀₅ is the tabled value for the nearest given df.

TABLE 3. Summary of results of critical difference (C.D.) tests for significance of differences between mean two-point discrimination limen values for selected oral and extra-oral locations.[*]

Locations													
Tm	Tr	Tl	FT	Lm	Ll	Lr	Pm	Rm	Pl	Pr	Rr	Rl	TH
1.70	1.72	1.82	2.09	2.31	2.47	2.49	2.64	2.66	2.95	3.06	3.20	2.39	5.60

[*]Any mean values underscored by the same line are not significantly different from each other at the $p = .05$ level (C.D. $= .46$).

noted that the three tongue tip locations (Tm, r, l) are significantly more discriminate to the experimental stimuli than any other oral or extra-oral structure studied, regardless of position, with the exception of the finger tip (FT). In addition, the three lip positions (Lm, l, r) were significantly more discriminate than either of the left or right aspects of the alveolar ridge (Rl, r) and soft palate (Pl, r), but not significantly different from the midline region of these structures (Rm, Pm). Also, the right and left regions of the alveolar ridge (Rr, l) yield significantly greater limen values than the midline area of the alveolar ridge or soft palate (Rm, Pm, respectively).

Further inspection of Table 3 with regard to laterality reveals certain consistent data tendencies. Specifically, in those instances where the right, left, and midline regions of a particular structure were stimulated, the midline was always the most discriminate. This observation, however, while consistent, reached the level of statistical significance only for the alveolar ridge. No consistent pattern was noted among comparisons of thresholds determined for right and left aspects of the various oral structures.

When extra-oral sites are considered, it is reported that the finger tip (FT) is significantly more capable of the required discrimination than the other non-oral structure (TH) and the three aspects of the two palatal structures. The thenar region (TH) yielded significantly larger limen values than any of the other regions studied.

It has been hypothesized that the discriminatory ability of an area varies directly with the size of its cortical and thalamic projection areas (Mountcastle and Powell, 1959; Ruch, 1951). It has also been reported that the relative volume of tissue of the thalamic relay nuclei and of the post-central cortical gyrus which is devoted to a given peripheral area is directly related to the density of peripheral neural innervation of that region and inversely related to the size of the receptive fields contained within this peripheral area (Mountcastle and Powell, 1959; Granit, 1962). It appears thus that areas of maximal tactile sensitivity exhibit relatively large thalamic and cortical projection areas, dense peripheral neural innervation, and small receptive fields.

These observations are of interest with respect to the presently reported findings. The progression of discriminatory capacity for the selected structures, presented earlier in this paper, approximates the progression obtained when these structures are ordered on the basis of the relative size of their cortical and thalamic projection areas. This progression is also consistent with that obtained from the interpretation of Ruch's findings (1951). In addition, it has been reported that structures such as the finger tip and those found in the oral region exhibit relatively dense neural networks and small receptive fields when compared to areas like thenar eminence (Greishiemer, 1963). The finding of significance of differences among structures such as tongue, lip, and palate is consistent with the observation that a correspondence exists between the mobility of a structure and its discriminatory ability (Silverman, 1961; Shewchuk and Zubek, 1960).

The literature does not contain data concerning the absolute value of the two-point limen for all the regions tested in this investigation. For those structures that have been evaluated by other researchers, however, the present findings are generally compatible. Specifically, interpretation of Ruch's data reveals limen values of 1-2mm for the tongue tip, 2-3mm for the finger tip, and approximately 4mm for the upper lip (1951). Silverman (1961) presents threshold values in the order of 1.4mm and 2.0mm for the tongue tip and finger tip respectively. Grossman (1964) has also reported tongue tip two-point discrimination values of 2-3mm. The small discrepancies in values may be related to variation in the force exerted by the contactor upon the skin (mucosa) surface in the various investigations.

The observation that the two-point limen value is generally greater for the lateral aspects of a specific structure than for its midline plane is also consistent with previous research findings. Both Ruch (1951) and Grossman (1964) have reported greater limen values for the lateral aspects of the tongue tip when compared to measurements made along the axis of the lingual raphe.

The present authors were unable to find neurophysiologic or histologic data from a primary source that would explain these latter findings. Grossman (1964) has concluded, however, based upon his review of the histologic literature, that these results are compatible with regional variations in the density of neural elements. Explanations of this data, in addition to/or in lieu of the "density theory" may involve concepts based upon the existence of a facilitory effect when bilateral somato-sensory systems are stimulated simultaneously.

SUMMARY

The first in a series of experiments designed to gather normative data for selected parameters of oral region tactile perceptivity was conducted. These investigations were prompted by the belief that knowledge of the perceptual abilities of certain oral structures may yield greater insights into the role of tactile feedback in the total speech monitoring system. In addition, it was hypothesized that certain problems of speech output may be related to disturbed tactile—input signals from the oral sensing mechanisms.

For this study of two-point discrimination, instrumentation and procedures were developed that facilitated the evaluation of relatively inaccessible oral structures under controlled contactor—skin (mucosa) force and stimulus point separation. Results suggest the following statements.

(1) The progression from maximal to minimal discrimination of two-point stimulation involves the tongue tip, finger tip, lip, soft palate, alveolar ridge, and thenar regions in that order, respectively.

(2) Significant differences exist among the values representing the two-point limens for various oral and/or extra-oral structures.

(3) The midline aspect of a specific structure consistently yields a smaller limen value than either of its lateral aspects.

(4) The findings are generally consistent with previously reported neurophysiologic and histologic data and theory.

(5) The instrumentation and procedures developed for use in this study appear to be appropriate for this, and subsequent, investigations.

(6) Finally, the normative data presented may serve as a body of comparative information for future investigations with speech deviant populations.

This investigation was supported by Public Health Service Research Grant No. 3-TI-DE-103 from the National Institute of Dental Research, and by a Wisconsin Alumni Research Foundation Grant. The assistance of William Sturlaugson is acknowledged with appreciation.

REFERENCES

BARTLEY, S., Principles of Perception. New York: Harper (1958).

BERRY, M., and EISENSON, J., Speech Disorders: Principles and Practices of Therapy. New York: Appleton-Century-Crofts (1956).

FAIRBANKS, G., Systematic research in experimental phonetics. I. A theory of the speech mechanism as a servosystem. J. Speech Hearing Dis., 19, 133-140 (1954).

FORSTER, F., Synopsis of Neurology. St. Louis: Mosby (1962).

CAIRNS, F., The sensory nerve endings of the human palate. Quart. J. exper. Physiol., 40, 40-48 (1955).

GELDARD, F., The Human Senses. New York: Wiley (1953).

GRANIT, R., Receptors and Sensory Perception. New Haven: Yale University (1962).

GREISHIEMER, E., Physiology and Anatomy. Philadelphia: Lippincott (1963).

GROSSMAN, R., Methods for evaluating oral surface sensation. J. dent. Res., 43, 301 (1964).

JENKINS, W., Somesthesis. In S. S. Stevens (Ed.), Handbook of Experimental Psychology, New York: Wiley (1951).

LORENZE, E., SOKOLOFF, M., and CRUZ, R., Prognosis for deficiencies in speech accompanying cerebral palsy. Arch. phys. Med., xliii, 621-626 (1962).

MCCROSKEY, R., The relative contribution of auditory and tactile cues to certain aspects of speech. South. Speech J., 24, 84-90 (1958).

MCDONALD, J., and CHUSID, J., Correlative Neuroanatomy and Functional Neurology. California: Lange (1962).

MOUNTCASTLE, V., Some functional properties of the somatic afferent system. In W. A. Rosenblith (Ed.), Sensory Communication, New York: Wiley (1961).

MOUNTCASTLE, V., and POWELL, T., Neural mechanisms subserving cutaneous sensibility. Bull. Johns Hopkins Hosp., 105, 201-232 (1959).

370

MYSAK, E., A servo model for speech therapy. *J. Speech Hearing Dis.*, **24**, 144-149 (1949).
NAFE, J., and KENSHALO, D., Receptive capacities of the skin. In Hawkes, G. (Ed.) *Symposium on Cutaneous Sensitivity*, U.S. Army Med. Res. Lab. Report No. 424 (1960).
PALMER, M., WURTH, C., and KINCHELOE, J., Evaluation of selected variables in relation to articulatory deviations. *Asha*, **5**, 784 (1963).
RINGEL, R., and STEER, M., Some effects of tactile and auditory alterations on speech output. *J. Speech Hearing Res.*, **6**, 369-378 (1963).
RUCH, T., Sensory mechanisms. In S. S. Stevens (Ed.), *Handbook of Experimental Psychology*, New York: Wiley (1951).
SHEWCHUK, L., and ZUBEK, J., Discriminatory ability of various skin areas as measured by a technique of intermittent stimulation. *Canad. J. Psych.*, **14**, 244-248 (1960).
SILVERMAN, S., *Oral Physiology*. St. Louis: Mosby (1961).
STEVENS, S., Mathematics, measurement and psychophysics. In S. S. Stevens (Ed.), *Handbook of Experimental Psychology*, New York: Wiley (1951).
VAN RIPER, C., and IRWIN, J., *Voice and Articulation*. New Jersey: Prentice-Hall (1958).
WIENSTIEN, S., Weight judgment in somesthesis after penetrating injury to the brain. *J. comp. and physiol. Psych.*, **47**, 31-35 (1954).
WIENSTIEN, S., Tactile size judgment after penetrating injury to the brain. *J. comp. and physiol. Psych.*, **48**, 106-109 (1955).

371

ORAL TWO-POINT DISCRIMINATION: FURTHER EVIDENCE OF ASYMMETRY ON RIGHT AND LEFT SIDES OF SELECTED ORAL STRUCTURES[1]

NORMAN J. LASS, CYNTHIA L. KOTCHEK, JODELLE F. DEEM

Summary.—2-point discrimination thresholds were established on 13 test sites (the midline, right, and left sides of the upper lip, lower lip, tongue tip, and tongue dorsum, and on the finger tip) in each of 14 Ss. A total of 10 thresholds, 5 ascending and 5 descending, were obtained at each site. It was found that all Ss exhibited evidence of asymmetry in their 2-point limen values between the right and left sides of at least one of the 4 oral structures tested. The results provide further support for McCall and Cunningham's (1971) proposed theory of "sensory sidedness" as a normal neurological phenomenon of the tactile sensory system.

The current increased interest in the role of the tactile feedback system in the speech production process has led to the development of a variety of tests for assessment of tactile skills in the oral cavity. One such test is the test of oral two-point discrimination, which measures the minimum separation of two punctiform stimuli that an individual can perceive as two points.

From administration of this test to various groups of normal and speech defective individuals have come many interesting observations and consequently increased knowledge of oral sensory functioning. Ringel and Ewanowski (1965), employing a device called an "oral esthesiometer," explored the two-point discrimination capacity of a group of normal Ss on the tongue tip, alveolar ridge, soft palate, upper lip, and two extra-oral sites (thenar eminence and finger tip). Testing of the intra-oral structures included thresholds on midline, right, and left areas of each structure. They found that: (1) significant differences exist among two-point limen values for the oral and extra-oral structures; (2) the progression from maximal to minimal discrimination of two-point stimulation is as follows: tongue tip, finger tip, upper lip, soft palate, alveolar ridge, and thenar eminence; and (3) the midline region of a specific structure consistently yields a smaller limen value than either of its lateral margins. These findings have been corroborated by other investigators of oral two-point discrimination thresholds in normal Ss[2] (Grossman, 1964; Olroyd, 1965; Henkin & Banks, 1967; Addis, 1968).

However, a surprising observation was made in a study by McCall and Morgan (1966). Employing a modified caliper system for testing two-point

[1]This research was supported by an Institutional General Research Support Grant from the School of Medicine, West Virginia University.
[2]G. N. McCall & N. R. Morgan. Two-point discrimination: two-point limens on the tip and lateral margins of the tongue. (Unpublished manuscript, Louisiana State University Medical Center, 1966)

limen values on the tongue, they found that not only did their normal *S*s exhibit differences in thresholds on the lateral and midline regions of the tongue, but that in some *S*s the two-point limens for one lateral margin differed from those obtained on the other lateral margin. This observation had never been reported in previous studies concerned with oral two-point discrimination. In a follow-up study (McCall & Cunningham, 1971), they established two-point limen values on the left and right tongue margins of a group of 25 normal *S*s, considered to be representative of adult individuals with normal anatomical and physiological bodily mechanisms. They discovered that 14 of the 25 *S*s presented evidence of asymmetry in two-point discrimination ability. Of these 14 *S*s, nine exhibited lower limen values on the left side of the tongue, while five showed lower values on the right side.

This finding of asymmetry in two-point discrimination thresholds in 56% of their *S*s has led McCall and Cunningham (1971, p. 370) to suggest that ". . . 'sensory sidedness' may be a normal neurological phenomenon for the tactile sensory system."

McCall and Cunningham's (1971) observations of asymmetry were made only on the tongue region. Furthermore, their thresholds were obtained without controlling, other than through visual inspection of tissue deformation, for the pressure applied to the skin surface upon testing. The purpose of the present investigation was to pursue the study of symmetry of two-point limen values on the lateral margins of the tongue of normal individuals, and to extend such observations to include other oral structures in an attempt to corroborate or refute this proposed theory of sensory sidedness as a normal neurological phenomenon for the tactile sensory system.

METHOD

Eight sessions were required of each *S*: one screening and seven experimental sessions. In the screening session *S*s were selected. The seven experimental sessions were used for obtaining two-point limens at various test sites. The sessions were held in the Speech and Hearing Sciences Laboratory at West Virginia University.

Subjects

Fourteen individuals, 10 females and 4 males, served as *S*s. All were students at West Virginia University. They ranged in age from 18 to 24 yr., with a mean age of 20 yr. All *S*s had normal hearing, articulation, oral cavity structure, superficial tactile sensation, and neurological history and status. Eleven *S*s were right-handed, right-footed, and right-eyed, while three were left-handed, left-footed, and left-eyed.

Screening Session

The following tasks were included in the screening session: (1) a hearing screening evaluation; (2) the reading of a standard prose passage; (3) an oral peripheral examination; (4) two tests of superficial tactile sensation; (5) a questionnaire on neurological history and status; and (6) a series of tests to assess lateral dominance.

The hearing screening evaluation was performed on a Beltone Model 12-D portable audiometer from 500 through 8000 Hz at 20 dB (re: ISO, 1964). Individuals who failed any of the tested frequencies were excluded from the study.

The prose passage employed in the study was Van Riper's (1963) "My Grandfather" passage. The articulatory characteristics of each S were determined from the reading of this passage. Those with articulation defects were not included as Ss in the study.

The oral peripheral examination was used to assess the structural integrity of the oral cavity. Individuals with structural abnormalities of the oro-facial region were eliminated from the study.

The "Test of Light Touch" and "Test of Tactile Agnosia" (Mayo Clinic and Mayo Foundation, 1963) were employed to exclude individuals with defects in superficial tactile sensation. In the former test, S was instructed to close his eyes and to report by saying "yes" when he felt a wisp of cotton on his skin. Random presentations of a cotton wisp were made to the right and left hands, forearms, and face. A cotton-tipped applicator was used to assess sensation on the tongue. Individuals who reported no sensation on any single stimulus presentation were excluded from the study. In the latter test, S closed his eyes and was asked to identify by touch several common objects (spoon, watch, key, pencil, fork, and cup) which were placed in his right and left hands. Individuals who failed to identify any of the objects were not included in the study.

The questionnaire on neurological history and status was employed to eliminate individuals with any central nervous system disturbances.

The Harris Tests of Lateral Dominance (Harris, 1958) were used to determine the lateral dominance, including hand dominance, eye dominance, and foot dominance, of each S in the study.

Experimental Sessions

Test of two-point discrimination.—A specially constructed oral esthesiometer was used to obtain Ss' two-point discrimination thresholds. Fig. 1 shows the device used. It consists of a set of forceps attached to a dynamometer, thus allowing for the amount of pressure being applied by the forceps on any given skin surface to be measured. The dynamometer component on the esthesiometer was calibrated using a Torsion Balance Model DRX balance and Ohaus Model 5601 weights. In addition, the dynamometer was periodically calibrated during the study to assure correctness of dynamometer readings.

In administering the test of oral two-point discrimination, the examiner touched the two points of the forceps to S's skin, and S was required to report whether he felt one or two points. A modification of the psychophysical technique referred to as the "method of limits" (Stevens, 1951) was employed in

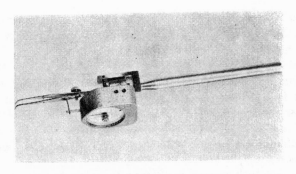

FIG. 1.   Oral esthesiometer used to establish Ss' two-point discrimination thresholds

determining each S's two-point discrimination thresholds.   An ascending threshold was established by beginning with the two points of the forceps approximated and gradually moving the two points apart until S perceived two distinct points when touched.   A descending threshold was established by beginning with the two points far enough apart that they were perceived as two points and gradually moving them together until they were identified by S as one point.

Experimental procedure.—A set of instructions describing the nature of the study and the required task was orally presented to each S.   After the instructions were given, a pre-testing training period was provided to orient and familiarize S with the experimental task prior to data collection.   One ascending and one descending series were administered on the palmar surface of one of S's hands.   However, if, after the two series the examiner felt that S did not adequately understand the task, an additional ascending and descending series were established.

When the examiner was satisfied that S understood the required task, the experimental procedure was begun.   S was seated in a dental chair and blindfolded.   The specific anatomical areas under investigation were marked with a dye (1% Gentian Violet) to ensure consistency of location for placement of the two points of the forceps across stimulus presentations for each S and across all Ss.   S was reminded to indicate whether he felt one or two stimulus points by saying "one" or "two" after each stimulus presentation.   In all ascending series, S was cautioned to report two points only when he was absolutely certain that he felt two points, and not simply when he felt a departure from one point.   In descending series, he was told to report one point only when he was absolutely certain that he felt one point, and not simply when he felt a departure from two points.   These cautions were made in view of the concept that clear duality is the true two-point limen and that the transition from one to two points is not perceptually clear-cut, but rather passes through a series of intermediate stages (point, line, circle, oval, etc.) before it becomes two clearly distinct points (Jenkins, 1951; Ellender, 1968).

The test of two-point discrimination was administered to the selected regions in discrete steps of 0.5 mm. The stimulus points of the forceps were left in contact with the skin surface for approximately a 2-sec. period. The initial presentation of the stimulus points in a series was always made directly on the marked site, with all subsequent presentations made with the points opened lateral to the marked site. A total of 5 randomized ascending and 5 descending series were administered to each S at each test site. A criterion of three consecutive identical responses was required for termination of a particular series (Bolton, 1969). Therefore, in an ascending series, when S reported feeling two points in three consecutive presentations, that series was terminated and the next one begun. A descending series was terminated when S reported feeling only one point for three consecutive presentations. Each series was randomly begun at one of four possible points: at the point of the third consecutive identical response in the previous series, or at a point 0.5, 1.0, or 1.5 mm beyond the third consecutive identical response of the previous series. This procedure was employed to prevent the use of a specific "pattern" in testing and thus eliminate any additional cues for the subject.

"Threshold" was defined as the midpoint between the first of the three consecutive identical responses and the preceding response (Dember, 1960). Therefore, if S reported feeling one point at 1.5 mm and two points at 2.0-, 2.5-, and 3.0-mm presentations, his threshold for that series would be the midpoint between 1.5 and 2.0 mm, or 1.75 mm. In scoring the test of two-point discrimination, a single threshold value was used to represent the two-point limen score for each test site. This score was the average of the 5 ascending and 5 descending thresholds obtained at each site tested.

The above procedures were employed to test each S's two-point discrimination ability at each of the following test sites: (1) upper lip: right, left, and midline regions; (2) lower lip: right, left, and midline regions; (3) tongue tip: right, left, and midline regions; (4) tongue dorsum: right, left, and midline regions; and (5) finger tip of the middle finger of S's dominant hand. Testing of upper lip sites was performed at a point 1.0 mm superior to the vermilion border of the upper lip; lower lip sites were tested at a point 1.0 mm inferior to the vermilion border of the lower lip. Measurements on the tongue tip were made at a point 5.0 mm posterior to the leading margin of the tongue; tongue dorsum measurements were made at a point 30.0 mm posterior to the leading margin of the tongue. Finger tip thresholds were obtained at the core of the cutaneous ridges which comprise the finger print; testing on the finger tip was performed from the core superiorly toward the tip of the finger. "Right" was defined as 2.5 mm from the right lateral extremity of the structure being tested; "left" was defined as 2.5 mm from the left lateral extremity of each structure. Thus, a total of 13 test sites were included in the study. To prevent fatigue in the experimental tasks, no more than two sites (i.e., 20 threshold series) were tested in any single experimental session. In addition, the order of sites tested was randomized for each S.

RESULTS AND DISCUSSION

Table 1[3] contains the mean two-point discrimination thresholds based on all 14 Ss for each of the 13 test sites included in the study. The table indicates the following: (1) the most sensitive structure is the tongue tip, and the least sensitive structures are the tongue dorsum and lower lip; (2) for all structures tested, the midline thresholds are lower than those obtained on the lateral regions; and (3) some differences exist between right and left two-point discrimination thresholds on the structures tested.

TABLE 1

MEANS, STANDARD DEVIATIONS, AND RANGE VALUES FOR TWO-POINT
DISCRIMINATION THRESHOLDS BASED ON 14 SUBJECTS AT EACH OF 13 TEST SITES

Structure		Two-point Thresholds		
		Left	Midline	Right
Upper Lip	M	2.88	2.44	3.61
	SD	1.07	0.76	1.80
	Range	2.05–6.15	1.50–4.00	0.85–6.85
Lower Lip	M	4.52	3.14	4.57
	SD	1.89	2.01	1.32
	Range	2.00–8.85	0.55–8.20	3.00–6.50
Tongue Tip	M	1.97	1.41	2.36
	SD	0.72	0.43	0.94
	Range	1.00–3.10	0.85–2.45	0.85–4.15
Tongue Dorsum	M	4.19	2.96	3.68
	SD	2.06	1.53	1.89
	Range	1.25–9.40	1.05–6.75	1.20–7.00
Finger Tip	M		2.08	
	SD		0.90	
	Range		0.50–3.70	

To evaluate the differences between right and left two-point discrimination thresholds in each S, t tests (Guilford, 1965) were computed. Results indicate that all 14 Ss showed statistical evidence of asymmetry in two-point limen values (critical value of $t = 2.26$, $p < .05$, $df = 9$) on at least one of the four oral structures tested. Only one S showed asymmetry on all four structures, while four exhibited asymmetry on three of the four structures, and seven manifested asymmetry on two of the four structures.

---

[3]A table of individual Ss' data is in Document NAPS-01819. Order from ASIS National Auxiliary Publications Service, c/o CCM Information Corp., 866 Third Ave., New York, N. Y. 10022. Remit $2.00 for microfiche or $6.90 for photocopy.

Table 2 summarizes the findings obtained from the t tests. It indicates that of the 14 Ss in the study, 7 showed asymmetry on the upper lip, 10 on the lower lip, 6 on the tongue tip, and 9 on the tongue dorsum. However, across all structures tested, no consistent trend is evident in the table regarding the side exhibiting the lower thresholds. Furthermore, except for the tongue tip, there is no evident trend within a given structure. For the tongue tip, all Ss who exhibited significant differences between their right and left two-point discrimination thresholds showed better sensitivity on the left side.

TABLE 2

Ss EXHIBITING SIGNIFICANT DIFFERENCES BETWEEN RIGHT AND LEFT TWO-POINT
DISCRIMINATION THRESHOLDS ON EACH OF FOUR ORAL STRUCTURES AND THE
SIDE MANIFESTING LOWER THRESHOLD

Side of Lower Threshold	Upper Lip	Lower Lip	Tongue Tip	Tongue Dorsum
Right	4	5	0	6
Left	3	5	6	3
Total	7	10	6	9

The finding of asymmetry in two-point discrimination ability in all 14 Ss on at least one of the four oral structures tested provides further support to McCall and Cunningham's (1971, p. 370) suggestion that ". . . 'sensory sidedness' may be a normal neurological phenomenon for the tactile sensory system." At the same time, the current findings disagree with those obtained by Ringel and Ewanowski (1965) and Olroyd (1965). However, both of these studies were concerned only with group data and not with comparisons of right vs left thresholds for individual Ss. Perhaps upon reanalysis of their data, evidence of asymmetry would be found in some of their Ss' two-point limens. However, it should be noted that direct comparisons with the above-mentioned studies are difficult to make in light of the procedural differences, including analysis of data, that exist among the studies.

Furthermore, the group data in the present investigation show only slight differences between right and left two-point discrimination thresholds, while comparisons of thresholds based on the performance of each S individually provide evidence of asymmetry. The present authors are aware of the consequent rise in the a level and the resultant increase in the number of Type I errors as a result of the use of a large number of t tests in the present study. However, the finding of such extensive significant right-left differences, with all 14 Ss in the study exhibiting asymmetry in their two-point limens on at least one of the four oral structures tested, provides us with more confidence in our assertions of evidence of asymmetry in the data.

The other findings in the present study are consistent with those reported in all previous investigations on oral two-point discriminatory capacity in normal *Ss*. The finding that the midline thresholds of the structures tested were usually more sensitive than those obtained on the lateral regions is in agreement with the results of Grossman (1964), Olroyd (1965), Ringel and Ewanowski (1965), McCall and Morgan (1966), Henkin and Banks (1967), and Addis (1968). Furthermore, the finding that the tongue tip was frequently the most sensitive structure tested is also in agreement with previous results (Ringel & Ewanowski, 1965).

It was found that all but one *S* in the present study who manifested asymmetry in their two-point limen values did not do so for all four structures tested. This finding, which implies differential laterality effects on the different structures in the oral cavity, is not readily explainable by the present authors. It is suggested that future research explore this issue in an attempt to discover the reason for such differences in asymmetry.

Since it has been found in McCall and Cunningham's (1971) earlier investigation that some normal individuals exhibit asymmetry in their spatial discrimination ability while others do not, and since all but one *S* in the present study did not show asymmetry for all structures tested and since the findings of studies concerned with laterality differences in the general tactual domain have been inconsistent (Semmes, *et al.*, 1960; Ghent, 1961; Weinstein & Sersen, 1961; Fennell, Satz, & Weiss, 1967; Carmon, Bilstrom, & Benton, 1969), future research should continue to explore the issue of asymmetry in tactual discrimination and perception in an attempt to discover those factors which are responsible for, or related to, this phenomenon. One specific suggestion is to study the auditory and visual perceptual characteristics of individuals exhibiting tactual asymmetry in an attempt to determine whether a meaningful relationship exists in such individuals among all three modalities. Perhaps such information will help to locate the factors involved in such laterality differences.

REFERENCES

ADDIS, M. G. Oral perception: an evaluation of normal and defective speakers. Unpublished Master's thesis, Purdue Univer., 1968.

BOLTON, M. L. Two-point discrimination and oral stereognosis testing in normal males ages 45 to 70. Unpublished Master's thesis, Univer. of Kansas, 1969.

CARMON, A., BILSTROM, D. E., & BENTON, A. L. Thresholds for pressure and sharpness in the right and left hands. *Cortex*, 1969, 5, 27-35.

DEMBER, W. N. *The psychology of perception.* New York: Holt, Rinehart, & Winston, 1960.

ELLENDER, E. Z. A methodological investigation of the transition from one to two-point perception. Unpublished Master's thesis, Louisiana State Univer., 1968.

FENNELL, E., SATZ, P., & WEISS, R. Laterality differences in the perception of pressure. *Journal of Neurology, Neurosurgery, and Psychiatry*, 1967, 30, 337-340.

GHENT, L. Developmental changes in tactual thresholds on dominant and nondominant sides. *Journal of Comparative and Physiological Psychology*, 1961, 54, 670-673.

GROSSMAN, R. C. Methods for evaluating oral surface sensations. *Journal of Dental Research*, 1964, 43, 301.

GUILFORD, J. P. *Fundamental statistics in psychology and education.* New York: McGraw-Hill, 1965.

HARRIS, A. J. *Harris Tests of Lateral Dominance: manual of directions for administration and interpretation.* New York: Psychological Corp., 1958.

HENKIN, R. I., & BANKS, V. Tactile perception on the tongue, palate and the hand of normal man. In J. F. Bosma (Ed.), *Symposium on oral sensation and perception.* Springfield, Ill.: Thomas, 1967. Pp. 182-187.

JENKINS, W. Somesthesis. In S. S. Stevens (Ed.), *Handbook of experimental psychology.* New York: Wiley, 1951. Pp. 1172-1190.

MAYO CLINIC AND MAYO FOUNDATION. *Clinical examinations in neurology.* Philadelphia: Saunders, 1963.

MCCALL, G. N., & CUNNINGHAM, N. M. Two-point discrimination: asymmetry in spatial discrimination on the two sides of the tongue, a preliminary report. *Perceptual and Motor Skills,* 1971, 32, 368-370.

OLROYD, M. H. Lingual somesthetic sensibilities of normal nine and eleven year old children. Unpublished Master's thesis, Louisiana State Univer., 1965.

RINGEL, R. L., & EWANOWSKI, S. J. Oral perception: 1. Two-point discrimination. *Journal of Speech and Hearing Research,* 1965, 8, 389-398.

SEMMES, J., WEINSTEIN, S., GHENT, L., & TEUBER, H. L. *Somato-sensory changes after penetrating brain wounds in man.* Cambridge, Mass.: Harvard Univer. Press, 1960.

STEVENS, S. S. Mathematics, measurement and psychophysics. In S. S. Stevens (Ed.), *Handbook of experimental psychology.* New York: Wiley, 1951. Pp. 1-49.

VAN RIPER, C. *Speech correction: principles and methods.* Englewood Cliffs, N. J.: Prentice-Hall, 1963.

WEINSTEIN, S., & SERSEN, E. Tactual sensitivity as a function of handedness and laterality. *Journal of Comparative and Physiological Psychology,* 1961, 54, 665-669.

ORAL TWO-POINT DISCRIMINATION: CONSISTENCY OF TWO-POINT LIMENS ON SELECTED ORAL SITES[1]

NORMAN J. LASS AND WILLIAM E. PARK

Summary.—20 Ss participated in 3 experimental sessions; 10 thresholds, 5 ascending and 5 descending, were obtained on each of 2 oral sites (tongue tip and tongue dorsum) in each session. Results indicate that Ss' two-point limens are very consistent across sessions when obtained on the tongue tip. However, they exhibited poor reliability on the tongue dorsum. A relationship between degree of sensitivity of an oral site and the consistency of two-point thresholds at that site is offered to explain the differences in the present study, and suggestions for testing this proposed relationship are offered.

The current increased interest in the role of the tactile feedback system in the speech production process has led to the development of a number of tests for assessment of tactile skills in the oral cavity. One such test is the test of oral two-point discrimination, which measures the minimum separation of two punctiform stimuli that an individual can perceive as two distinct points (Ringel & Ewanowski, 1965).

From administration of this test to various groups of normal and speech defective individuals have come some interesting observations and, consequently, increased knowledge of oral sensory functioning. However, there appears to be a dearth of information on the consistency of Ss' two-point thresholds. The purpose of the present investigation was to study systematically the consistency of Ss' two-point limens on several selected oral sites.

Method.—Ss, 11 females and 9 males, were students who ranged in age from 19 to 23 yr. ($M_{age} = 21$ yr.). All Ss had normal hearing, articulation, oral cavity structure, superficial tactile sensation, and neurological history and status. Each S participated in three experimental sessions. At each session, 10 thresholds, consisting of 5 ascending and 5 descending series, were obtained on each of two oral structures: the tongue tip and tongue dorsum. All testing was performed in the midline region, i.e., along the median sulcus of the tongue. The order of testing of the two sites was randomized. Measurements on the tongue tip were made at a point 5.0 mm posterior to the leading margin of the tongue; tongue dorsum measurements were made at a point 25.0 mm posterior to the leading margin of the tongue. The test of two-point discrimination was conducted with an oral esthesiometer in discrete steps of 0.5 mm for all ascending and descending series. The device and details of the procedure are described elsewhere (Lass, Kotchek, & Deem, 1972). Each session lasted approximately 50 min.

Results.—Discrepancy scores were calculated for each S's two-point limens based on data from three sessions. These scores reflect the variability in S's performance; they are computed by obtaining the difference between S's lowest and highest two-point thresholds for the three sessions.

The discrepancy scores indicate that Ss' two-point thresholds are highly consistent across sessions when tested on the tongue tip; the group mean discrepancy score of 0.27 is evidence of a very small amount of variability. On the average, less than one step (0.50

[1]This research was partially supported by an Institutional General Research Support Grant from the School of Medicine, West Virginia University.

mm) separated Ss' two-point limens across the three sessions. However, the consistency of their two-point thresholds was much lower on the tongue dorsum; the group mean discrepancy score for the dorsum is 0.67. These differences between discrepancy scores on the tongue tip and tongue dorsum are statistically significant ($t = 3.46$, $df = 19$, $p < .01$).

It is interesting to note that Ss showed high reliability on the tongue tip, the area typically found to be the most sensitive in the oral cavity and to yield the lowest two-point thresholds (Ringel & Ewanowski, 1965; McCall, 1969; Lass, Kotchek, & Deem, 1972), while they exhibited poor reliability on the tongue dorsum, an area found to have much less sensitivity (Lass, Kotchek, & Deem, 1972). Thus, it appears that Ss' two-point limens are more reliable on the more sensitive oral areas. However, this statement needs to be verified through further testing of other oral sites, including the upper lip, alveolar ridge, and soft palate, before a very definite relationship between sensitivity and reliability of structure is established. Furthermore, since sensitivity to two-point stimulation varies at different regions of the same structure in the oral cavity (Ringel & Ewanowski, 1965; McCall & Cunningham, 1971; Lass, Kotchek, & Deem, 1972), it is suggested that midline, right, and left sides of oral structures be included in the reliability testing. If the proposed relationship between sensitivity and reliability holds, the two-point limens on the midline region would be expected to be more reliable than those obtained on the lateral regions of the same structure. However, this has yet to be proven.

The finding that Ss' two-point limen values on the tongue dorsum vary considerably from session to session leads us to conclude that caution must be exercised in interpretation of, and generalization from, the data on the tongue dorsum. Furthermore, if such poor reliability is obtained on other oral structures, it is suggested that further exploration of the test of oral two-point discrimination and of the variables pertinent to performance on this test be undertaken.

REFERENCES

LASS, N. J., KOTCHEK, C. L., & DEEM, J. F. Oral two-point discrimination: further evidence of asymmetry on right and left sides of selected oral structures. *Perceptual and Motor Skills*, 1972, 35, 59-67.

McCALL, G. N. The assessment of lingual tactile sensation and perception. *Journal of Speech and Hearing Disorders*, 1969, 34, 151-156.

McCALL, G. N., & CUNNINGHAM, N. M. Two-point discrimination: asymmetry in spatial discrimination on the two sides of the tongue, a preliminary report. *Perceptual and Motor Skills*, 1971, 32, 368-370.

RINGEL, R. L., & EWANOWSKI, S. J. Oral perception: 1. Two-point discrimination. *Journal of Speech and Hearing Research*, 1965, 8, 389-398.